# Interventions for Anti-Oppressive Clinical Supervision

*Interventions for Anti-Oppressive Clinical Supervision* reimagines the current landscape of clinical supervision training and praxis by offering 50 transformative interventions grounded in the principles of anti-oppression.

Designed for interdisciplinary mental health professionals across roles and contexts, it provides dynamic tools to dismantle systems of oppression and embrace liberatory, intersectional approaches to supervision. More than a resource, this book inspires a paradigm shift by blending theory, research, and praxis to cultivate critical reflexivity, critical consciousness, and collaboration.

This book provides readers with the foundation to create brave supervision spaces and processes that foster healing, equity, and personal to societal change, setting a new standard for liberating mental health professionals and their communities.

**Harvey Charles Peters**, PhD, NCC, is an associate professor in the Department of Counseling at Montclair State University.

**Melissa Luke**, PhD, LMHC, NCC, ACS is a dean's professor in the unit of Counseling and Human Services at Syracuse University.

"Peters and Luke have transcended layers of colonization and oppression to name the oppressive structures within our pedagogical traditions, articulating anti-oppression as a transtheoretical means of re-organizing counselor supervision. In this book, they articulate the Anti-Oppression Supervision Model (AOSM) as the foundation of this new supervisory praxis, and then, with each chapter addressing one tenet of the AOSM, they present various supervisor interventions that meet that tenet. This book represents a new wave of anti-oppression in counseling; as new clinicians are trained using anti-oppression, it will be easier for them to practice anti-oppression in their counseling and in their communities. We can now become the change we have been waiting for."

**Dr. Colette T. Dollarhide,** *professor, retired at Ohio State University.*

"This essential book is a transformative read for clinical supervisors dedicated to anti-oppression work. The authors expertly intertwine the concepts of supervision and social justice, delivering insights that are both enlightening and actionable. Through robust theoretical frameworks, this text empowers future clinical supervisors with the essential skills to effectively support counselors who work with clients facing oppression. A powerful resource for anyone committed to fostering social change in their practice!"

**Manivong J. Ratts, PhD, LMHC, LPC, NCC,** *is a professor of counseling at Seattle University.*

"I am grateful to see this this text, as it is an important advancement in defining anti-oppressive practices in supervision. The editors and authors have provided key practical next steps so mental health professionals serving in supervisory roles can create more equitable, just, and liberatory environments."

**Anneliese Singh, PhD, LPC,** *is the chief diversity officer and professor at Tulane University.*

"This book remains a resounding answer to the complicated dilemma of unbinding from oppression and power hierarchies that still unfortunately underlie supervision practices. In vexing sociopolitical times facing multiple health disciplines, this long-awaited collection of voices is a vision of the future of supervision, but more importantly, it is the hope we need to sustain us."

**Christian D. Chan, PhD, NCC,** *is an assistant professor at the University of North Carolina at Greensboro*

# Interventions for Anti-Oppressive Clinical Supervision

## Navigating Critical Praxis

*Edited by Harvey Charles Peters and Melissa Luke*

Routledge
Taylor & Francis Group

NEW YORK AND LONDON

Designed cover image: Getty Images

First published 2026
by Routledge
605 Third Avenue, New York, NY 10158

and by Routledge
4 Park Square, Milton Park, Abingdon, Oxon, OX14 4RN

*Routledge is an imprint of the Taylor & Francis Group, an informa
business*

ISBN: 978-1-032-74741-5 (hbk)
ISBN: 978-1-032-74411-7 (pbk)
ISBN: 978-1-003-47065-6 (ebk)

DOI: 10.4324/9781003470656

Typeset in Bembo
by Apex CoVantage, LLC

# Contents

# About the Editors

**Harvey Charles Peters,** PhD, NCC is Associate Professor in the Department of Counseling at Montclair State University. Prior to his position at Montclair State University, he was the co-coordinator of the counseling doctoral program at The George Washington University. Dr. Peters has served in a variety of leadership positions across professional organizations, including the Association for Counselor Education and Supervision (ACES), Chi Sigma Iota (CSI), Counselors for Social Justice (CSJ), and the North Atlantic Association for Counselor Education and Supervision (NARACES). Dr. Peters has published more than 40 publications and delivered over 60 presentations across interdisciplinary and international contexts. He also teaches the doctoral clinical supervision course and supervises doctoral supervisors-in-training at his university. Dr. Peters' scholarship and clinical practices center on expanding culturally sustaining, critical, and anti-oppressive identity development and practices across counseling, leadership and advocacy, scholarship, supervision, and teaching across mental health professions.

**Melissa Luke,** PhD, LMHC, NCC, ACS is a Dean's professor in the Department of Counseling & Human Services at Syracuse University. She is a National Certified Counselor (NCC), an Approved Clinical Supervisor (ACS), and both a Licensed Mental Health Counselor (LMHC) and certified School Counselor in the state of New York. Dr. Luke is an international leader in counselor education with over 200 publications and has delivered presentations and workshops in seven countries to date. Dr. Luke is the 2024 recipient of the American Counseling Association's Extended Research Award. In addition, Dr. Luke currently serves as the Associate Editor of Counselor Education and Supervision and previously served as the Editor of the Journal of Counselor Leadership and Advocacy.

Dr. Luke has held numerous servant leadership positions in the American Counseling Association's divisions and sister organizations, including the Association for Counselor Education and Supervision (ACES), the Association for Specialists in Group Work (ASGW), Counselors for Social Justice (CSJ), the Society for Sexual, Affectional, Intersex, and Gender Expansive Identities (SAIGE), and Chi Sigma Iota (CSI). She also teaches the doctoral clinical supervision course as well as provides supervision to doctoral supervisors-in-training at her university. Dr. Luke's scholarship and clinical practices focus on effective and anti-oppressive practices to increase equity, inclusion, and accessibility in counseling, clinical supervision, and faculty professional development, in addition to incorporating critical qualitative and quantitative methodologies and andragogies.

# Contributors

**Rehman Abdulrehman**, PhD, is an assistant professor at the University of Manitoba.

**Rawan Atari-Khan**, PhD, LP, is an assistant professor at Marquette University.

**Mina Attia**, PhD, NCC, is an assistant professor at The George Washington University.

**Clark D. Ausloos**, PhD, is an assistant professor at Oakland University.

**Casey Barrio Minton**, PhD, NCC, is a professor at The University of Tennessee, Knoxville.

**Lindsey M. Bell**, MS, is a doctoral student at The University of New Mexico.

**Kenya G. Bledsoe**, PhD, LPC-S NCC, NCSC, BC-TMH, is an assistant professor at The University of Mississippi.

**Susan Branco**, PhD, LPC, NCC, ACS, BC-TMH, is an associate professor at Palo Alto University.

**Theodore R. Burnes**, PhD, is a professor at the University of Southern California.

**Janice A. Byrd-Badjie**, PhD, is an associate professor at The Pennsylvania State University.

**Peggy L. Ceballos**, PhD, NCC, is a professor at the University of Texas at San Antonio.

**Philippa Chin**, PhD, LPC, LMFT, NCC, is an assistant professor at Barry University.

**Devika Dibya Choudhuri,** PhD, LPC (MI/CT), ACS, is a professor at Eastern Michigan University.

**Karina Crescini**, M.A., LMHC, LPC, RPT, NCC, is a doctoral student at the University of North Texas.

**Tahani Dari**, PhD, LPC, NCC, is an assistant professor at the University of Detroit Mercy.

**Bagmi Das**, PhD, LMFT, is an assistant professor at The George Washington University.

**Cirleen DeBlaere**, PhD, is a professor and interim associate provost for faculty affairs at Georgia State University.

**Mary DeRaedt**, PhD, LPC, is a clinical assistant professor at The George Washington University.

**Kirsis A. Dipre**, PhD, is an assistant professor at Northeastern Illinois University.

**Melissa J. Fickling**, PhD, LCPC, CADC, ACS, is an associate professor at Northern Illinois University.

**Michael M. Gale**, PhD, LP, is an assistant professor at Springfield College.

**Diana Gallardo**, PhD, is an associate professor at the Northeastern Illinois University.

**Katie Gamby**, PhD, LPCC-S, is the founder and a licensed professional clinical counselor and supervisor at The Wellife, LLC.

**Kristopher Goodrich**, PhD, is Dean of the College of Education and Human Sciences at The University of New Mexico.

**Darius A. Green**, PhD, LPCC, NCC, is an assistant professor at the University of Colorado.

**Sravya Gummaluri**, MA, LAC (NJ), NCC, is a doctoral candidate at The George Washington University.

**Natoya Haskins**, PhD, LPC, NCC, is an associate professor at the University of Virginia.

**Joshua N. Hook**, PhD, is a professor at the University of North Texas.

**Arpana G. Inman**, PhD, is a distinguished professor at Rutgers University.

**Connie T. Jones**, PhD, LCMHCA, LCAS, NCC, ACS, is an associate professor at The University of North Carolina at Greensboro.

**Kavita Khara**, M.S.C.P, LCPC, NCC, is a doctoral student at Northern Illinois University.

**Thomas Killian**, PhD, is an assistant professor at Montclair State University.

**Kelly M. King**, PhD, LPCC, LMHC, NCC, is an assistant professor at California State University, Sacramento.

**Ah Ram Lee**, PhD, NCC, is an assistant teaching professor at Syracuse University.

**Dan Li,** PhD, NCC, LSC (K-12, NC), is an associate professor at the University of Oklahoma Health Sciences.

**Yanhong Liu**, PhD, NCC, is an associate professor at Syracuse University.

**Melissa Luke**, PhD, NCC, ACS, LMHC, is a dean's professor at Syracuse University.

**Krista M. Malott**, PhD, LPC, is a professor at Villanova University.

**Jeff Moe**, PhD, LPC, NCC, CCMHC, is an associate professor at Old Dominion University.

**Kelly Moore**, PsyD, is a director for the Center for Psychological Services and a clinical associate professor at Rutgers University.

**Deepika Raju Nantha Kumar**, M.Ed, NCC, is a doctoral student at The Pennsylvania State University.

**Sylvia Nassar**, PhD, is a professor at North Carolina State University.

**Jane E. Atieno Okech**, PhD, is a professor and vice provost for faculty affairs at the University of Vermont.

**Tina R. Paone**, PhD, LPC, ACS, RPT-S is a professor at Monmouth University.

**Dilani Perera**, PhD, LPCC-S, LICDC-S, NCC, MAC, BC-TMH, is a professor at Fairfield University.

**Harvey Charles Peters**, PhD, NCC, is an associate professor at Montclair State University.

**Alex L. Pieterse**, PhD, LP, is an associate professor of counseling psychology at Boston College.

**Stacy A. Pinto**, PhD, is a clinical associate professor at the University of Denver.

**Maria Reyna**, PhD, LPC-S (TX), is an assistant professor at the Seminary of the Southwest.

**David P. Rivera**, PhD, is an associate professor at Queens College, City University of New York.

**Madison Rowohlt**, MA, is a doctoral student at Montclair State University.

**Rochele Royster**, PhD, ATR-BC, is an assistant professor of art therapy in the Department of Creative Arts Therapy at Syracuse University.

**Deborah Rubel**, PhD, is a professor at Oregon State University.

**Jordan Shannon**, PhD, NCC, is an assistant professor at Seattle University.

**Elyssa B. Smith**, PhD, LPC, RPT, NCC, ACS, leads a private practice focused on psychodynamic and depth-informed psychotherapy and play therapy at The Inner Canvas Collective.

**Jaimie Stickl Haugen**, PhD, LPC, NCC, ACS, is a clinical assistant professor in counselor education at William & Mary.

**Cassandra A. Storlie**, PhD, LPCC-S, NCC, is a professor at Kent State University.

**L. Xochitl Vallejos**, PhD, LPC, is an advocate, educator, and consultant for the Rocky Mountain Counseling and Psychological Association.

**Ahmad Rashad Washington**, PhD, is an associate professor at The University of Louisville.

**C. Edward Watkins, Jr.**, PhD, is a professor at the University of North Texas and Institute of Psychotherapy, Psychological Counselling, and Clinical Supervision (Reşiţa, Romania).

**Melanie M. Wilcox**, PhD, ABPP, LP, is an associate professor at the University at Albany.

**Monnica T. Williams**, PhD, ABPP, is a professor at the University of Ottawa.

**Laura Wood**, PhD, LMHC, LPC, RDT/BCT, is an associate professor at Lesley University.

# Acknowledgments

Our book is dedicated to the contributing authors, supervisors, supervisees, and students whose development will be enhanced through the anti-oppressive content, as well as the clients, community partners, and community members who will also benefit. We are indebted to our mentors and personal and professional communities, supervision and anti-oppressive scholars, and practitioners whose support, research, and practice laid the foundation for this work to take root. We also honor the next generation of supervisors and scholars who will carry this work forward into new contexts in the future.

# Book Overview

In an effort to support the theorization and praxis of anti-oppressive supervision, the book includes 12 distinct chapters. Chapter 1 provides an overview of anti-oppression and the 10 guiding principles, clinical supervision, and anti-oppressive supervision, thereby ensuring professionals across the globe and stages of their careers have a shared understanding of each of the core constructs. Next, Chapters 2 through 11 present a range of clinical supervision interventions grounded in the existing literature, scholarship, and theoretical farmworkers addressing various facets of anti-oppressive supervision. The interventions presented in each chapter provide essential information contextualizing the processes and practices of anti-oppression supervision as well as account for multiplistic identities and various supervision foci (e.g., documentation, evaluation, skill development, theory development, professional identity, advocacy, etc.). The format for the interventions across these 10 chapters include: (a) proposed supervision format and modality, (b) proposed supervisee developmental level, (c) supervisory goals and learning objectives, (d) time requirements, (e) materials requirements, (f) instructions, (g) supervisory alliance and relationship considerations, (h) legal and ethical considerations, (i) references, and (j) reflective questions.

Each of these chapters aligns with one of the 10 principles of anti-oppression (Peters & Luke, 2022). Chapter 2 presents clinical supervision interventions focused on *developing critical consciousness through critical reflexivity* (Peters & Luke, 2022). Chapter 3 provides clinical supervision interventions focused on *overcoming comfort and fragility through unlearning privilege and domination* (Peters & Luke, 2022). Chapter 4 presents clinical supervision interventions focused on *centering the margins through empowerment and liberation* (Peters & Luke, 2022). Chapter 5 provides clinical supervision interventions focused on *wellness and self-care through acts of compassion and vigilance* (Peters & Luke, 2022). Chapter 6 presents clinical supervision interventions focused on *co-constructing a brave space through relationships and community* (Peters & Luke, 2022). Chapter 7 provides clinical supervision interventions focused on *developing goals and assessing outcomes through stakeholder investment* (Peters & Luke, 2022). Chapter 8 presents clinical supervision interventions focused on *challenging and disrupting oppression through broaching and accountability* (Peters & Luke, 2022). Chapter 9 provides clinical supervision interventions focused on *identifying and addressing barriers through resistance and opposition* (Peters & Luke, 2022). Chapter 10 presents clinical supervision interventions focused on *socioecological advocacy and activism through collective action* (Peters & Luke, 2022). Chapter 11 provides clinical supervision interventions focused on *redistributing social, cultural, and political capital through access and opportunity* (Peters & Luke, 2022). Chapter 12 concludes the book by synthesizing each of the chapters, issuing a call to action, and outlining implications for the future of anti-oppressive clinical supervision research and praxis.

Collectively, the book can aid clinical supervisors in grounding themselves in the current and evolving practice of anti-oppressive supervision. Through the intentional use of supervision interventions, clinical supervisors across the globe can enhance and revitalize the development of practices and facilitation of anti-oppressive supervision. The interventions can also provide clinical supervisors with a framework and tools to continuously reflect, guide, and refine supervisors' and supervisees' anti-oppressive attitudes and beliefs, knowledge, skills, and actions (Killian et al., 2023; Ratts et al., 2016) through the continuous and iterative process of anti-oppressive clinical supervision praxis.

# Introduction

Within counseling and clinical supervision exists a noticeable disparity between theoretical frameworks and practical implementation, particularly within the context of anti-oppression (Lee, 2023; Legha, 2023a, 2023b; Peters et al., 2022). While the contemporary counseling and supervision literature has increasingly embraced the paradigms of multiculturalism and social justice (Asakura & Maurer, 2018; Dollarhide et al., 2021; Falender et al., 2014; Hair, 2015; Hardy & Bobes, 2016; Kemer et al., 2022; Spowart & Robertson, 2024), the translation of principles grounded in anti-oppression and related constructs (e.g., equity, empowerment, liberation, activism, decolonization, anti-racism) within clinical praxis remains a persistent challenge for trainees, practitioners, and supervisors alike (Bussey, 2024a, 2024b; Legha, 2023b; Mitchell & Butler, 2021; Musson Rose & Baffour, 2023; Okech et al., 2023a; Peters et al., 2022; Pieterse & Gale, 2023; Ramírez Stege et al., 2020; Torres Rivera & Torres Fernández, 2024; Williams et al., 2023b). Thus, the chasm between theory and customary contemporary practice, hereafter referred to as praxis, becomes particularly pronounced when considering the imperative of anti-oppressive clinical praxis. As the need and demand for anti-oppressive clinical approaches and practices continue to gain momentum and prominence within mental health (Legha, 2023a, 2023b; Okech et al., 2023a; Peters et al., 2022), bridging these concerning clinical, structural, content, and research gaps become a theoretical aspiration and a practical necessity for all mental health professionals (Lee, 2023; Legha, 2023b; Peters & Luke, 2022). One vital approach to addressing this disparity and fulfilling professional and societal needs lies within clinical supervision (Burnes & Manese, 2019; Watkins et al., 2022; Wilcox et al., 2022a, 2022b; Zhang et al., 2022), which is the primary tool for supporting, mentoring, and training professionals across each of the mental health professions (Bernard & Goodyear, 2019; Borders & Brown, 2022; Borders et al., 2023; Calderwood & Rizzo, 2023; Falender & Shafranske, 2021; Kadushin & Harkness, 2014).

The exigency for additional techniques and interventions to facilitate the integration of anti-oppression into clinical supervision cannot be overstated (Luke & Goodrich, 2015a, 2015b; Okech et al., 2023a). Current supervision models and frameworks mostly fall short of providing supervisors with actionable anti-oppressive strategies and interventions that empower them to navigate, train, and supervise the next generation of mental health professionals to efficaciously attend to sociocultural identities as well as the structural and systemic ramifications of power, oppression, discrimination, subjugation, and disempowerment across cultures and contexts (Ali & Lee, 2019; Bradley et al., 2023; Howard et al., 2023; Lee, 2023; Legha, 2023a, 2023b; Okech et al., 2023a; Peters et al., 2022). Accordingly, the aim of our book is to support clinical supervisors across mental health professions (e.g., counselors, marriage and family therapists, psychologists, social workers) and professional settings and contexts (e.g., private practice, community centers, inpatient and outpatient clinics, non-profit organizations, higher education, pK–12 schools) in conceptualizing and implementing clinical supervision within the paradigm of anti-oppression; thereby, bridging the gap between the theory and praxis of anti-oppressive supervision.

To support supervisors across all stages (Kemer, 2020) of their career (e.g., novice, mid, late, expert) in the practice of anti-oppressive supervision (Okech et al., 2023a), we utilize Peters and Luke's (2022) 10 principles of anti-oppression to operationalize and situate clinical supervision as an anti-oppressive theory and practice. The 10 principles of anti-oppression, operationalized in what follows, are contemporary, consistent with, and further illuminate each mental health profession's multicultural, social justice, and/or anti-oppressive standards, competencies, and guidelines (American Psychological Association [APA], 2017; Knudson-Martin et al., 2019; National Association of Social Workers [NASW], 2015; Ratts et al., 2016; Toporek & Daniels, 2018). Moreover, applying these 10 principles to clinical supervision complement and extend each profession's supervision standards and competencies (APA, 2014; Borders, 2014; Henriksen et al., 2019; NASW, 2013; Ogbeide & Bayles, 2023), literature (Dollarhide et al., 2021; Fickling et al., 2019; Kemer et al., 2022; Middleton et al., 2023; Mitchell & Butler, 2021; Peters, 2017; Peters & Luke, 2021a; Peters et al., 2022; Wilcox et al., 2022b), and calls to actions (Chang et al., 2009; Legha, 2023b; Peters & Luke, 2022; Okech et al., 2023a) by moving beyond theoretical discussions to interrogating and transforming the praxis of clinical supervision to anti-oppressive clinical supervision (Lee,

2023; Legha, 2023a, 2023b). Consistent with existing books (Luke & Goodrich, 2015a, 2015b; Pope et al., 2020; Singh, 2018, 2019) that target transnational professionals committed to upholding each mental health profession's anti-oppressive commitments and aims (APA, 2014; Borders, 2014; NASW, 2013), we seek to address the disconnection concerning the theory and praxis of anti-oppressive supervision by calling all clinical supervisors across professions to action and supporting them through the implementation of anti-oppressive supervisory interventions guided by the anti-oppressive theory and literacy.

In pursuit of anti-oppressive clinical praxis, our book includes a range of supervisory interventions organized by Peters and Luke's (2022) 10 principles of anti-oppression to illuminate and guide clinical supervisors with multiplistic privileged and marginalized identities working with diverse local to international stakeholders across professional and socioecological contexts in the practice of anti-oppressive supervision. Given the documented dearth of scholarly and clinical support in moving the theoretical into the actionable (Luke & Goodrich, 2015a, 2015b; Peters et al., 2022), we include anti-oppressive supervision interventions informed by the extant literature and best practices as an ideal and long overdue support for clinical supervisors. We intentionally sought out a range of diverse critical scholars and practitioners for input on as well as the development of anti-oppressive supervision interventions. Such contributions are essential, given contemporary scholars (Luke & Goodrich, 2015a, 2015b; Pope et al., 2020) argue that both mental health and supervisee trainees and highly skilled practitioners, supervisors, and educators need additional guidance and support in implementing theoretically-and empirically-driven techniques and interventions to move clients and supervisees towards mutually agreed-upon culturally situated and anti-oppressive goals. Furthermore, scholars (Ali & Lee, 2019; Bradley et al., 2023) suggest there exists a dearth of interventions present within the extant scholarship and frameworks within clinical supervision, particularly those focused on anti-oppression. Much of the current scholarship and ancillary resources on supervisory interventions, at best, focus on multicultural supervision or are detached from social justice and anti-oppressive perspectives (Ali & Lee, 2019; Bradley et al., 2023; Okech et al., 2023a). The clinical, structural, content, and research gaps concerning the theory and praxis of anti-oppressive supervision present a significant barrier for supervisors, supervisees, and the communities they serve at the local, state, national, or international levels. Arguably, the practice of anti-oppressive clinical supervision is a global imperative as diverse societies continue to face longstanding and evolving issues concerning human rights, oppression, capitalism, inequity, and injustice (Gutierrez, 2018; Hernández & McDowell, 2010; Lee, 2023; Legha,

2023a, 2023b), and mental health professionals are tasked with supporting and advocating with, and on behalf of those at the center of marginalization (Chang et al., 2009; Fickling et al., 2019; King & Jones, 2019; Peters, 2017; Storlie et al., 2019). Thus, this unique and timely book is aimed at supporting new and advanced clinical supervisors, supervisees-in-training, supervisor educators, and scholars across the globe in the theorization and praxis of anti-oppressive supervision.

CHAPTER 1

# Interventions for Anti-Oppressive Clinical Supervision

## Navigating Critical Praxis

*Harvey Charles Peters and Melissa Luke*

## THE FOUNDATION OF ANTI-OPPRESSIVE CLINICAL SUPERVISION

The confluence of multiculturalism, social justice, and anti-oppression serves as a significant influence across the fields of counseling and counselor education, psychology, social work, marriage and family therapy, and creative arts therapies (Peters & Luke, 2022; Singh et al., 2020). Given the unique and inextricably linked nature of these three overarching constructs, it is essential that mental health professionals understand the evolution of multiculturalism, social justice, and anti-oppression, as they account for the fourth (i.e., multiculturalism; Arredondo et al., 1996; Sue et al., 1982, 1992), fifth (i.e., social justice; Peters & Luke, 2021a; Ratts, 2009; Thrift & Sugarman, 2019), and sixth (i.e., anti-oppression; Peters & Luke, 2022) forces of counseling and psychological theory and praxis (Peters & Luke, 2022). Of the existing paradigms, Peters and Luke (2022) only recently called for and coined anti-oppression as the sixth force. Each force provides mental health professionals, educators, and supervisors with a historical and current cartographic map of modern-day mental health, as well as the potential to help envision and construct a more equitable future (DeBlaere et al., 2019; Hansen, 2014; Peters & Luke, 2022; Singh et al., 2020).

Considering the proverbial map, mental health professionals and trainees should not be surprised that the origins of mental health practices across disciplines developed around values that prioritize hierarchy, neutrality,

DOI: 10.4324/9781003470656-1

monolithic representations of privileged and hegemonic cultures, and limited understanding of the subjective and culturally situated nature (Goodman & Gorski, 2015; Johnson et al., 2022) of philosophy, ontology (i.e., the nature of truth and reality), and epistemology (i.e., the nature of knowledge and knowledge acquisition). Singh et al. (2020) argued that the history of mental health was situated within "North American and European colonist ideologies related to power, marginalization, and oppression" (p. 261). Thus, mental health professions do not consider or account for the rich, complex, and dynamic nature of concepts such as identity, culture, power, equity, privilege, and oppression. Consequently, mental health scholars and practitioners, particularly those from marginalized communities (e.g., race, gender identity, affectional orientation, disability, etc.), sought to advance mental health by advocating for and developing the fourth (i.e., multiculturalism), fifth (i.e., social justice), and sixth (i.e., anti-oppression) forces of counseling and psychological theory and praxis.

## MULTICULTURAL, SOCIAL JUSTICE, AND ANTI-OPPRESSION

Multiculturalism is an approach to mental health practice that seeks to recognize and respect the sociocultural diversity of individuals from different cultural backgrounds, such as ethnic, racial, religious, or socioeconomic. A dominant perspective of multiculturalism was developed by Sue et al. (1982) and Sue et al. (1992) and later advanced by Arredondo et al. (1996), who defined multiculturalism through mental health professionals' attitudes, beliefs, knowledge, and skills. Related concepts, such as cultural knowledge, cultural sensitivity, cultural empathy, cultural guidance, cultural responsivity, and cultural humility, were connected to the theory and practice of multiculturalism (Hook et al., 2013; Peters & Luke, 2021a; Peters et al., 2022; Placeres et al., 2024; Tseng & Streltzer, 2004). Collectively, these concepts guide mental health professionals in seeking to understand, value, and respect the unique and dynamic sociocultural backgrounds of all persons we seek to serve through understanding how their sociocultural identities, values, and practices inform their worldviews, needs, relationships, and mental health and wellness (Arredondo et al., 1996; Sue et al., 1982, 1992).

Following multiculturalism, social justice emerged as the next dominant force, building upon and extending the existing focus on sociocultural attitudes, beliefs, knowledge, and skills (Finn, 2020; Killian et al., 2023; Peters & Luke, 2021a; Ratts, 2009; Ratts et al., 2016). Although a large range of interdisciplinary definitions, models, and practices exist, social justice serves as an approach to mental health practice that seeks to "rec-ognize and address issues of power, privilege, oppression, and inequity through actions such as advocacy and activism" (Peters & Luke, 2021a, p. 3). Social justice also extends beyond multiculturalism through actions such as advocacy to challenge and disrupt issues of equity and oppres-sion that impede people personally, professionally, familially, and cultur-ally (DeBlaere et al., 2019; Ratts, 2009) across socioecological systems (e.g., micro, meso, macro; Ahmed et al., 2018; Bronfenbrenner & Mor-ris, 1998; Brutzman et al., 2022; Peters et al., 2022). Across these aspects exist multiple facets of social justice, such as associational, cultural, deco-lonial, distributive, emancipatory, intergenerational, procedural, retribu-tive, and restorative justice (Peters & Luke, 2021a), each with overlapping and distinctive definitions, foci, and scope. Despite the diverse schol-arship on social justice across mental health disciplines, several scholars have employed content analyses to examine the literature and suggested that there is a dearth of research and praxis outlining the implementation of social justice, limited interventions, and a lack of focus on outcome research and scholar-practitioner partnerships (Clark et al., 2022; Gantt-Howrey et al., 2023; Graybill et al., 2018; Pieterse et al., 2009; Seedall et al., 2014). Moreover, these results parallel Killian et al.'s (2023) findings that mental health professionals report greater social justice competence at the individual and interpersonal levels than at the community and systems levels.

Anti-oppression can arguably serve as a framework and practice to address the gaps associated with multiculturalism and social justice. Accordingly, anti-oppression has surfaced as a force grounded in liberation and emanci-pation across the mental health disciplines that build on and augment the multiculturalism and social justice forces of mental health theory and praxis (Morgaine & Capous-Desyllas, 2020; Peters & Luke, 2022; Pieterse et al., 2016). Although anti-oppression encapsulates multiple related concepts and/or theories, including but not limited to liberation, empowerment, anti-racism, intersectionality, abolitionism, anti-capitalism, anti-ableism and decolonization, it serves an approach that supports mental health pro-fessionals in actively seeking to disrupt and ameliorate all singular and mul-tiplistic forms of oppression, discrimination, and subjugation that occur on individual, structural, and societal levels (Bussey, 2024a, 2024b; Calhoun et al., 2023; Johnson et al., 2022; Morgaine & Capous-Desyllas, 2020; Peters & Luke, 2022; Ramírez Stege et al., 2020). For example, using community engagement and civil disobedience to call attention to and fight against the multiple types of harm and discrimination faced by those at the intersections of racial, ethnic, queer, and migrant status marginaliza-tion (e.g., queer migrants of color). Peters and Luke (2022), using critical analytic synthesis (CAS) methodology and the interdisciplinary literature on anti-oppression, define anti-oppression as follows:

> A framework and practice that addresses the process and outcomes of challenging and combating oppressive and inequitable forces, structures, and systems while simultaneously supporting the empowerment and liberation of those within the margins from the distorted, unjust, and hegemonic foundations of a society.
>
> (p. 336)

Thus, anti-oppression provides mental health professionals with an essential transtheoretical framework to deconstruct the problematic history of oppression within mental health and society and to reconstruct our professional identities and clinical practices to highlight, center, and achieve newfound equity for all marginalized communities.

## Principles of Anti-Oppression

Despite the evolving understanding of and commitment to anti-oppression across mental health professions and contexts (Grant et al., 2023; Liu & Li, 2023; Luke et al., 2023; Okech et al., 2023a; Shaikh et al., 2024), a substantial gap exists between professionals' shared operationalization, commitment, and clinical practice. Accordingly, Peters and Luke (2022) employed a critical, intersectional, and poststructural qualitative CAS methodology to redress the gaps. Given that the theorization and practice of anti-oppression across mental health professions remain nascent, the authors' CAS study enabled them to comprehensively review, synthesize, and analyze existing interdisciplinary scholarship on anti-oppression. Peters and Luke's (2022) CAS study resulted in 10 guiding principles of anti-oppression detached from a specific theory, context, or clinical modality, which include:

1. *Developing critical consciousness through critical reflexivity:* Anti-oppression represents dynamic, iterative, and dialogic processes wherein one examines their values, worldviews, multiplistic social locations, positions, identity development, and biases concerning the interlocking forces, structures, and systems of power, resulting in increased anti-oppressive knowledge and complexity.
2. *Overcoming comfort and fragility through unlearning privilege and domination:* Anti-oppression requires an evolving personal and professional practice wherein one actively works to address, unlearn, and overcome issues of socialization and privilege grounded in domination and oppression meant to uphold oppressive forces, structures, and systems

maintained and weaponized through discomfort, silence, objectivity, apathy, neutrality, bias, and fragility.

3. *Centering the margins through empowerment and liberation*: Anti-oppression prioritizes the voices, narratives, and experiences of minoritized populations and communities by counteracting the dominant and majoritarian forces, structures, and systems by repositioning to center historically excluded persons and perspectives while championing emancipation and liberation.

4. *Wellness and self-care through acts of compassion and vigilance*: Anti-oppression emphasizes the centrality of self-care, wellness, and somatic regulation as an act of resistance against the biopsychosocial impact of oppression and is essential in remaining vigilant and accountable in one's anti-oppressive commitments and actions.

5. *Co-constructing a brave space through relationships and community*: Anti-oppression necessitates co-developing relationships and brave spaces to equitably meet the needs of all through a bottom-up approach to justice and equity while fostering difficult dialogues, courage, compassion, and owning the impact people have on one another.

6. *Developing goals and assessing outcomes through stakeholder investment*: Anti-oppression values the cyclical process of developing, overseeing, and evaluating short-and long-term anti-oppressive goals and objectives across personal and professional stakeholders.

7. *Challenging and disrupting oppression through broaching and accountability*: Anti-oppression requires engaging in intra-, interpersonal, and group-systems actions that name, address, and counter exploitation, erasure, interpersonal violence, marginalization, powerlessness, cultural imperialism, and subjugation, here as means to take responsibility for and redressing harm.

8. *Identifying and addressing barriers through resistance and opposition*: Anti-oppression acknowledges the multifaceted barriers that disempower and disarm community, collective, and systemic change, asserting the need to anticipate and resist compliance and counteract these obstacles.

9. *Socioecological advocacy and activism through collective action*: Anti-oppression catalyzes transformation through deliberate community engagement and collaborative actions aiming to decenter, dismantle, and ameliorate oppressive and inequitable forces, structures, relationships, and policies across the microsystem, mesosystem, exosystem, macrosystem, and chronosystem.

10. *Redistributing social, cultural, and political capital through access and opportunity*: Anti-oppression seeks to identify and address historic inequities in the distribution of capital, resources, access, and opportunity and repair the adverse effects, harm, and consequences through redistribution and/or reparations (p. 343-344).

These 10 principles can be used across mental health professions to (a) develop one's anti-oppressive professional identity, (b) conceptualize and theorize the process of anti-oppressive mental health services, and (c) develop one's anti-oppressive skills, techniques, and interventions across socioecological systems (e.g., micro, meso, and macro) and professional contexts (e.g., counseling, social work, and supervision). However, given the documented issues faced by professionals in moving the theoretical into practice, there remains an essential need to support mental health practitioners and trainees in implementing anti-oppressive skills and practices (Pope et al., 2020). Such issues exist despite a robust body of scholarship (Clark et al., 2022; Gantt-Howrey et al., 2023; Graybill et al., 2018; Pieterse et al., 2009; Seedall et al., 2014) and the existence of many interdisciplinary competencies, such as the Multicultural and Social Justice Counseling Competencies (MSJCC; Ratts et al., 2016), Multicultural Guidelines: An Ecological Approach to Context, Identity, and Intersectionality (APA, 2017), National Association of Social Workers (NASW) standards and indicators for cultural competence in social work practice (NASW, 2015), guidelines for socioculturally attuned family therapy (Knudson-Martin et al., 2019), and American Counseling Association (ACA) advocacy competencies (Toporek & Daniels, 2018). Thus, the 10 principles of anti-oppression (Peters & Luke, 2022) serve as the first set of interdisciplinary mental health principles focused on anti-oppression, which can be used to bridge the gap between theory and praxis, particularly relevant in the context of supervision.

## SUPERVISION

Interdisciplinary scholars have developed a robust literature over the past five decades, distinguishing clinical supervision as a unique intervention, separate from counseling, teaching, consultation, and administrative supervision (Bernard & Luke, 2015; Luke, 2019). In the most frequently cited definition of supervision, Bernard and Goodyear (2019) defined supervision as

> an intervention provided by a more senior member of a profession to a more junior colleague or colleagues who typically (but not always) are members of the same profession. This relationship is evaluative, extends over time, and has the simultaneous purposes of enhancing the professional functioning of the more junior person(s); monitoring the quality of professional services offered to the clients that she, he, or they see; and serving as a gatekeeper for the particular profession the supervisee seeks to enter.
>
> (p. 9)

Increasingly, supervision has been acknowledged as the primary and signature pedagogy (Shulman, 2005a, 2005b) for the training and professional development of all mental health practitioners (Bernard & Goodyear, 2019; Luke & Peters, 2020). As an inherently andragogical and interpersonal intervention with a hierarchical and evaluative structure (Bernard & Goodyear, 2019), supervision also incorporates experiential knowledge, the only type of learning that Carl Rogers (1957) accepted as directly related to counseling (Mullen et al., 2007). More recently, scholars have described andragogical empathy as a multidimensional disposition (Baltrinic & Luke, 2022); in this case wherein the supervisor's experiential and empathic attunement extend across affective, cognitive, behavioral, systemic, and cultural learning domains. Consequently, accreditation bodies (i.e., APA, 2006; Commission on Accreditation for Marriage and Family Therapy Education [COAMFTE], 2014; Council for Accreditation of Counseling and Related Educational Programs [CACREP], 2023; Council on Social Work Education [CSWE], 2022), licensing boards (Henriksen et al., 2019), and credentialing agencies (e.g., Commission on Rehabilitation Counselor Certification [CRCC], 2023; National Board for Certified Counselors [NBCC], 2016) each address mandatory participation in supervision as part of the education and training of mental health practitioners.

To date, there is no interdisciplinary consensus on the requisite supervisory training or supervision competencies (APA, 2014; Borders, 2014; Henriksen et al., 2019; Ogbeide & Bayles, 2023); however, theories of mental health practitioner development and supervision models across psychology, counseling, social work, marriage and family therapy, and medical fields (e.g., nursing, psychiatry) recognize three major functions of supervision; these include:

> administrative (e.g., monitoring case documentation, legal/ethical issues), supportive/restorative (e.g., providing support for emotional impact of clinical work, developing confidence), and educational/formative (e.g., fostering clinical skill development) (Holloway, 1995; Kadushin, 1985; Proctor, 1994). However, little is known about the relative emphasis given to these functions.
>
> (Accurso et al., 2011, p. 89)

There is also interdisciplinary agreement that integral to competent, ethical, and effective supervision are multicultural, social justice, and ecological proficiencies (Dollarhide et al., 2021; Fickling et al., 2019; Mitchell & Butler, 2021), increasingly represented in "supervision practices, models, and paradigms" (Peters et al., 2022, p. 520) over the past 20 years.

Supervision models and frameworks have long provided a theoretical scaffold and conceptual template for both supervisors and supervisees, grounding the requisite supervisory content, and guiding the intra-and interpersonal processes (Watkins, 2020). Supervision has also been recognized as a socialization process that acculturates the supervisee to professional values, dispositions, cognitive patterns, and problem-solving strategies (Luke, 2008b). Therefore, it is not surprising that psychotherapy-based supervision models (e.g., *psychodynamic, humanistic relationship, cognitive behavioral, systemic,* and *feminist;* Bernard & Goodyear, 2019) were the first developed (e.g., Ekstein & Wallerstein, 1958), wherein the supervisor served as a theoretical expert and transferred their knowledge about the processes and procedures within a distinct and shared theoretical orientation. These were followed by developmental models (e.g., *systemic cognitive-developmental supervision* model [Rigazio-DiGilio & Anderson, 1995] and *integrated developmental model* [Stoltenberg et al., 1998; Stoltenberg & McNeil, 2010]) of supervision (e.g., Littrell et al., 1979; Stoltenberg, 1981) which recognized differing supervisee needs and goals across distinct stages throughout the growth of the supervisee. Process models (e.g., *discrimination model* [Bernard 1979, 1997] and *systems approach to supervision* model [Holloway, 1995, 2016]) of supervision appeared next (e.g., Bernard, 1979), outlining the differing supervisory focus, goals, functions, styles, and roles. More recently, second-generation models of supervision have emerged (e.g., Peters & Luke, 2021a; Peters et al., 2022), integrating two established supervision models or combining an established model with a specific population, target issue, or counseling context (Bernard & Goodyear, 2019). While most established supervision models were developed for in-person, individual supervision with students or nascent clinicians, numerous integrated models focus specifically on triadic (i.e., one supervisor with two supervisees) or group (i.e., one supervisor with three or more supervisees) supervision in live and computer-mediated online settings, and some with more seasoned post-graduate and post-licensure practitioners as part of ongoing professional development (Bernard & Goodyear, 2019).

Despite the increased number of supervision models that address differing supervisory content, contexts, and configurations (Luke et al., 2011) and the expansion of individual, triadic, and group supervision across live, in-person, and computer-mediated or online deliveries, there has been an underlying assumption that supervision is the largely the same across these domains (Luke, 2019). That said, there is minimal evidence to support the notion that supervision across specialty area, development, and setting should be treated as ubiquitous or that addresses supervisory processes and effectiveness (Accurso et al., 2011; Keum & Wang, 2020; Merlin &

Brendel, 2017; Zhu & Luke, 2022). In addition, although most mental health practitioners will supervise at some point in their careers (Bernard & Goodyear, 2019), a considerable number of supervisors are not trained in supervision, and when they are trained, it is primarily in established psychotherapy-based, developmental, and process-focused models of supervision (Keum & Wang, 2020; Luke, 2019). Supervisors with little to no training; however, should identify a psychotherapy-based, developmental, and process model of supervision, which can include second generation models to support supervisee development. Moreover, despite the interdisciplinary commitments to multiculturally-focused, social justice-oriented, and ecological-responsive supervision approaches, most supervisory theories and frameworks do not specifically address the contemporary understanding of anti-oppression (Peters et al., 2022).

In their content analyses of the supervision literature, Bernard and Luke (2015) identified a diminishing focus on multiculturalism between 2005–2014 and minimal attention to social justice and ecology. More recently, Kemer et al. (2022) identified similar patterns in the supervision literature, with a primary emphasis on multiculturalism and less so on social justice. Of note is that despite growing attention to the layered cultural and systemic processes (Wilcox et al., 2021) as well as the role of intersectionality and power in supervision (Mitchell & Butler, 2021; Gutierrez, 2018; Hernández & McDowell, 2010), there has been minimal attention to theoretically grounded and developmentally responsive supervisory interventions. Although several scholars have sought to address the gap by describing creative approaches (L. Bradley et al., 2023), experiential approaches (Luke, 2008a; Mullen et al., 2008), relational-cultural approaches (N. Bradley et al., 2019), and group activities (Luke & Goodrich, 2015a, 2015b), the presentation and discussion of these supervisory interventions and techniques was circumscribed. While most of the approaches and interventions presented assume an in-person supervisory context (Bean et al., 2014), there have been isolated discussions of the recent contextual shifts in supervision, with a focus on moving from in-person and retrospective supervision to live supervision that requires increased digital systemic competence (Sherbersky et al., 2021). Nonetheless, supervisors seeking a comprehensive understanding of the background and rationale for supervisory interventions remain under-prepared and in need of step-by-step information for the implementation of the techniques (Bean et al., 2014; Prasath & Copeland, 2021), as well as more detailed support for the processing and evaluation of the interventions. Moreover, none of the identified interventions directly consider anti-oppression. Therefore, there is an emergent need for increased attention to anti-oppression in supervision (Peters & Luke, 2022, 2023). Given that research has indicated prior experience as a supervisor did not correlate with increased supervisor development (Vidlak, 2002), but that training in supervision (DeKruyf & Pehrsson, 2011) and access to supervisory resources was correlated with both efficacy and effectiveness (Bean et al., 2014), there is also a need for supervisory resources that address anti-oppression (Okech et al., 2023a).

## ANTI-OPPRESSION IN SUPERVISION

The myriad benefits of supervision include but are not limited to interdisciplinary documentation of an extended and deepened understanding of theoretical, developmental, and relational principles, an augmented ability to recognize and effectively manage the intra-and inter-personal dynamics as well as the systemic and structural forces impacting counseling and supervision, and an improved ability to select and implement interventions leading to positive change for clinicians and clients (Bernard & Goodyear, 2019; Castonguay & Hill, 2023; Friedlander & Heatherington, 2023; Hill & Norcross, 2023). Throughout the last decade, supervision models, frameworks, and paradigms incorporating multiculturalism, social justice, and ecology have emerged as part of best practice (Fickling et al., 2019; Kemer, 2024; Middleton et al., 2023; Wilcox et al., 2022b), with increasing empirical support (Social Justice Supervision Model [Dollarhide et al., 2021]; The Multicultural Integrated Supervision Model [Mitchell & Butler, 2021]; Supervision of Leadership Model [Peters & Luke, 2021a]; Integrated Supervision Framework [Peters et al., 2022]; Queer People of Color Resilience-Based Model of Supervision [Singh & Chun, 2010]). Arguably, the call for the inclusion of contemporary data and "big ideas that are relevant to diverse learning and supervision experiences" described by Castonguay and Hill (2023, p. 3) should integrate anti-oppression; however, there is limited inclusion of anti-oppression in the supervision literature, except for Okech et al. (2023a).

In their application of Peters and Luke's principles of anti-oppression (2022, 2023) to group work supervision, Okech et al. (2023a) described the goals of anti-oppressive supervision to involve identifying and addressing oppression as it arises in counseling and supervision, as well as optimizing counseling and supervision to be both internally and externally, anti-oppressive. The supervisor, and increasingly the supervisee, need to develop an ability to distinguish and understand varied forms of singular and multiplistic oppression, engage reflexivity and self-awareness to understand their contributions to upholding and enacting oppression, as well as "have the skills to intervene and challenge oppressive structures"

(Okech et al., 2023a, p. 90) to accomplish this. Unfortunately, problematic supervisory experiences that fail to address these and other goals are far too common (Bernard & Goodyear, 2019).

The growing research on inadequate and harmful supervisory experiences includes supervisors engaging in unresponsive and neglectful behaviors that fail to create a safe and supportive supervisory environment, providing inappropriate feedback that is callous and does not reflect accountability or ethical practices, and demonstrating limitations to the basic knowledge and skills that are part of ongoing development (Coleiro et al., 2023; Hutman et al., 2023). To date, scholars have not framed problematic supervision through an anti-oppressive lens; however, much of the research in this area evidence oppressive supervisory practices. For example, scholars suggest that when a supervisor's development lags behind a supervisee's development in a particular area, in this case, related to multicultural or social justice orientation and anti-oppressive principles, the regressive pairing not only stymies the growth of the supervisee but this may also increase the likelihood of their non-disclosure putting the supervisee, clients, and the supervisor at risk (Bernard & Goodyear, 2019). Because supervision can be oppressive or anti-oppressive within a particular moment, session, or at large, based in part on the competence of the supervisor, it is imperative for supervisors to intentionally consider how to systematically infuse and center anti-oppression into their preparation for, implementation of, and assessment used within supervision. Accordingly, Okech et al. (2023a) posit that supervisors need to attend to three intersecting elements when applying the anti-oppression principles to supervision, namely the target of anti-oppressive, the supervision modality, and supervision models and processes.

Similarly, Legha (2023b) argues that clinical supervisors must move beyond the sidelines and be active participants and advocates for anti-oppressive supervision and training, especially given the scant number of codified strategies used to practice anti-oppressive supervision. Accordingly, Legha's tenets of anti-oppressive supervision suggest the need to (a) recognize the historical inheritance of oppression, (b) recognize and name oppression as an enduring public health crisis, (c) acknowledge when one is being oppressive to be anti-oppressive, (d) amplify critical consciousness to disrupt and challenge all systems and structures of oppression, (e) cultivate anti-oppressive knowledge, skills, and actions, and (f) dismantle oppression in clinical supervision and client care. We argue that clinical supervisors must attend to these overarching tenets of anti-oppressive supervision across socioecological levels, including intrapersonal (e.g., internalized oppression), interpersonal (e.g., microaggression, implicit bias, myside bias), institutional and structural (e.g., racial and queer discrimination within housing and employment), policy (e.g., oppressive laws, policies, regulations), and ideology (e.g., superiority or inferiority based on a social location). Taken collectively, Okech et al.'s (2023a) and Legha's (2023b) works provide essential contributions to framing the processes and practices associated with anti-oppressive supervision.

## Anti-Oppressive Supervision Model

One way to continuously work towards these aims is by employing a second-generation supervision model that specifically addresses the principles of anti-oppression. While we acknowledge there are undoubtedly many possible supervisory frameworks and approaches (Li et al., 2018; Mitchell & Butler, 2021; Zhou et al., 2020) that can accomplish this (see Chapter 12), for illustrative purposes, we have developed the Anti-Oppressive Supervision Model (AOSM). We ground our decision to extend the atheoretical discrimination model (DM, Bernard, 1979, 1997) in the fact that the DM is among the most researched and widely used models of supervision (Luke et al., 2011; Peters & Luke, 2021b). The three foci (e.g., intervention, conceptualization, personalization) by three roles (e.g., instructor, facilitator, consultant) matrix of the DM does not ever prescribe a specific foci-role combination and instead offers the supervisor and supervisee both structure and flexibility to approach arising supervisory material through developmental, theoretical, and contextual lenses (Luke & Peters, 2020). Further, the DM has been extended into many multicultural and social justice second-generation models (Bernard & Goodyear, 2019; ISF Peters et al., 2022), making it the logical supervision model in which to initially integrate the 10 research-derived principles of anti-oppression (Peters & Luke, 2022, 2023).

The use of the AODM is organized by three primary and sequential decisions. First, the supervisor, ofttimes with input from the supervisee, determines the domain for the current point of entry (Luke & Bernard, 2006), in this case, one of the 10 principles of anti-oppression. This initial decision is based upon prioritizing which of the 10 principles the supervisory material arises from. While it is possible that a supervisory circumstance may transcend more than one principle, the supervisor and supervisee should establish the domain they will first address. Secondly, the supervisor has a choice between the three supervisory foci, basing their selection of an intervention, conceptualization, or personalization focus on the supervisee's presentation and development, as well as the unique

*Table 1.1* AODM point of entry Principle 1: *Developing critical consciousness through critical reflexivity*

|  | Instructor | Facilitator | Consultant |
|---|---|---|---|
| Intervention | The supervisor demonstrates how to use reframing and externalization to support a client with marginalized social locations in expanding their critical consciousness and critical reflexivity. | The supervisor validates the supervisee's engagement of critical reflexivity on the intent and outcome of raising a discrepancy with the client. | The supervisor invites the supervisee with predominately privileged identities to brainstorm additional ways to integrate critical consciousness and critical reflexivity into supervision and counseling. |
| Conceptualization | The supervisor reviews the definitions of critical consciousness and critical reflexivity with the supervisee for clarity. | The supervisor explores the supervisee's understanding of the role of critical consciousness and critical reflexivity in the client's presenting circumstance. | The supervisor and supervisee discuss the challenges, benefits, and need for engaging in critical consciousness and critical reflexivity in assessment and treatment planning. |
| Personalization | The supervisor labels the supervisee's frustration, disappointment, and guilt in missing an opportunity to engage critical consciousness and critical reflexivity. | The supervisor guides the supervisee in identifying how their own identities and social locations influence their experience of critical consciousness and critical reflexivity in counseling and supervision. | The supervisor and supervisee examine how critical consciousness and critical reflexivity within their relational dynamics may parallel that evidenced in the counseling relationship. |

case material needs of the supervisee and client (Bernard, 1979, 1997; Luke & Peters, 2020; Peters & Luke, 2021a). While it is possible that all three foci are relevant to the supervisory material, the supervisor needs to prioritize one to start. Thirdly, the supervisor must decide which of the three supervisory roles (e.g., instructor, facilitator, consultant) through which to first engage. The supervisor considers counseling and supervision theories of practice and contexts, as well as the intersections of individual differences and positional, relational/social, and cultural ascriptions, as well as other related clinical judgments when selecting the role posture

*Table 1.2* AODM point of entry Principle 2: *Overcoming comfort and fragility through unlearning privilege and domination*

|  | Instructor | Facilitator | Consultant |
| --- | --- | --- | --- |
| Intervention | The supervisor directs the supervisee to re-examine the client's non-verbal behavior when discussing privilege and oppression in the counseling session. | The supervisor facilitates the supervisee to connect their own discomfort and fragility with privilege and domination and their ability to address clients. | The supervisor provides a resource list related to overcoming comfort and fragility for the supervisee to consider and discuss in the subsequent supervision session. |
| Conceptualization | The supervisor evaluates the supervisee's client assessment, including how the supervisee incorporates the client's experiences of privilege and domination. | The supervisor uses Socratic questioning to help the supervisee identify themes of comfort and fragility across their caseload. | The supervisor offers the supervisee an opportunity to list congruencies across their theory of practice and the role of unlearning privilege and domination. |
| Personalization | The supervisor takes responsibility for failing to prioritize opportunities to unlearn privilege and domination in their feedback on the supervisee's clinical documentation. | The supervisor uses creative interventions to assist the supervisee in understanding how their sociocultural privilege and unexamined comfort and fragility are manifesting in both counseling and supervision. | The supervisor and supervisee discuss potential ways the supervisee can identify their own discomfort and fragility in session to increase their opportunity to respond. |

through which they will intervene as supervisor (Bernard, 1979, 1997; Luke & Peters, 2020).

Like other second-generation process models of supervision, the AODM is predicated on the belief that once the point of entry is determined, the majority of supervisory material can be effectively addressed through any of the available foci-role combinations (Luke & Bernard, 2006). In fact, supervisor competence includes the flexibility to utilize the full range of foci-role combinations (Luke et al., 2011), as opposed to identifying a match between supervisory foci-role combination and a specific supervisory presentation or circumstance. That said, there is agreement that

Table 1.3 AODM point of entry Principle 3: *Centering the margins through empowerment and liberation*

| | Instructor | Facilitator | Consultant |
|---|---|---|---|
| Intervention | The supervisor explains the importance of client empowerment and liberation by connecting them back to professional competencies, standards, and literature. | The supervisor rehearses with the supervisee how they can raise discrepancies about the client's goal to center non-dominant perspectives in their journey of racial healing (Singh, 2019) and their resistance when the supervisee attempts to center the margins. | The supervisor and supervisee review anti-oppressive interventions to identify examples that can be used to center the margins and help empower and liberate the client's voice. |
| Conceptualization | The supervisor describes how the supervisee can determine the client's readiness for (e.g., pre-contemplation, contemplation, action) and the appropriateness of a shift to include a more liberatory counseling approach. | The supervisor investigates the supervisee's rationale for not wanting to discuss empowerment and liberation in counseling or supervision with a client who has multiple marginalized identities. | The supervisor and supervisee take turns identifying process goals for empowerment and liberation that can lead to an outcome goal of the client independently centering the margins (e.g., identifying an alternative view). |
| Personalization | The supervisor instructs the supervisee about how to address the client's values, biases, and assumptions related to empowerment and liberation in a therapeutic space, given their socialization. | The supervisor uses immediacy to explore the supervisee's countertransference related to centering the margins (e.g., the use of abolitionist and Indigenous resources). | The supervisor suggests the supervisee consider writing a letter to client empowerment and liberation to discover more about its meaning in their work and professional development. |

supervisory decisions should prioritize using one point of entry with one foci and role at a time, without combining or shifting across these to avoid confusion for the supervisee (Bernard, 1997; Hilts et al., 2022; Luke & Peters, 2020). While we acknowledge that most of the 90 potential

*Table 1.4* AODM point of entry Principle 4: *Wellness and self-care through acts of compassion and vigilance*

|  | Instructor | Facilitator | Consultant |
|---|---|---|---|
| Intervention | The supervisor reviews the Chi Sigma Iota Wellness Competencies (or other similar documents), asking the supervisee to develop two wellness-related supervisory goals informed by critical theory (e.g., queer theory, critical race theory, dis/crit) to incorporate into their supervision. | The supervisor requests the supervisee's permission to interrupt and address instances where the supervisee may be missing opportunities to extend self-compassion and self-care within the supervisory session. | The supervisor and supervisee collaboratively review the supervisee's treatment notes and identify instances where the topics or client wellness and self-care arose and how they were and were not responded to in session because of cultural similarities. |
| Conceptualization | The supervisor leads the supervisee in identifying the salience of and links between the client's social location and presenting concerns, wellness, and the supervisee's theoretical framework. | The supervisor facilitates the supervisee to consider potential ways in which the supervisor can more vigilantly and compassionately incorporate more wellness informed by decolonial theory into the supervisory space. | The supervisor offers a potential link between the supervisee's sociocultural understanding of wellness and that of their clients and then asks them to identify three more. |
| Personalization | The supervisor provides feedback to the supervisee about their observations of the counseling working alliance during the implementation of a wellness intervention with a client who was socialized to take care of others and not themselves. | The supervisor processes the supervisee's intra-personal, inter-personal, and cultural associations with wellness given their unique experiences, including identities and social locations. | The supervisor suggests that the supervisee may want to consider how they can incorporate self-compassion and self-care into their own wellness plan, given their reported ongoing personal experiences with oppression and battle fatigue. |

*Table 1.5* AODM point of entry Principle 5: *Co-constructing a brave space through relationships and community*

|  | Instructor | Facilitator | Consultant |
|---|---|---|---|
| Intervention | The supervisor asks the supervisee to review their counseling recording and identify instances where there is evidence of them co-constructing a brave space with their client. | The supervisor reinforces the supervisee's excitement about client feedback related to the counseling working alliance, including the client's identification of the impact of brave space. | The supervisor invites the supervisee to bring a supervisory activity for use in their next supervision session that may positively contribute to their co-construction of a brave supervisory space to explore issues of racism within the queer community and heterosexism within BIPOC communities. |
| Conceptualization | The supervisor asks the supervisee to explain their conceptualization of how a brave space differs from a safe space and in what ways they see their role in co-creating such. | The supervisor helps the supervisee identify how the client's development (e.g., including their multicultural, social justice, and anti-oppressive development) may be influencing their interpersonal engagement in counseling. | The supervisor and supervisee discuss their differing thoughts and perceptions of what constitutes a brave space, attending to the ways identities, social locations, and positionality may influence subjectivity. |
| Personalization | The supervisor points out to the supervisee that they repeatedly bypass the supervisor's queries about family, community, and stakeholder relationships as part of a brave space. | The supervisor explores the supervisee's affirming and disaffirming experiences related to a brave supervisory space, given previous negative experiences that felt performative. | The supervisor collaborates with the supervisee in locating instances when they each took intra-and inter-personal risks in supervision, as well as instances when they did not. |

*Table 1.6* AODM point of entry Principle 6: *Developing goals and assessing outcomes through stakeholder investment*

|  | *Instructor* | *Facilitator* | *Consultant* |
|---|---|---|---|
| Intervention | The supervisor shows the supervisee how to use linking and blocking when developing anti-oppressive goals in anticipation of the supervisee independently leading their first meeting with stakeholders. | The supervisor reflects the supervisee's awareness that they have struggled to incorporate the client's family and community in-session when setting and assessing process goals within client treatment, given their training solely focused on individualism and not collectivism. | The supervisor shares one way they might involve stakeholders in developing anti-racist goals and assessing outcomes and asks the supervisee to suggest another option. |
| Conceptualization | The supervisor provides the supervisee with a handout on assessing and measuring goals that promote positive health outcomes for clients from marginalized communities. | The supervisor explores the supervisee's theoretical and developmental rationales for using a traditional and non-western framing of client goals and the level of stakeholder investment in the outcome assessment processes. | The supervisor asks the supervisee to make a list of culturally responsive and anti-oppressive professional resources (including professional relationships) that can be referred to in the future for goal setting and outcome assessment. |
| Personalization | The supervisor stops the counseling recording, replays a short segment, and asks the supervisee to describe what they are experiencing as they consider how the segment relates to the client's goals of identity exploration and self-community empowerment. | The supervisor uses Interpersonal Process Recall (IPR; Kagan, 1976; Kagan & Kagan, 1990) to support the supervisee in sharing their experiences of a recent treatment team meeting where they didn't understand the impact of social determents of health on marginalized communities. | The supervisor shares information about an upcoming professional conference on decolonial counseling, reviewing with the supervisee the sessions that may be related to goal setting, outcome assessment, or stakeholder engagement. |

*Table 1.7* AODM point of entry Principle 7: *Challenging and disrupting oppression through broaching and accountability*

|  | Instructor | Facilitator | Consultant |
|---|---|---|---|
| Intervention | The supervisor explains the purpose of broaching offers to role play opportunities to disrupt oppression with the supervisee. | The supervisor introduces a sculpting activity (Satir et al., 1991) to assist the supervisee in expressing how their use of culture broaching and accountability impacted the clients. | The supervisor offers themselves as a sounding board for the supervisee to consider their ambivalence about taking accountability with their peers for not challenging and disputing oppression on site. |
| Conceptualization | The supervisor offers a potential interpretation of the client's response when the supervisee tried to take accountability for a microaggression. | The supervisor notes a potential discrepancy between the supervisee's theoretical orientation and the premises underlying challenging and broaching behaviors and asks the supervisee to reflect on this. | The supervisor displays the principles of oppression and engages the supervisee in thinking about how the 10 principles can be understood as developing separately and in relation to one another. |
| Personalization | The supervisor reviews a recording where the supervisee stops mid-way through broaching cultural norms with their older White female client, pointing out that this is quite different than the supervisee's prior use of broaching. | The supervisor validates and normalizes the supervisee's struggle to challenge systemic authority and broach oppressive behaviors with supervisors and faculty. | The supervisor broaches a conversation with the supervisee, taking accountability for their role in upholding structural oppression in supervision, and creates space for the supervisee to share how they want the supervisor to be accountable. |

*Table 1.8* AODM point of entry Principle 8: *Identifying and addressing barriers through resistance and opposition*

|  | Instructor | Facilitator | Consultant |
|---|---|---|---|
| Intervention | The supervisor requires the supervisee to prepare a transcript of their counseling session to identify how they addressed and missed opportunities to identify and address oppressive barriers related to the client's presenting concerns. | The supervisor asks the supervisee to reflect on the possibility that they can identify the structural and systemic barriers the client is facing and empathize with the client's resistance to taking action. | The supervisor encourages the supervisee to consider alternative counseling skills that could be used with the client to support and direct their resistance and opposition to oppressive behaviors. |
| Conceptualization | The supervisor reviews the mid-term evaluation form with the supervisee, informing them that they will add the supervisory goal of conceptual skills related to identifying and addressing barriers faced by clients from lower socioeconomic statuses when seeking and attending counseling during the second half of the semester. | The supervisor assists the supervisee in clarifying their understanding of the definitions of resistance and opposition within an anti-oppressive framework. | The supervisor offers a few interpretations of the client's initial reaction to the supervisee, raising the possibility of resistance and opposition, and asks the supervisee to determine which fits their understanding of the client's social locations and supervisee's theory (e.g., relational cultural theory informed by intersectionality). |
| Personalization | The supervisor notices that the supervisee is starting to become somatically activated in their seat while discussing their responsibilities to ensure the virtual counseling space and process is equitable and accessible for persons with disabilities and suggests that the supervisee may be experiencing anxiety, guilt, and embarrassment. | The supervisor notices the supervisee's embarrassment about mis-identifying a client barrier and then uses self-disclosure to illustrate a similar example from their own developmental trajectory. | The supervisor provides the supervisee with an opportunity to review training resource videos (e.g., challenging authority and using opposition) within supervision and then asks the supervisee if and how they wish to incorporate the material into their supervisory goals given the power differentials. |

*Table 1.9* AODM point of entry Principle 9: *Socioecological advocacy and activism through collective action*

|  | Instructor | Facilitator | Consultant |
|---|---|---|---|
| Intervention | The supervisor affirms the supervisee's selection of Bronfenbrenner's theory (Bronfenbrenner & Morris, 1998) through which to intervene across the socioecological system (e.g., the micro, meso, and macro levels). | The supervisor asks the supervisee to examine different ways to address advocacy and activism in session with a queer, Black, and deaf client, experimenting with varied linguistic choices. | The supervisor introduces a sociogram and collaboratively works with the supervisee to identify opportunities for advocacy and activism within the client's socioecological system. |
| Conceptualization | The supervisor reviews systems theory (Luke, 2016) with the supervisee and explains the purposes of advocacy and activism at the intrapersonal, interpersonal, and group as a whole levels. | The supervisor facilitates the supervisee's examination of the similarities and differences in advocacy and activism across individual and collective action. | The supervisor suggests that the supervisee locate literature on theoretically congruent examples of socioecological advocacy and activism with queer migrant populations and explores how they can work with the client to incorporate collective action. |
| Personalization | The supervisor outlines common developmental struggles that the supervisee may experience as they expand their skills related to socioecological and anti-racist advocacy and activism through collective action. | The supervisor uses reframing to identify and normalize the supervisee's concerns about upholding boundaries grounded in privilege and domination when using collective action while also expanding the supervisee's awareness of possibilities for advocacy and activism. | The cisgender supervisor and supervisee unpack the supervisee's recent experience advocating for a transgender teenager in a high school and state where anti-trans rhetoric and legislation exist. |

*Table 1.10* AODM point of entry Principle 10: *Redistributing social, cultural, and political capital through access and opportunity*

|  | Instructor | Facilitator | Consultant |
|---|---|---|---|
| Intervention | The supervisor models how the supervisee can redistribute capital (e.g., social, cultural, political) in counseling by using their power and the think-aloud intervention ("I am saying/doing this because . . .") with a cross-cultural family struggling to understand and empathize with generational differences that can result reifying oppression within the family's household. | The supervisor uses motivational interviewing to gauge the supervisee's readiness to redistribute capital (e.g., social, cultural, political) within counseling and supervisory contexts. | The supervisor and supervisee take turns roleplaying how the supervisee can use their social and cultural capital to address and rectify a culturally inappropriate diagnosis for a client who is a transgender international student of color, given the sites concerning policy for diagnosis and billing. |
| Conceptualization | The supervisor asks the supervisee to label the capital (e.g., social, cultural, political) that appears and functions within supervision. | The supervisor assists the supervisee in describing how they understand the role of the working alliance as part of redistributing capital (e.g., social, cultural, political) within the recorded counseling session just reviewed. | The supervisor and supervisee process their experiences of redistributing capital (e.g., social, cultural, political) in supervision and ways to continue to develop new and innovative ways to do so moving forward. |
| Personalization | The supervisor assesses the supervisee's reaction to client resistance to the supervisor's attempt to disrupt the established counseling norms and redistribute social and cultural capital in their counseling session. | The supervisor invites the supervisee to use the sand tray to represent their real and ideal experiences (e.g., thoughts, feelings, behaviors) of social, cultural, and political capital in counseling and supervision. | The supervisor shares their ideas about what might be at the root of the supervisee's struggle with redistributing capital (e.g., social, cultural, political) in counseling due to social locations and previous political positions and invites the supervisee to discuss what resonates and what does not. |

AODM domain x foci x role combinations are operational to efficaciously address presenting supervisory material and circumstances, the supervisor should examine their choices throughout the course of supervision with each supervisee, as well as across supervisees at any point in time to ensure that these decisions are responsive to the needs and development of each individual supervisees and that they reflect the full range of principles of anti-oppression. Development of an anti-oppressive supervision instrument and future research that examines supervisory processes and outcomes associated with anti-oppressive supervision are warranted. Similarly, meta-supervision (Bernard & Goodyear, 2019), whether in the form of self-, peer-, or supervision of supervision, should also integrate contemporary research and practice-related resources, such as anti-oppressive supervisory activities and interventions like those included in this book.

CHAPTER 2

# Developing Critical Consciousness Through Critical Reflexivity

*Devika Dibya Choudhuri, Joshua N. Hook, Ah Ram Lee, Yanhong Liu, Melissa Luke, Harvey Charles Peters, Elyssa B. Smith, and C. Edward Watkins, Jr.*

## CHAPTER 2 INTERVENTIONS

### Intervention Title: Flip the Internalized Supervisory Script for Learned Agency

### Author(s) and Affiliation(s)

Melissa Luke, Ph.D., NCC, ACS, LMHC
Syracuse University

Harvey Charles Peters, Ph.D., NCC
Montclair State University

### Supervision Format and Modality

This supervision intervention was developed for in-person or virtual individual supervision, but it could be adapted for use within triadic and small group supervision with 6–10 supervisees.

DOI: 10.4324/9781003470656-2

## Supervisee Development

This supervision intervention can be used across all levels of supervisee development, but it is particularly useful when supervisees are feeling stuck and having difficulty identifying opportunities for advocacy within their counseling and/or supervision.

## Supervisory Goals and Learning Objectives

1. Supervisees will expand their critical consciousness and reflexivity.
2. Supervisees will articulate and explore their values, worldviews, multiplistic social locations, positions, identity development, and biases.
3. Supervisees will examine interlocking forces, structures, and systems of power that impact their counseling and supervision.
4. Supervisees will identify opportunities for agency and advocacy within counseling and supervision.

## Time Required

This anti-oppressive supervisory intervention is designed for use within a 50–60-minute supervision session.

## Materials

Supervisors refamiliarize themselves with the concept of learned helplessness (Abramson et al., 1978; Maier & Seligman, 1976; Seligman & Maier, 1976). They may find it helpful to prepare a few slides or handouts to outline learned helplessness (Overmier & Seligman, 1967) and define locus of control, self-efficacy (Bandura, 1977; Springer & Schimmel, 2015), and agency (Bandura, 1989), depicting the relationships between these constructs and learned agency (Goodrich & Luke, 2016), particularly in persons having experienced-isms and oppression. The supervisor also needs access to lateral thinking puzzles with answers, as well as a golf ball and paper bag.

## Intervention Instructions

1. The supervisor explains this is a tripartite anti-oppressive supervision intervention that contains psychoeducational, experiential, and interactive components. The supervisor reviews the primary goals of the intervention and explains how these support the supervisee's overall learning goals.

2. The supervisor introduces learned helplessness as first observed in experiments with dogs unable to escape electric shock and describes later research with humans exposed to unavoidable aversive stimuli and found to have lower motivation and increased passive acceptance (Overmier & Seligman, 1967; Seligman & Maier, 1976). The supervisor explains that it has been theorized that learned helplessness (and its concomitant external attribution or locus of control) can also result from vicarious learning (Bandura, 1989) through exposure to others' experiences "with aversive stimuli and uncontrollable events" (Goodrich & Luke, 2016, p. 71).

3. The supervisor invites the supervisee's reaction, exploring their understanding within their counseling and supervision. The supervisor asks the supervisee, "How are you making sense of this information right now?" or "How might your values, worldviews, multiplistic social locations, positions, identity development, and biases intersect with learned helplessness?" or "When you consider your counseling and supervision, where might systemic forces and power intersect with your identification of and perhaps experience with learned helplessness?"

4. The supervisor identifies the concept of self-efficacy (Bandura, 1989) and reviews its role within counselor development (Springer & Schimmel, 2015). The supervisor explains that "learned agency" can develop through similar processes of direct exposure and vicarious learning. The supervisor suggests the supervisee reflect on "What connections do you identify between these concepts and your own experiences?" or "How might the intersections of your values, worldviews, multiplistic social locations, positions, and/or biases facilitate and hinder the development of self-efficacy and learned agency?" or "What begins to look different when we start to account for the varied systemic and power dynamics within your counseling and supervision?"

5. The supervisor gauges the supervisee's willingness to take part in a brief experiential component of the supervision intervention. If the supervisee agrees, the supervisor provides a lateral thinking puzzle (see resources for examples) but provides minimal time for the supervisee to consider the conundrum before telling them it is time to move on to the next one. The supervisor provides one or two more lateral thinking puzzles without giving the supervisee adequate time, in effect creating an inescapable experience of low-risk failure within supervision. If the supervisee prefers not to directly engage in an experiential intervention, the supervisor can demonstrate a lateral thinking puzzle using a golf ball and paper bag (see Goodrich & Luke, 2016, p. 72).

6.  The supervisor explains the intention of the lateral thinking puzzle and processes the supervisee's experiences, attending to both intra-and inter-personal aspects. The supervisor asks, "What was your experience of the lateral thinking puzzle(s)?" or "How did you feel toward me during the tasks?" or "What intra-and inter-personal tensions can you identify?" or "How might our differing values, worldviews, multiplistic social locations, positions, and/or biases contribute?" or "When might your clients ever have experiences like this in counseling?"

7.  The supervisor explains the final component of this intervention includes a review of the supervisee's recording and/or case report through the lenses of learned helplessness and learned agency. The supervisor indicates that the supervisee and the supervisor will either stop the recording or interrupt the case report to identify instances when the counseling was stuck, the process stymied, or there is a lack of agency.

8.  The supervisor asks the supervisee to describe what's taking place, reflect on what might be contributing to agency or lack thereof, and examine how they could infuse learned agency. The supervisor inquires, "What stands out to you about what's taking place here?" or "In what ways might the earlier portion of our supervision be influencing your thinking now?" or "How might the concepts we have discussed be playing out between you and/or your client?" or "In what ways might your or your client's values, worldviews, multiplistic social locations, positions, and/or biases as well as the systems of power and privilege be contributing?" or "What might happen if you identified and/or reinforced resiliency, efficacy or agency?" or "How can you model this for your client or transfer some of what we have done in supervision?"

9.  The supervisor helps the supervisee consolidate their learning, examining what the supervisee is taking away and how the new concepts can be used to redress prior conceptualizations and future work using reflective questions.

## Supervisory Alliance and Relationship

Supervisees can experience an increased vulnerability as they examine their values, worldviews, and biases, as well as the ways they have and have not enacted agency within their own work. Depending upon the supervisee's attachment style, prior experiences with feedback, and propensity toward shame, they may have difficulty remaining open and receptive to exploration with the supervisor. As such, the supervisor needs to carefully monitor and respond to the supervisee's capacity for engagement and provide a balance of challenge and support to promote their reflexivity and increased understanding of the complexities related to interlocking forces, structures, and systems of power within anti-oppressive work.

## Legal and Ethical Considerations

This intervention frequently elicits new supervisee insights and behaviors; however, supervisees frequently encounter difficult thoughts and feelings, particularly with respect to their previously unrecognized but longstanding personal, familial, and cultural patterns. Given that the lateral thinking puzzle component of the supervision intervention may elicit supervisee frustration, the supervisor should attend to any interpersonal or relational breach and make efforts to repair the supervisory alliance if so.

## Reflective Questions

1.  What did you learn about yourself today?
2.  How can you apply the concepts we examined today in your future counseling, and what will you need to support this?
3.  When have/do you experience learned helplessness (and learned agency) in our supervisory work, and how might systems of power help and hinder our attention to this?
4.  How can your interventions for learned agency further your goals toward anti-oppressive counseling and supervision?
5.  What remains challenging with respect to learned agency?

## Intervention Title: Creating Circle: Journey of Critical Reflexivity

## Author(s) and Affiliation(s)

Elyssa B. Smith Ph.D., LPC, RPT, NCC, ACS

## Supervision Format and Modality

The intervention is designed primarily for in-person supervision. This anti-oppressive, (re) Indigenous supervision model synthesizes the practice of Creating Circle (Whyte & Toll, 2023) to engage supervisees on their journey of developing critical reflexivity and is intended for group supervision (up to 10 supervisees). With modifications, this activity could be implemented in individual and triadic supervision.

## Supervisee Development

The intervention is primarily intended for master's or doctoral-level trainees in practicum or internship; however, it can be adapted for postgraduate, pre-licensure, and post-licensure clinicians. The intervention is designed to occur within each supervision session spanning the semester, with attention to each developmental stage across the supervisee's journey and process.

## Supervisory Goals and Learning Objectives

1. Supervisees will identify at least three ways their roots, ancestry, and intersectional identities present vulnerabilities and strengths in supervision and counseling.
2. Supervisees will collaborate with supervisor(s) and other supervisee(s) to *Create Circle* as a safe and anti-oppressive supervisory space/community for an effective supervisory alliance.
3. Supervisees will enact their critical reflexive skills during supervision to sit with their discomfort and fragility by describing at least two occasions of this during the supervision intervention process.
4. Supervisees will increase critical consciousness and attend to the ongoing process of engaging in critical reflexivity.
5. Supervisees will identify two actions taken to enact critical reflexivity within current and ongoing counseling practice.

## Time Required

The intervention takes 45–50 minutes per supervision session, depending on the number of supervisees, across a semester or a 12 to 16-week period of time.

## Materials

A private and confidential space for group supervision is needed, and it is recommended that supervisors create a circle with desks/chairs/furniture or encourage supervisees to join them by sitting on the floor/ground in a circle.

## Intervention Instructions

As the intervention is intended to span the semester across supervisees' development, the prompts that follow engage critical reflexivity across each stage of the supervision process and journey.

# STEPPING INTO (CREATING) CIRCLE

<u>Foundation</u>: Start Here (Used within Pre-group session; Orientation; Ongoing) *Steps for Creating Circle for Safety, (Re) Indigenization, & Anti-oppression* (please see Whyte & Toll, 2023 for an example and further details on how to go about this process): To start, the supervisor introduces the activity by explaining the concept of Creating Circle and invites each member to take turns engaging in the following three steps by sharing and speaking aloud. The other group members validate and affirm their entry into the circle (space) as each member speaks:

1. Validate: Acknowledge what we carry with us into the space; validate the enoughness of the group and its members.
2. Imagine: Imagine multiple ways of knowing with "allies to listen and witness; to make individual change."
3. Collaborate: Foster a collaborative culture that acknowledges a desire for the safety of all persons.

# SUPERVISION PROCESS

### Begin (Mind/Nucleus): Weeks 1–5

Although the supervisor does not need to follow the prompts sequentially, they may initiate this process in supervision sessions 1–5 by stating that this phase is the beginning of the journey. Supervisees are invited to go inward in the safe space created and begin to understand self, others, and community to build the foundation for their engagement with critical reflexivity. The supervisor needs to help the group understand that this process occurs both individually (internally) and across the group dynamic/members (collectively). To do so, the supervisor may ask:

*Root (Within: Self)*

- What roots and perspectives do we bring into the space?
- How will we step into the circle (see illustrative examples from Whyte & Toll, 2023)?
- What do we need to feel safe and to be seen, heard, and validated?

*Ground (Outside: Other)*

- Where can we locate ourselves within the conversation regarding oppression (i.e., unequal treatment on individual, systemic, interpersonal levels, overt and covert forms of oppression)?
- When in counseling practice and supervision, have we been shocked or surprised by what we have observed (Smith & Luke, 2021)?

*Water (Community: Self/Other/Context)*

- What are our strengths and areas of growth concerning systems of oppression and discrimination?
- How do these impact our counseling and supervision processes?

## In Medias Res (Body/Heart/Spirit): Weeks 6–10

To move into this phase, the supervisor acknowledges that this phase involves the engagement of critical reflexivity with body, heart, and spirit. For example, they can indicate that the group is in the middle of things, and that can be disorienting but also rewarding and profound. The supervisor may facilitate the process by asking:

*Seeding*

- Where and how does each person locate themselves in the conversation around oppression based on their roots (ancestry) and intersectional identity?

- What assumptions do we hold regarding perceived notions of what seems "normal" and what does not (Smith & Luke, 2021)?

*Rising*

- What about the counseling and supervision process related to oppression was (is) comfortable?
  - Where/When/Why do we feel discomfort (uncomfortable)?
  - How can we honor and sit with this discomfort?

*Envisioning*

- What do we believe is our role as change agents, advocates, and activists?
- Where do our ethics, morals, and values lie? How do these shape our practice?

## Recycle (Soul): Weeks 11–14

At this point, the supervisor indicates that the group is moving toward the final supervision sessions, and the supervisor may want to encourage supervisees to embrace this transformative stage of their journey. To do so, the supervisor might ask:

*Bloom / Transformation*

- How can we turn toward spaces of discomfort and explore deeper?
- What is needed to create community spaces for belonging and circles for healing?
- What can we do to face uncomfortable and painful truths and foster a spirit of deep respect, allyship, solidarity, and liberation?

*Fertilization*

- How can we lean into complexity and hold space for both/and (i.e., holding the tension of opposites (Smith, 2019)?
- What moves us toward action and change?
- How can we inspire others to Create Circle?

*Flower/Spread Seed*

- How can we collaborate with others to foster a desire for safety and validation for all persons?
- What is needed to build the alliances necessary to move forward and create lasting change within our practice and community?
- Who are we becoming as part of this process?

## Supervisory Alliance and Relationship

Group safety and cohesion are foundational aspects of the group alliance. Reflexive group supervisors must possess supervisory skills for building trust, listening, and deepening, along with strong group facilitation and management abilities (Heffron et al., 2016). Group supervisors serve as models of personal growth and awareness through demonstrations of humility and transparency and encourage supervisees to do the same (Mastoras & Andrews, 2011). Competent group supervisors partner with members to create, establish, and enforce emotional safety through a group community contract. The contract provides an opportunity for the group to state expectations, rules, and a frame for the group process and outcome (Bernard & Goodyear, 2019). Ruptures in the group are inevitable (Heffron et al., 2016); Supervisors attend to ruptures that surface in the group and further elicit feedback from members throughout the entire process.

## Legal and Ethical Considerations

As supervisors are responsible for adhering to best practices in clinical supervision (Bernard & Goodyear, 2019), they must possess training, professional dispositions, skills, competency, and experience in group supervision to conduct this intervention (Luke, 2019). Group supervisors ought to remain sensitive to the power differential within group supervision and acknowledge it transparently. Supervisor feedback must be direct and clear, with attention to each member's professional development and group dynamic/stage. Group supervisors must consider dual relationships (Bernard & Goodyear, 2019) and refrain from engaging in social interaction that would comprise the professional nature of the group and supervisory relationship. Although confidentiality cannot be guaranteed in a group setting, supervisors should reiterate and impress upon supervisees the importance of confidentiality concerning clients of focus and members (Bernard & Goodyear, 2019). Group supervision often evokes unconscious emotions within both members and leaders. Thus, the group may evoke unexpected reactions within the supervisor. When this occurs, supervisors are encouraged to engage in supervision of supervision or peer support.

## Reflective Questions

1. What roots, perspectives, and experiences are you bringing into the Circle today, and how do they shape the way you perceive safety and belonging within this space?
2. How can we collectively imagine a Circle that honors multiple ways of knowing, and what role can you play in supporting an environment where all voices feel heard and validated?
3. What specific actions can you take to foster a collaborative culture within the Circle, where each member feels safe and acknowledged?

## Intervention Title: A Narrative Supervision Intervention Using Letter Writing

### Author(s) and Affiliation(s)

Ah Ram Lee Ph.D., NCC
Syracuse University

Yanhong Liu, Ph.D., NCC
Syracuse University

### Supervision Format and Modality

This supervision intervention is developed primarily to be implemented in individual supervision in in-person or virtual settings. With modifications, it can be used in triadic and group supervision.

### Supervisee Development

This intervention is designed to be used with intermediate- and advanced-level supervisees.

This intervention can be adapted for all supervisees across developmental levels and social locations.

### Supervisory Goals and Learning Objectives

1.  Supervisees will expand their critical consciousness and reflexivity.
2.  Supervisees will be able to practice a narrative supervision intervention grounded in anti-oppressive principles.
3.  Supervisees will implement feedback from their supervisor on their case conceptualization skills and the use of the narrative intervention.

### Time Required

This intervention requires approximately 45 minutes within a series of supervision sessions across a semester, or the length of the supervision agreement contract.

## Materials

In preparation, supervisors should be familiar with the core concept of narrative therapy, supervision, and the use of letter writing in counseling spaces (Bjorøy et al., 2016).

1. Supervisees will bring letters they wrote to their clients based on the supervisor's instructions.
2. Supervisees will bring a recording of a session in which they read their letter to the client as a counseling intervention to receive feedback and increase reflexivity.
3. Supervisees will bring their reflective artifacts, such as a letter to themselves, journals, or artistic expressions, for further processing and reflection.

## Intervention Instructions

1. The supervisor begins by introducing the intervention structure that involves multiple phases of the supervisee writing letters to their clients, receiving feedback, reading the letters to the clients, and engaging in their own personal reflection of the processes.
2. The supervisor operationalizes and models critical consciousness by inviting the supervisee to discuss how their various sociocultural locations may inform their counseling (and supervisory) work and any challenges that they might face in working with diverse clients/students. Additionally, to foster critical consciousness through reflexivity, the supervisor invites the supervisee to reflect on nuances of cultural encounters in client-counselor relationships and how they may inform and/or be informed by intersecting dynamics of systemic oppression and privilege (Peters & Luke, 2022).
3. The supervisor emphasizes that Narrative Theory embraces horizontal relationships with clients and discusses the applicability of the theory to empowering clients/students to be authors of their own stories and to take ownership of their meaning-making (Combs & Freedman, 2012). They share the principles of anti-oppression practice (Peters & Luke, 2022) as a guideline for further reflection, noting that ultimate goals for changes occur in the supervisee's counseling practice. Additionally, the supervisor explains how letter writing can create a space for the supervisee to reflect on their work with clients/students and their conceptualization.
4. The supervisor invites the supervisee to engage in letter writing with multiple clients with different presenting issues, sociocultural locations,

and stages in counseling relationships. The supervisor can discuss with the supervisee to decide on the first 2–3 clients to write the letters to, based on the progression of their counseling relationships and supervisees' growth areas related to specific clients. The supervisee writes letters that address the following areas as their homework and brings it to the following supervision meeting.

a.  Identify at least three of the client's sociocultural locations and communicate their understanding of how these locations intersect with each other within the client's current societal context. Communicate how they understand that the client's intersecting social locations inform their personhood and experiences of privilege and/or oppression and the presenting issues.

b.  Identify one metaphor that can represent the supervisee's understanding of the client's presenting issues, their strengths, or critical progress achieved through counseling. The supervisee uses the metaphor to communicate empathic understanding in a creative and therapeutic manner.

c.  Communicate how the supervisee may have experienced the development of their counseling relationship with their client.

5.  The supervisee brings the letters to their next supervision meeting. The supervisor starts by providing feedback at the content level. For example, the supervisee may be asked to highlight key words and phrases included in the letter and the meaning that they intend to convey to their clients. The supervisor then shifts focus to cultivate the supervisee's critical consciousness through self-reflexivity. For example, the supervisor might suggest that the supervisee identify a specific dynamic in their counselor-client relationship informed by pervasive social biases connected to their identities and the social systems that embody. The supervisor invites the supervisee to reflect on how systems of power and marginalization are embedded in the sociocultural identities and the counseling relationship. The supervisor invites the supervisee to engage in critical reflexivity (see Reflective Questions).

6.  Through feedback and critical reflexivity, the supervisee and the client co-conceptualize and contextualize the client's presenting issues linked to their intersecting identities embedded in the systems of power and marginalization. The supervisor invites the supervisee to reflect on the principles of anti-oppression in light of their counselor-client relationship. The supervisor empowers the supervisee to expand upon their conceptualizations; they may encourage revisions of letters to bring critical awareness to systemic influences on client issues.

7.   To promote supervisee agency, the supervisor may suggest that the supervisee engage in additional independent reflective processes outside of supervision through one of the activities: letter to self, reflective journaling, and art expression. The reflection should be grounded in elements listed in Phase 4.

8.   The supervisor provides reiterative feedback on the letter till it reaches therapeutic quality. The supervisor models critical consciousness by holding themselves accountable for how their relationships with social structures may inform their sense of power and privilege. Upon the finalization of the letter, the supervisor invites the supervisee to identify a symbol (e.g., specific animal, plants, a character from a story) that can represent what is communicated through the letter. The supervisor recommends the supervisee share their letter and their symbol with the client and bring the recording of the session.

9.   The supervisor reviews the recorded counseling session and provides feedback on the supervisee's use of the narrative intervention. The supervisor invites the supervisee to reflect on their process of sharing the letter, the perceived effectiveness of the intervention, and new discoveries on self-consciousness and their understanding of the client. The supervisor asks the supervisee to identify a symbol that can represent their own learning and increased awareness gained through letter-writing, letter-sharing, and critical reflexivity. Additionally, the supervisor selects and shares their own symbol that represents what they have observed in the supervisee's development through the processes.

## Supervisory Alliance and Relationship

When introducing the intervention, the supervisor needs to consider the cultural backgrounds of their supervisees. If/when assessing barriers in written communication, the supervisor may consider incorporating other expressive arts (e.g., drawing, painting, selection of symbols) in lieu of writing to convey an in-depth understanding of their clients. The supervisor is expected to model critical consciousness in learning and understanding the supervisee's social-cultural background.

## Legal and Ethical Considerations

Professional ethics include the necessity for clinical supervisors to simultaneously monitor client welfare and facilitate the growth and development of the supervisee. The intervention aims to challenge supervisees' critical consciousness and encourage consistent self-reflexivity through writing letters to clients from diverse backgrounds; however, sensitivity should be directed to the client's unique situations, welfare, and therapeutic changes.

## Reflective Questions

1. What did you enjoy about writing the letter? Was there a particular client/student and/or issues that you were more excited about or more comfortable writing about? If so, reflect on what you and your client contributed to your experience.
2. Was there a particular client/student and/or issues that felt more stressful to identify or that you were more uncomfortable addressing in the letter? If so, reflect on what about you and your client and/or the issues that informed your experience.
3. Describe a new discovery in how you understand your clients/students and your work after writing the letters. What did you learn about yourself, particularly related to critical consciousness and reflexivity?
4. How might your social locations have informed your experience of letter writing? How might these things influence your understanding of your clients, of yourself, or of me as your supervisor?

## Intervention Title: Centering Critical Reflexivity in Trauma-Focused Supervision

### Author(s) and Affiliation(s)

Devika Dibya Choudhuri, PhD, LPC (MI/CT), ACS
Eastern Michigan University

### Supervision Format and Modality

The group supervision format and modality can be conducted either in person or through synchronous virtual sessions.

### Supervisee Development

The introductory or intermediate-level supervision intervention is designed to support the development of post-graduate and pre-licensed professionals.

### Supervisory Goals and Learning Objectives

1. Develop a safe supervisory group space where supervisees can actively integrate critical reflexivity into their clinical work.
2. Facilitate a developmental process that enables supervisees to explore intersectional identities and their influence on clinical development.
3. Cultivate authenticity and ease in discourse as supervisees critically examine and discuss anti-oppressive clinical practices.

### Time Required

The time required is 15 minutes per supervisee for a group of 6–8, spanning 3–4 initial group sessions; larger groups may require more time or break down into triads.

### Materials

The materials for the intervention include Self-Reflective Questions and a Trauma-Focused Supervision Approach handout.

## Intervention Instructions

As Menakem (2017) said, traumatic responses stripped of context might look like aspects of personality, just as in marginalized groups of peoples, survival adaptations to transgenerational oppression can emulate culture. For supervisees to be able to use group supervision to develop anti-oppressive practice, a space must be created where it is both safe to explore vulnerability while being sensitive to trauma resulting from historical oppression. Essentially, it starts with the supervisor's critical self-reflexivity as sharing vulnerability to help equalize the power imbalance, while modeling the need to maintain constant awareness of intersectional identities and their impacts.

1.  At the first group supervision meeting, the supervisor welcomes participants and distributes a disclosure and informed consent form outlining their clinical experience, credentials, stance, expectations, ethical guidelines, and complaint procedures. They introduce themselves, state their preferred name and pronouns, and share their identities, starting with those of privilege. This process sets the stage for a transparent, inclusive, and ethically grounded supervision process.
    The supervisor might say, "While some of this might be obvious, other identities might not so let me disclose that I currently identify as a middle-class, middle-aged, queer cisfemale of Asian Indian origin who is an immigrant, Buddhist, disabled mother in the privilege of a longstanding marriage." Supervisees then share their identities in as much detail as they feel comfortable. The supervisor provides the group with the trauma-focused supervision handout to read and prepare for discussion at the following meeting.
    Group supervision follows a set format: participants share weekly highlights and indicate if they need time for specific issues, such as, "Had three no-shows this week. . . . No crisis, but I have a client I'd like to discuss who no-showed after an intense session." The supervisor facilitates the discussion, combining or scheduling topics as needed.
2.  At the second meeting, after the first go around and addressing crises, if any, the supervisor will ask for responses and discussion on the handout. After that discussion, the supervisor can make connections between the survival styles by disclosing their own areas of vulnerability. A supervisee might share, "I've realized that what I thought was cultural humility and harmony was, in part, placating or fawning. After 500 years of British colonization, we instinctively say sorry, even when we are the ones hurt. I can't attune to my oppressors while

also attending to my own needs. In counseling, my ability to listen while bracketing my reactions was a form of subtle dissociation. It felt impossible to focus on my needs while attending to others, and my body often ached—especially my neck and shoulders—after sessions." This reflection highlights the complex intersection of cultural conditioning, trauma, and self-awareness, encouraging deep, critical reflexivity in supervision.

This models for supervisees that it is both possible and helpful to connect the survival style as adaptive, linked to oppression, and analyze how it might impact clinical work. To begin that process, the supervisor hands out the Self-Reflective Responses for folks to think about individually and prepare to share in a following session.

3.  In the third meeting, supervisees will discuss their responses to the Self-Reflective Responses, focusing on connections between their adaptive survival styles and interactions with clients. This includes examining how intersecting identities of marginalization and privilege affect these dynamics. Although the discussion may conclude here, future sessions can revisit these styles. The supervisor can use this framework to initiate interventions and identify response patterns while supervisees gain insight into their development. This approach encourages critical reflexivity without causing feelings of shame, promoting growth in a supportive and non-judgmental environment.

## Supervisory Alliance and Relationship

For this intervention, supervisors must be comfortable using authenticity and vulnerability to foster the same qualities in supervisees. Familiarity with trauma-informed supervision is beneficial, as the process aligns with trauma treatment stages: establishing safety, processing, and reintegration. In a group format, informing participants of these principles helps them become resources for each other, fostering supportive relationships that enable deeper, more meaningful work.

## Legal and Ethical Considerations

Supervision disclosure and informed consent forms are ethical necessities. Disclosures should outline the supervisor's stance, theories, expertise, style, and evaluation criteria. Informed consent should specify evaluation grounds, required artifacts, timelines, confidentiality limits, reporting obligations, and vicarious liability. When exploring critical consciousness, supervisors must remind the group to share only their personal insights and not disclose others' private information.

# APPENDIX

## Appendix 1 Self-Reflective Reponses to Think Through and Prepare (adapted from Kennard, 2020)

1. What is one of your greatest strengths?
2. What are you most proud of?
3. What is difficult for you to do?
4. What do you do when under stress?
5. How do you handle extreme pressure?
6. How are you with deadlines?
7. How do you get your "way"?
8. How easy is it for you to say "no"?
9. What do you do when you are upset?
10. Do you cry easily? Do you cry in front of others?
11. Would you call yourself a "rule follower"?
12. How do you deal with conflict?
13. In a crisis situation, how are you likely to react?
14. How easy is it for you to ask for or accept help?
15. How convincing are you at pretending? How easy is it to carry it off?
16. What are you likely to do when someone tells you "no"?

## Appendix 2 Neuroaffective Relational Model for Trauma-Informed Supervision (adapted from Heller & LaPierre, 2012)

Developed by Heller and LaPierre (2012), NARM integrates object relations, ego state, attachment, and body-centered theories to address complex trauma. This approach is resiliency-based, moves bottom-up and top-down to help practitioners recognize what they feel about their thoughts and what they think about their feelings when it comes to the therapeutic relationship. It seeks to promote creativity, curiosity, and connection. These five core needs are considered essential to physical and emotional well-being. When these core needs are met, persons feel safe, trusting of the world, and connected to their bodies and emotional selves. As helpers, we can address these needs effectively in ourselves and others.

| Core Need | Core Capacity |
|---|---|
| Connection | Capacity to be in touch with our bodies and emotions<br>Capacity to be in connection with others |
| Attunement | Capacity to attune to our needs and emotions<br>Capacity to reach out for and take in emotional nourishment |
| Trust | Capacity for health dependence and interdependence |

*(Continued)*

| Core Need | Core Capacity |
| --- | --- |
| Autonomy | Capacity to set appropriate boundaries |
| | Capacity to speak our minds without guilt and fear |
| Love-Sexuality | Capacity to live with an open heart |

In oppressive systems, unmet core needs lead to adaptive survival styles that help individuals cope with discrimination, marginalization, and trauma. These survival responses, while life-saving during difficult times, can distort present experiences if they persist. These patterns often emerge in counseling and should be addressed in supervision for the supervisee's long-term growth. For instance, a supervisee with a connection survival style might emotionally disconnect and use interpersonal distancing for comfort. An attunement survival style often involves devaluing and rejecting one's own needs. Trust styles can lead to "acting as if" behaviors, hiding true motives, and risking betrayal. Autonomy styles may associate love with obligation and foster a fear of criticism. In the love-sexuality survival mode, helpers might feel unlovable and rejected, often preemptively rejecting others to protect against hurt.

## Appendix 3 Supervisee Response Form

| CORE NEED | Adaptive Survival Style | Adaptive Supervisee Response | Professional Goal | Your Thoughts |
| --- | --- | --- | --- | --- |
| Connection | Overvalues rationality, disconnects from emotion as too vulnerable | Distances emotionally or invalidates client feelings as deficient | Develops self-trust and improves capacity for emotional connection | |
| Attunement | Caretakes others, neglecting personal needs for a sense of indispensability | Feels client distress as failure, devalues self, and prioritizes caretaking | Recognizes and expresses personal needs, increasing tolerance for fulfillment | |
| Trust | Pretends to connect but conceals motives, risks betraying or abusing | Performs for trust, unable to see clients as individuals, fosters dependence | Cultivates vulnerability, accepts help with healthy boundaries | |

*(Continued)*

| CORE NEED | Adaptive Survival Style | Adaptive Supervisee Response | Professional Goal | Your Thoughts |
|---|---|---|---|---|
| Autonomy | Over-generous, fears criticism but depends on pleasing others | Avoids confrontation, lies to please clients, and reacts rather than responds | Builds personal authority, learns to set limits and say no | |
| Love-Sexuality | Feels unlovable, rejects others to avoid being rejected | Assumes resistance or rejection is personal, fears and anticipates rejection | Embraces bodily experience and appreciates diverse beliefs | |

## Appendix 4 Chart of Possible Supervisory Responses Validating What the Supervisee Needs to Hear

| CORE NEED | Core Capacity | Adaptive Survival Style | Possible supervisee adaptive response | Supervisory response when supervisee shares |
|---|---|---|---|---|
| Connection | To connect with emotions and others | Overvalues rationality; disconnects from emotion as too vulnerable | Emotionally distances; invalidates client feelings as deficient | It is safe to connect. Invite somatic noticing of emotion held in the body. Validation: "It can be difficult to see other people break down with ease when you had to be strong." |
| Attunement | To recognize personal needs and take in emotional support | Caretakes others, avoiding own needs; seeks value in being indispensable | Views client distress as failure, prioritizes caretaking over self-care | You can feel safe when you are safe. Invite supervisee to notice that client distress preceded counseling, and they are not responsible for fixing it. Validation: "You can get your own needs met and you don't have to earn belonging for that." |

(Continued)

| CORE NEED | Core Capacity | Adaptive Survival Style | Possible supervisee adaptive response | Supervisory response when supervisee shares |
|---|---|---|---|---|
| Trust | To be healthily interdependent | Acts connected but conceals motives; risks betraying others | Performs to gain trust, fosters dependence | *You deserve to be supported.* Invite noticing vulnerability and tension around it. Explore concerns around asking for help when looking weak or helpless would be used against them. Validation: "Being able to ask for and receive help makes you strong." |
| Autonomy | To set flexible boundaries and speak without fear | Over-gives, fears criticism, seeks to please others | Avoids confrontation, lies to please, reactive rather than responsive | *You can say no.* Invite the supervisee to replay client confrontation or imagine setting boundaries. What would that look like? What would it feel like? Validation: "When you set a boundary, you do it for yourself and to benefit the other." |
| Love-Sexuality | To love without fear of rejection | Feels unlovable, rejects others to avoid being rejected | Assumes resistance is personal; fears and anticipates rejection | *Daring to love.* Invite the supervisee to imagine themselves in a relationship with their client. What parallels are there between the therapeutic relationship and their personal ones? Are there patterns? Validation: "The more generous your care, the less you are anxious about its loss. Every connection is a strength." |

## Intervention Title: Using the Cultural Genogram to Promote Cultural Self-Awareness

## Author(s) and Affiliation(s)

Joshua N. Hook, PhD
University of North Texas

C. Edward Watkins, Jr., PhD
University of North Texas and Institute of Psychotherapy, Psychological Counselling and Clinical Supervision (Reșița, Romania)

## Supervision Format and Modality

This supervision intervention was developed for use within group supervision (in-person or virtual), but the intervention is flexible and can also be used in individual, triadic, or peer supervision.

## Supervisee Development

This supervision intervention can be used across all levels of supervisee development, but it is particularly useful for beginning supervisees who are starting their journey of growth toward being a culturally competent and anti-oppressive clinician. Thus, the intervention is probably most appropriate for master's and doctoral practicum. It can also be used for professional development and remediation plans related to cultural competence.

This supervision intervention is appropriate for all levels of supervisee development but is aimed at supervisees at the introductory or intermediate levels (i.e., level 1 or 2 in the Integrative Developmental Model; McNeill & Stoltenberg, 2016) who have not engaged in much critical reflection on one's cultural identities and worldview.

## Supervisory Goals and Learning Objectives

1. Supervisees will develop critical consciousness and critical reflexivity.
2. Supervisees will increase their awareness of their and their family of origin's cultural background and identities.
3. Supervisees will identify how various aspects of their cultural identities relate to experiences of power, privilege, and marginalization.

4.  Supervisees will articulate the cultural beliefs, values, and attitudes of their family of origin, as well as how their own personal beliefs, values, and attitudes may have shifted over time.
5.  Supervisees will be able to identify how they can transfer their learning into their counseling practice with current and future clients.

### Time Required

This supervision intervention involves personal reflection and journaling (approximately 3–5 hours), as well as a group presentation and discussion (approximately 30 minutes)

### Materials

Supervisors may find it helpful to prepare a handout or brief PowerPoint presentation to discuss the purpose, expectations, and key steps of the cultural genogram project. Supervisors may find it helpful to review journal articles that discuss the cultural genogram (e.g., Hardy & Laszloffy, 1995; Hook et al., 2016). These articles can provide a foundation for the activity, which can then be tailored to the preferences of the supervisor and the needs of the supervisee.

### Intervention Instructions

1.  The supervisor begins by introducing the purpose of the cultural genogram project. Namely, cultural self-awareness is an important foundational component of becoming a culturally competent and anti-oppressive therapist. For example, the tripartite model of cultural competence (Sue et al., 1992) notes the importance of developing awareness of one's assumptions, values, and biases. Similarly, the multicultural orientation model (Owen, 2013) notes the importance of cultural humility and awareness of one's cultural limitations. Cultural self-awareness is also foundational to the principles of anti-oppression and developing critical consciousness through critical reflexivity. Completing the cultural genogram is designed to help supervisees understand their cultural background and identities in a deeper way, as well as how their identities intersect with experiences of power, privilege, and marginalization.

2.  The supervisor will then walk through the key steps and instructions for completing the cultural genogram project. (Supervisors should provide a copy of this handout.)

    a.  Write out the first names of all family members for at least two or three generations. Include gender identity and approximate age.
    b.  Fill in the cultural background and identities for each person in your genogram using your own symbols. Possible cultural identities include (but are not limited to) race, ethnicity, language, sexual orientation, religion, political affiliation, ability status, and socioeconomic status. Also, identify interracial/ethnic marriages and relationships.
    c.  For each of your cultural identities, think about its relationship to power, privilege, and marginalization in our society. Note the level of privilege that each part of your cultural identity affords you in society (e.g., low, medium, high).
    d.  Reflect on the important beliefs, values, and attitudes that were taught to you by your family. If you are having trouble thinking about these, here are some topics that could be interesting to explore: money/possessions, gender roles, education, work, religion, politics, and diversity.
    e.  As you have grown up and become an adult, what important beliefs, values, and attitudes that were taught in your family growing up have stayed consistent over time? What important beliefs, values, and attitudes have changed over time? How have your beliefs, values, and attitudes changed thus far throughout your counselor training and development?

3.  Supervisees will then be given time to work on their cultural genogram project. Ideally, supervisees would have at least two weeks to think about and complete this project.
4.  Supervisees will then present their cultural genogram projects to the supervision group. There are different ways to organize these presentations based on the supervisor's preference. For example, the supervisor can set a time during each meeting for one supervisee to present their project or have all supervisees present their projects during one or two meetings. The time allotted for the presentations will depend on time constraints, but ideally, at least 20–30 minutes for each presentation. After each supervisee finishes their presentation, there could be a short amount of time for questions and discussion. Thank each supervisee after their presentation.

5.  If the supervisor desires, there can also be a short paper assignment (5–10 pages) associated with the cultural genogram project. The paper can have multiple sections:

    a.  Section 1: Narrative description of the cultural genogram.
    b.  Section 2: Describe your cultural worldview, including key beliefs, values, and attitudes. Compare and contrast your cultural worldview with the cultural worldview taught to you by your family growing up.
    c.  Section 3: Discuss your cultural worldview using a relevant model of racial/ethnic identity development. (Note: If another aspect of culture is more salient for you [e.g., gender or sexual identity], you may choose a different cultural identity development model.)
    d.  Section 4: Connect your growing awareness of your cultural identity and worldview to your role and identity as a culturally competent and anti-oppressive clinician.
    e.  Section 5: Identify 3–5 areas that you will continue to reflect upon post-assignment to support ongoing critical reflexivity.

### Supervisory Alliance and Relationship Considerations

Sharing about one's family and cultural worldview with the supervisor and group can be a vulnerable experience and may be challenging for some students if they do not have a strong supervisory working alliance with the supervisor or do not have trusting relationships with fellow group members. Some students may be more private and feel less comfortable sharing information about their families. Supervisors should encourage supervisees to share what they are comfortable with sharing. There is a balance here, given that this is a supervision group (not therapy), so it is reasonable that supervisees have limits on what they feel comfortable sharing. Conversely, we are training culturally competent and anti-oppressive clinicians, and it may be difficult for therapists-in-training to competently address culture with their clients if they are not willing to explore and share vulnerably about their own cultural identities and worldviews.

### Legal and Ethical Considerations

Completing this assignment does ask supervisees to share vulnerably about their beliefs, values, and attitudes, which may feel uncomfortable for some supervisees. Supervisors should attend to supervisees' reactions and work to mend any alliance ruptures. Supervisors should remember that supervision is different from therapy and keep in mind the goals of the supervision experience. Also, supervisors are encouraged to monitor any personal reactions to the content that supervisees share and engage in supervision or consultation.

## Reflective Questions

1.  What was it like to complete this project? Did you have any reactions that surprised you?
2.  What was it like to share about your cultural genogram and worldview in front of me and the group? How do you think your clients might feel about sharing vulnerable information about their cultural background with you?
3.  What was it like to hear your fellow group members share their cultural genogram and worldview with you? Do you feel more or less connected with them after they share?
4.  How can you use this experience to help work toward anti-oppression in your counseling work?

# Overcoming Comfort and Fragility Through Unlearning Privilege and Domination

*Thomas Killian, Melissa Luke, Krista M. Malott,
Tina R. Paone, Harvey Charles Peters,
Madison Rowohlt, Jordan Shannon,
C. Edward Watkins, Jr., and L. Xochitl Vallejos*

## CHAPTER 3 INTERVENTIONS

**Intervention Title: Love It-Hate It: Establishing Intra-and Inter-Personal Processes to Overcome Comfort and Fragility and Unlearn Privilege and Domination in Triadic Supervision**

### Author(s) and Affiliation(s)

Melissa Luke, Ph.D., NCC, ACS, LMHC
Syracuse University

Harvey Charles Peters, Ph.D., NCC
Montclair State University

### Supervision Format and Modality

This activity is an extension of Lee and Luke's (2018) first group supervision activity and was developed specifically for anti-oppressive triadic supervision. The activity can be adapted for use within in-person or online individual and group supervision with up to 12 supervisees.

DOI: 10.4324/9781003470656-3

## Supervisee Development

This supervisory activity can be implemented with master's and doctoral students in training, as well as with practicing pre- and post-licensed professional counselors. Intentional consideration is given to supervisee development when pairing supervisees to enhance the supervisee working alliances and minimize regressive supervisory pairings (Lawson et al., 2010).

## Supervisory Goals and Learning Objectives

1. Supervisees will articulate and explore intra-and inter-personal processes connected to their counseling and supervision.
2. Supervisees will co-construct triadic supervisory norms for an effective supervisory working alliance.
3. Supervisees will examine how socialization and privilege grounded in domination and oppression may be upholding oppressive forces, structures, and systems that impact clients, counselors, and supervisors.
4. Supervisees will expand their skills to address, unlearn, and overcome discomfort, silence, objectivity, apathy, neutrality, bias, and fragility in their counseling and supervision.

## Time Required

This activity is designed for a 60-minute triadic supervisory session.

## Materials

The supervisor prepares a set of cards for the intervention, each containing an anti-oppressive 'love it' and 'hate it' prompts, ensuring there are at least 2–3 more prompts than will be used.

We encourage the supervisor to continually refine and add to their list of prompts; however, sample prompts include:

1. To develop our triadic supervisory norms, I would love it if . . . and I would hate it if . . .
2. In my first recorded session this semester, I would love it if . . . and I would hate it if . . .
3. When I present a case in triadic supervision, I would love it if . . . and I would hate it if . . .
4. In sharing intra-and inter-personal processes, I would love it if . . . and I would hate it if . . .

5. In responding to my peer's intra-and inter-personal processes, I would love it if . . . and I would hate it if . . .
6. When examining my socialization, I would love it if . . . and I would hate it if . . .
7. To improve my counseling competencies, I would love it if . . . and I would hate it if . . .
8. When discomfort and fragility, I would love it if . . . and I would hate it if . . .
9. As I encounter ethical issues, I would love it if . . . and I would hate it if . . .
10. When observing apathy, neutrality or bias, I would love it if . . . and I would hate it if . . .
11. If I work with client in crisis, I would love it if . . . and I would hate it if . . .
12. When my supervisor addresses silence, I would love it if . . . and I would hate it if . . .
13. If I knew what my peer thinks of me, I would love it if . . . and I would hate it if . . .
14. As I observe my supervisor's or peer's lack of objectivity, I would love it if . . . and I would hate it if . . .
15. As I recognize how my identities and social locations impact and are impacted by domination and oppression, I would love it if . . . and I would hate it if . . .
16. In developing skills to identify and counter domination and oppression, I would love it if . . . and I would hate it if . . .
17. When conceptualizing cases using an anti-oppressive framework, I would love it if . . . and I would hate it if . . .
18. In receiving supervisory feedback, I would love it if . . . and I would hate it if . . .
19. In receiving peer feedback, I would love it if . . . and I would hate it if . . .
20. When giving formative feedback, I would love it if . . . and I would hate it if . . .
21. During my final evaluation process, I would love it if . . . and I would hate it if . . .
22. As I reflect on progress toward my anti-oppressive goals at the end of triadic supervision, I would love it if . . . and I would hate it if . . .
23. When asked to offer additional prompts for use in this activity in the future, I would love it if . . . and I would hate it if . . .

## Intervention Instructions

1. The supervisor indicates that sharing intra-and inter-personal experiences are requisite processes toward the intersecting goals of clinical supervision.
2. The supervisor describes how intra-and inter-personal processes assist in the "transformative learning process and facilitate [supervisee] reflectivity" (Lee & Luke, 2018, p. 304) broadly, but in a triadic supervisory context, they can also be a stimulus to examine commonalities and uniqueness, validate and normalize developmental experiences, and build both group cohesion and the supervisee working alliance.
3. The supervisor discusses the strengths and limitations of the triadic supervisory context (Gerstenblith et al., 2022; Lawson et al., 2010), the role of the supervisory multicultural orientation (King et al., 2020), and the ways relational and power dynamics (Lee & Thackeray, 2023) intersect with anti-oppressive work.
4. The supervisor introduces the supervision intervention by name and notes that each supervisee will alternate in selecting a card from the pile of pre-made prompts and reading it aloud. After both supervisees have an opportunity to consider and respond to the prompt, the supervisor facilitates a discussion and processing of the content.
5. The supervisor explains that the prompts are short and open-ended with no pre-determined outcome. They include a statement of "I would love it if. . . . And I would hate it if . . ."
6. The supervisor offers that each prompt is designed to broach an aspect of anti-oppressive work and to begin to establish a supervisory context and processes that will assist in overcoming comfort and fragility and unlearning privilege and domination as they relate to counseling and supervision.
7. To illustrate, the supervisor offers to select the first card and reads the prompt aloud, "To develop our triadic supervisory norms, I would love it if . . . and I would hate it if . . ." The supervisor models authenticity in their intra- and inter-personal processes and answers the prompt aloud, supporting supervisees to do so as well, and then facilitates discussion and processing.
8. When discussing and processing each prompt, the supervisor can draw on their use of reflection, summarization, linking, blocking, immediacy, modeling, reframing, etc. The supervisor may also wish to use open questions, such as:

## Prompts

a. What connections do you see between the responses to this prompt?
b. How might socialization contribute to the uniqueness in responses to this prompt?
c. What aspects of privilege may be influencing your reaction to this prompt?
d. Where might domination and oppression contribute to our discussion of this prompt?
e. Which parts of the discussion and processing of this prompt remain unfinished for you?

*End of Activity*

a. What has it been like for you to share your intra-and inter-personal experiences?
b. How do you understand the commonalities and uniqueness identified?
c. Which aspects of this activity connect to your current/future counseling?
d. What do you take from this activity into our future triadic supervision?
e. In what ways might content from this anti-oppressive activity re-emerge for you?

## Supervisory Alliance and Relationship

Supervisors are encouraged to intentionally consider the impact of the triadic supervisory context on supervisees' experiences (Gerstenblith et al., 2022), including how the potential influences of social comparison and shame may impact the triadic supervisory working alliances. Relatedly, there is increasing evidence that relational processes, including discursive manifestations of power and privilege, hold import to the learning experiences of supervisees (Lee & Thackeray, 2023) and attend to these alliance and relationship factors within supervision.

## Legal and Ethical Considerations

As this anti-oppressive supervisory intervention seeks to disrupt the status quo and raise disequilibrium in an effort to support supervisees to overcome comfort and fragility and unlearn privilege and domination, supervisors are cautioned to proactively address these processes with supervisees.

Although the triadic supervisory informed consent documentation should include any limits to confidentiality, particularly the inability of the supervisor to guarantee that triadic supervisees adhere to the confidentiality of one another, the supervisor is advised to regularly remind supervisees of the importance of privacy and professional boundaries related to supervisory content. If using an online supervision context, adherence to state and federal laws and ethical standards is paramount, including but not limited to the use of HIPAA-compliant video conferencing platform as well as supervisee and client informed consent. In addition, specific training in and competency with online supervision is advised (Phillips et al., 2021).

## Reflective Questions

1. What did you learn about your intra-and inter-personal processes connected to your counseling and supervision, and how will you translate this into your future practice?
2. Which specific prompts or follow-up questions or discussion facilitated the supervisory or therapeutic working alliance, and which identified or contributed to a breach?
3. How did your (or your client's) socialization and privilege grounded in domination and oppression uphold oppressive forces, structures, and systems in counseling and supervision, and what resources and practices can disrupt this?
4. Where are the growth edges to address, unlearn, and overcome discomfort, silence, objectivity, apathy, neutrality, bias, and fragility in your counseling and supervision, and how, if unaddressed, might these re-emerge in your counseling and our triadic supervision?
5. As a future supervisor, how might you incorporate your learnings into your supervision?

**Intervention Title: Incorporating Cultural Humility Guidelines, Supervisee Version, Into the Supervision Relationship**

### Author(s) and Affiliation(s)

C. Edward Watkins, Jr., PhD
University of North Texas and Institute of Psychotherapy, Psychological Counselling and Clinical Supervision (Reşiţa, Romania)

### Supervision Format and Modality

This supervision intervention was developed for use with supervisees in individual supervision. These guidelines, however, are but one part of a tripartite set of guidelines, with parallel versions also available for the supervisor (Watkins, 2023) and supervision group (Watkins et al., 2022). This complementary package set—best seen as an introductory starter kit—privileges cultural humility and orients supervision accordingly.

This intervention is anchored in the guiding tenets that "cultural humility matters in supervision" (Zhang et al., 2022) and that, as supervisors, "We go first" (Watkins, 2023, p. 12), (a) introducing culture (defined broadly to include such variables as gender, race/ethnicity, sexual orientation, gender identity, and dis/ability status) into the supervision relationship, (b) opening space for culture to be considered, and (c) using the guidelines as one way to convey and model our cultural humility embrace and stimulate dyadic/group discussion.

### Supervisee Development

This supervision intervention, potentially applicable across the full developmental spectrum, is considered particularly useful for beginning supervisees, those starting to provide counseling. This supervision intervention is considered most useful for beginning supervisees, but it is perhaps limited in their cultural humility and anti-oppressive knowledge/understanding.

### Supervisory Goals and Learning Objectives

*Supervisees Will*

1. Develop knowledge/understanding about cultural humility as an anti-oppressive, emancipatory supervisory way of being.

2. Learn that exploring and examining their own personal/cultural identities (e.g., values, worldviews, privilege, biases) are critical to their development of a culturally humble, anti-oppressive treatment/supervision stance.
3. Demonstrate one way to apply cultural humility to their role as supervisee.
4. Receive support to transfer these learnings into counseling practice.

## Time Required

This dyadic supervisee intervention involves supervisor orientation of supervisee, supervisee reading/self-reflection, and supervisor-supervisee discussion (two to three hours).

## Materials

The Cultural Humility Guidelines, Supervisee Version, included as a part of the supervision agreement (copy of agreement available from the author upon request), read as follows:

*Table 3.1* Supervision-Adapted Supervisee Ground Rules Based on Cultural Humility for You to Consider Implementing (As Best You Can)

| No. | Rules |
| --- | --- |
| 1 | I will enter each individual supervision meeting with an open mind and possess an attitude of willingness to explore new concepts with you. |
| 2 | I will be aware of my own personal values, beliefs, and behaviors and respect that you, my supervisor, may not abide by the same values and belief system. |
| 3 | I will focus on your feelings and experiences as my supervisor as well as my own feelings and experiences as your supervisee. |
| 4 | I will enter each supervision meeting with a flexible and humble attitude and strive to not allow my ego to impede the supervision learning experience. |
| 5 | I will engage in healthy, supportive interactions with you to help foster an engaging learning environment. |
| 6 | I will engage in self-reflection as a lifelong counseling/psychotherapy learner and strive to critique my own thoughts, actions, and behaviors as I interact with you. |
| 7 | I will attempt to embrace conflicting viewpoints that are expressed in supervision by giving those viewpoints my full consideration. |

*(Continued)*

*Table 3.1 (Continued)*

| No. | Rules |
| --- | --- |
| 8 | I will support you throughout supervision as we engage in discussions and learning. |
| 9 | Recognizing supervision power differences and your pledged (supervisor) efforts to minimize them, I in turn will strive to enact the spirit of mutuality in (the asymmetry of) our supervisory relationship. |
| 10 | I will demonstrate respect for you and for the clients that I serve. |

Note. Adapted from Smith, A., & Foronda, C. (2021). Promoting cultural humility in nursing education through the use of ground rules. *Nursing Education Perspectives, 42*(2), 117–119. 3/4, | https://doi.org/10.1097/01.NEP.0000000000000594, with permission of Wolters Kluwer Health, Inc.

## Intervention Instructions

This intervention is a two-part endeavor: a process of "setting the stage (Part I) for setting the stage (Part II). Part I involves rolling out and introducing diversity/inclusion/advocacy (DIA) and cultural humility as central to anti-oppressive supervisory work. Part II concretizes that rollout and introduction, presenting the emancipatory, anti-oppressive supervision framework of cultural humility and using the cultural humility guidelines as framework exemplification.

## Setting the Stage: Part I (Session 1)

1. As supervisor and supervisee get to know one another, supervisors strive to delineate the crucial constituents of their supervision vision (e.g., to create a courageous, anti-oppressive, multiculturally-minded learning space).
2. Supervisors bring up three matters for discussion: intersectional identities, the supervision power differential, and their personal profession of "supervision conviction."
3. Supervisors "go first" (Watkins, 2023), sharing their primary affecting identities; acknowledging the supervision power differential and their efforts to moderate its impact; and professing their preeminent valuing of supervision.
4. Supervisors bring up DIA/cultural humility and the supervision agreement (SA), provide supervisees with a SA copy to read, explain that they view cultural humility as a framework/container for supervision going forward (reflected in the SA), and those matters will be discussed next meeting.

## Setting the Stage: Part II (Session 2)

1. As the discussion proceeds, supervisors provide education about cultural humility as a supervision construct, framework, and anchor. Cultural humility is defined (e.g., to understand other's cultural identities), its core framework features are explicated (e.g., considering power, privilege, and oppression inherent in social systems), and its anchoring, anti-oppressive nature is accentuated (e.g., lifelong learning about others).

2. Supervisors render discussion more concrete by taking up the cultural humility guidelines. Supervisors again "go first," presenting the supervisor cultural humility guidelines (Watkins, 2023) to the supervisee, offering their personal pledge and promise to live out the spirit of those guidelines in all supervisory work together. In going "first," the supervisor thereby anchors and launches the next step.

3. Supervisors take up the supervisee cultural humility guidelines (Table 3.1), presenting these as guidelines "to be considered," ways of thinking and acting that can help get supervision started off most favorably. The 10 supervisee guidelines are closely reviewed, how they capture important facets of a supervisee's culturally humble way of being are considered, and guideline words that reflect that very essence are highlighted: openness, respect, flexibility, humbleness, being supportive, a lifelong learner; working toward relational mutuality, and valuing self-awareness, self-reflection, and self-critique (of personal values, beliefs, and biases, power, positionality, and privilege).

4. Because supervisees are asked to consider living out the spirit of these guidelines, much space is left open for discussion. For instance, the supervisor can facilitate a discussion where these key issues are raised for review: how the guidelines will be implemented, the challenges to practicing and upholding them, and how guidelines accountability can be maintained.

5. Supervisors also accentuate that these guidelines are aspirational; may we as supervisors and supervisees do the best that we can in guidelines implementation, recognizing that we are both fallible human beings who will make mistakes and accepting the reality of our personal/professional fallibility (e.g., by sharing one of our own supervisor misses, mistakes, or failings).

## Supervisory Alliance and Relationship Considerations

Supervisors, while creating a courageous, anti-oppressive place for supervisees to talk about and share their cultural identities/worldviews, emphasize the following: being able to meaningfully address culture with clients begins with being able to meaningfully address culture within ourselves. Anti-oppressive practice has its beginnings in the studious enactment of a relentless process of self-scrutiny and self-reflection. Developing good enough cultural comfort, or "comfortable discomfort," is requisite for supervisees to engage in meaningful cultural self-exploration/self-critique, engage clients in meaningful cultural discussions, and carry that over to supervision (Watkins et al., 2019, 2022).

## Legal and Ethical Considerations

This intervention asks supervisees to begin the process of self-critique, targeting their own power, positionality, privilege, values, beliefs, and biases and implement a culturally humble way of being. Because such self-critique can provoke understandable discomfort, supervisors should remain mindful of that reality, attend accordingly to their supervisees, and support them throughout. A no coercion, no shaming stance is employed.

## Reflective Questions

1. What is your personal perspective about the supervisee cultural humility guidelines?
2. How might these guidelines be helpful to you in better enacting your supervisee role?
3. How do you see these guidelines as supporting anti–oppressive supervision practice?
4. How do you envision translating your cultural humility learnings into your current and future counseling practice?

## Intervention Title: Sociocultural Fragility Mapping

## Author(s) and Affiliation(s)

Thomas Killian, PhD
Montclair State University

Madison Rowohlt, MA
Montclair State University

## Supervision Format and Modality

Our intervention, crafted for individual supervision, can be adapted for triadic and group settings, accommodating up to 12 supervisees. This intervention is applicable to in-person and HIPAA-compliant virtual formats.

## Supervisee Development

This intervention, applicable at all stages of supervisee development, explores supervisors' and supervisees' privileged social positions and when the supervisor or supervisee recognizes sociocultural fragility, especially in addressing challenges while counseling marginalized clients. This intervention requires a foundation in critical perspectives and abstract concepts. The supervisee must actively engage with the interdisciplinary scholarship and be dedicated to fostering critical consciousness.

## Supervisory Goals and Learning Objectives

1. The supervisee will engage in critical self-reflection of the interplay of their hierarchical professional role and privileged social location(s) on recreating and reinforcing oppressive systems with marginalized clients.
2. The supervisee will identify, unpack, and challenge at least two aspects of their sociocultural fragility used to avoid awareness of the presence, relevance, degree, and/or impact of oppressive systems on their marginalized clients.
3. The supervisee will locate one example of defensiveness (i.e., cognitions, affect, and behaviors) that have arisen in supervision.

## Time Required

Each part of *Sociocultural Fragility Mapping* (*SFM*) can be employed within a 50–60-minute supervision session.

## Materials

Supervisors need to refamiliarize themselves with the concepts of inter-sectionality (see Collins & Bilge, 2020), fragility (see DiAngelo, 2018), Interpersonal Process Recall (IPR; see Kagan, 1980), and social identity mapping (see Jacobson & Mustafa, 2019). Supervisors need access to supervisee session recordings, client documentation, and supervisee process notes. Additionally, supervisors need to provide drawing paper and colored markers.

## Intervention Instructions

*SFM* is a multipart intervention, integrating adapted elements of social identity mapping and IPR, aimed at assisting supervisees in exploring their sociocultural fragility and its impact on the counseling process/outcome. The supervisor demonstrates *SFM* within the supervisory relationship and then guides the supervisee in applying *SFM* with a marginalized client. Across clinical contexts, *SFM* involves identifying a critical incident, recognizing associated sociocultural fragility, exploring cognitive, affective, behavioral, and interpersonal reactions and their potential impact, and collaborating to unlearn sociocultural fragility and embrace discomfort.

## Part 1: *SFM* Overview

1. The supervisor anchors *SFM* with mutually agreed-upon supervisory goals, fostering a brave space prioritizing safety, trust, and vulnerability, and communicates that self-disclosure of social locations is anonymous, optional, and has no impact on supervisee evaluation.
2. Prior to *SFM*, all participants should be familiar with foundational readings (see Collins & Bilge, 2020; DiAngelo, 2018; Jacobson & Mustafa, 2019; Kagan, 1980) and associated concepts addressed in this multipart intervention.
3. *SFM* incorporates highlighting both privileged and marginalized social locations; however, *SFM* rests on identifying and exploring privileged social locations.

4. The participant begins by writing their name in the center of a blank piece of paper along with orbiting social locations. The participant labels each social location as privileged or marginalized, accompanied by a rationale of their status.
5. The participant, focused on their privileged social locations, identifies supervisory or clinical context(s) that trigger sociocultural fragility (i.e., critical incident[s]). Based on time and foundational understanding, the participant may want to limit their focus to one to three salient privileged social locations.
6. The participant identifies a critical incident related to their privileged social location(s), where sociocultural fragility was initiated as a defense.
7. The participant identifies and labels their potential cognitive, affective, behavioral, and/or interpersonal reactions related to the previously identified triggering event.
8. The participant reflects on ways of unlearning sociocultural fragility and embracing discomfort through process-oriented questions.

## Part 2a: Supervisor Models *SFM*

1. The supervisor and supervisee identify, self-disclose, and label their own social locations. The supervisor (e.g., White [privileged], cisgender female [marginalized], straight/heterosexual [privileged]) and supervisee (e.g., Black [marginalized], cisgender male [privileged], queer [marginalized]), focus on their own privileged social locations.
2. The supervisor and supervisee collaboratively identify the potential context(s) within the supervisory relationship that triggered sociocultural fragility (i.e., critical incident[s]). The supervisor and supervisee identify a critical incident related to the supervisor's privileged identity, where sociocultural fragility was initiated as a defense (e.g., the supervisee recounted the client's racial microaggression).
3. The supervisor identifies and labels their potential cognitive, affective, behavioral, and/or interpersonal reactions related to the previously identified triggering event (e.g., the supervisor never broached race [behavioral], identified as colorblind [cognitive], felt anxious initiating a discussion on the supervisee's Black experience [affective], responded with own disclosure of microaggressions as a woman [behavioral]).
4. The supervisor initiates process questions, framed through intersectionality (Collins & Bilge, 2020), meant to access depth and defuse defensiveness by addressing power, social inequality, social context,

and relationships between social locations (e.g., "How I can help you feel more seen in supervision?"; "How do I perpetuate racism/homophobia in supervision?"; "What would you like me to know about your lived experience as a Black-queer-male clinician?").

## Part 2b: Supervisee's *SFM*

1. If the supervisor hypothesizes that sociocultural fragility is a contributing factor to the supervisee's challenges (e.g., relational dynamics, conceptualization issues, countertransference) of working with the identified client, the supervisor encourages the supervisee to consider the role of sociocultural fragility. The supervisor reiterates the presence and pervasiveness of sociocultural fragility in all interpersonal dynamics. *Note:* More than one critical incident can be observed for a client, not only incidents that initiate sociocultural fragility but those that remerge and reinforce sociocultural fragility.

2. The supervisor introduces an adapted form of IPR (see Kagan, 1980) and communicates the need for the supervisee to engage in session recall referenced with session recording, triangulated with related clinical progress and process notes.

3. The supervisor prompts the supervisee to recall a critical incident related to their difficulty in working with the client, and prior to the upcoming supervision session, identify and rewatch the specific session, identify the moment when the critical incident emerged, and replay pre-identified critical incident recording in the upcoming supervision session.

4. The supervisor references their previous *SFM* and its renewed application to the supervisee-client relationship, where the supervisee now attends toward therapeutic challenges instigated by sociocultural fragility within the confines of the counselor-client relationship and asks the supervisee to share their critical incident segment recording.

5. The supervisor and/or supervisee stop the recording at any point to process the identified incident. The supervisor assists the supervisee in identifying the critical incident, including where and how sociocultural fragility was initiated as a defense (e.g., cisgender male clinician deemphasizes or inaccurately reframes a cisgender female client's disclosure of gendered microaggressions in the workplace).

6. The supervisor and supervisee revisit and reference the supervisee's previous map, which can be modified based on evolving supervisee awareness and client conceptualization. After pausing the recording, the supervisor assists the supervisee in identifying and labeling cognitive, affective, behavioral, and/or interpersonal reactions related

to the critical event (e.g., clinician shifts focus from client perspective to microaggressor's perspective [behavioral], clinician subconsciously overidentified with microaggressor [cognitive], clinician felt irritated discussing topic [affective], counselor-client relationship (interpersonal).

7.  The supervisor facilitates non-judgmental questioning, framed through an intersectional lens, aimed at accessing depth while mitigating defensiveness (e.g., "What other emotions were underneath your irritation?"; "What does your client want from you?"; "What would it be like to discuss these microaggressions?"; "What additional identities do you see as influencing your reaction here?"), meant to assist in unlearning sociocultural fragility and embracing discomfort.

## Supervisory Alliance and Relationship

While *SFM* involves self-disclosure, supervisors must communicate clearly, respecting supervisees' rights to refuse or control the extent of self-disclosure, confidentiality, and expectations, thereby creating brave/safe spaces for self-exploration. Furthermore, supervisors should be aware of the inherent challenges associated with maintaining accountability within the context of power dynamics in supervisory and counselor-client relationships, requiring attention to both interpersonal dynamics concerning power and process.

## Legal and Ethical Considerations

Supervisees, assigned the responsibility of self-disclosure, need supervisors to clarify expectations, roles, confidentiality, and assessment procedures. Establishing a brave/safe space is vital for fostering self-disclosure and exploration, with supervisors affirming autonomy and avoiding coercion. *SFM* should align with supervisees' clinical responsibilities. Soliciting ongoing feedback is essential for adapting the intervention. Due to the self-disclosure involved, supervisors are encouraged to seek their own supervision-of-supervision.

## Reflective Questions

1.  What are some potential modifications to *SFM* in clinical experience courses (e.g., practicum, internship)?
2.  What are some perceived challenges in instituting *SFM*?
3.  How would you address a supervisee who is unable to recognize the impact of their own sociocultural fragility?

### Intervention Title: Being Real: Giving Space to Process Internalized Oppression and Privilege in Supervision

### Author(s) and Affiliation(s)

Jordan Shannon, PhD, NCC
Seattle University

L. Xochitl Vallejos, PhD, LPC
Rocky Mountain Counseling and Psychological Association

### Supervision Format and Modality

This intervention is designed to be delivered in individual supervision through in-person and live formats and can be adapted to triadic, peer, and group (3–4 members) supervision.

### Supervisee Development

This anti-oppressive intervention has utility across all levels of supervisee development. However, we emphasize its applicability for supervisees struggling to recognize how identities influence their worldviews and clinical approaches when working with diverse clients. Both supervisors and supervisees must be open to dialoging around oppression and have an understanding of identity development models (e.g., race, gender, cultural). This intervention can be used for the exploration of identities at the introductory level but is ideally utilized at intermediate and advanced levels for unpacking the internalization of dominant identities within systems of oppression.

### Supervisory Goals and Learning Objectives

*Supervisees Will*

1. Explore how their social identities interact with client identities.
2. Identify at least two ways their identity intersects with privilege.
3. Discuss how one or more internalizations of privilege affect the clinical and supervisory relationships.

### Time Required

This intervention requires approximately 50–60 minutes.

## Materials

Supervisors and supervisees should familiarize themselves with the different cultural identity models, particularly earlier stages (conformity, internalization, awareness, etc.) of models; examples include integrated racial identity development (e.g., Hoffman & Hoffman, 2004) and sexual affectional identity development (e.g., Cass, 1979). Supervisors should have familiarity with the Integrated Developmental Model of supervision (IDM; McNeill et al., 1992) to differentiate the intervention use across supervisee development. Supervisees at levels 1 and 2 will need to create a paper or digital copy ADDRESSING model (Hays, 2022) worksheet for initial discussion of dominant and marginalized identity status, and supervisees at level 3+ will utilize the social identity wheel worksheet for advanced discussion of dominant and marginalized identities. Supervisors should prepare to revisit these interventions throughout the supervisory relationship as counselor reflections deepen. Copies of this wheel are available for free at Boston University Center for Community and Diversity (https://www.bu.edu/diversity/resource-toolkit/social-identity-wheel-activity/) and the University of Michigan Center for Equitable Teaching (https://sites.lsa.umich.edu/inclusive-teaching/wp-content/uploads/sites/355/2018/12/Social-Identity-Wheel-3–2.pdf).

## Intervention Instructions

★We chose not to capitalize dominant identities throughout the intervention as ways to decenter privileged social locations.

1. **For Level 1 & 2 supervisees**: Supervisors explain to supervisees how this intervention is designed to build awareness of anti-oppression and how our identities are influenced by greater sociocultural structures. Supervisors will explain the use of the ADDRESSING model, which stands for Age, Developed or other Disabilities, Race, Ethnicity, Social status, Sexual orientation, Indigenous heritage, National origin, and Gender (Hays, 2022). Supervisors should also discuss and respond to intrapersonal and interpersonal reactions (e.g., discomfort, silence, guilt, anger) that may emerge from conversing around internalized socialization. For instance, supervisors use this intervention to reflect on how identities are situated on privilege and oppression (see step 3).

2. **For Level 3:** Supervisors introduce the social locations wheel worksheet to supervisees. Supervisees should expect to identify their social locations as well as the clients. Together, they will critically examine how those social locations and the inherent power dynamics impact

therapy and what underlying factors may be present in the room. For example, a *white, cis, hetero clinician would identify that they understand that based on their social locations such as, "as a white, cis, hetero man, I will never fully understand the ways in which your identities have impacted you, but I commit to exercising empathy and self-awareness to do my best. If, and when, I mess up, please know that I want you to feel comfortable telling me immediately so I can take accountability, make repairs, and adjust."

The supervisor is then encouraged to ask questions of the supervisee based on the matched and unmatched areas of identity. For example, the supervisor might say, "Based on the wheel, you noted you tend to think about your gender identity most often; how might those thoughts be impacting your work with this client who holds a different race, gender, and ability status than you?"

3. **For Level 1 & 2 supervisees**: The supervisor proposes three process-oriented questions:

   a. What does it mean for you as the clinician to engage in anti-oppressive work?
   b. Which identities do you observe as privileged/oppressed in yourself and the client?
   c. What reactions emerge for you in processing these identities?

The first question is designed for supervisees to dialogue about the concept of anti-oppression and how it ties to their work. The supervisor can then share how they define anti-oppression (see Chapter 1). It is important for the supervisor to be grounded in discussing power dynamics, resource allocation, and how they relate to social identities. Supervisors should provide examples of oppressive clinical power dynamics, such as,

   • Specialize in working with marginalized communities (e.g., race, gender, socioeconomics, national origin), but not having alternative formats to in-person sessions, no provision of sliding scales, or understanding of policies that affect marginalized clients.
   • Readily advocate on behalf of causes that affect their identities, such as White feminism, but are silent on issues that affect multiply marginalized clients, such as Black Queer Women or international persons, such as Palestinian citizens.

4. Closing: After providing a definition and examples of oppression in clinical work, the supervisor encourages supervisees to assess their clinical approach with questions like the following,

   a. Who developed and researched the approaches I utilize with the client?

b. Do the theorist(s)' social identities reflect that of my own?

c. Do the interventions of choice attempt to address power-related/inequity issues?

5. **For Level 3+ supervisees:** Using the identities from the social identities wheel, the supervisor proposes five process-oriented questions for review with the supervisee when working with clients,

   a. How do your identities, whether dominant or marginalized, relate to power in the counseling room?

   b. How is power enacted in the counseling room?

   c. How does having multiple marginalized identities as a counselor impact the relationship with clients who have privileged identities?

   d. How can we begin broaching these dynamics?

   e. What feeling arises as you process any power imbalances you've experienced as a client or perpetuated as a clinician?

6. Supervisors should encourage conversation about the very real impact of marginalized locations on life. For supervisees who have mixed distributions of power/oppressed identities, how do the social locations impact counseling others? For instance, a Black Woman counselor who is married to a wealthy partner experiences both race and gender oppression but socioeconomic and role power.

7. Closing: Reflection should explore how supervisees' identities, both similarities and differences, influence their approach to working with clients. For supervisees who hold majority privilege identities, supervisors should encourage them to unpack ways that unconscious privilege and bias impact their clients.

   a. An example of this can be assisting a supervisee who is both White, middle class, heterosexual, able-bodied, and Christian, exploring how their own conscious and unconscious conformity to those identities and dominant societal status affects how they validate clients who identify as Christian, Queer, and Persons of Color.

## Supervisory Alliance and Relationship

Sue (2016) has established that conversations about race and other social locations can be difficult, leading to feelings of anger, frustration (for oppressed people), and anxiety and shame for others (privileged people). The supervisor needs self-awareness and self-regulation abilities throughout the intervention while practicing compassion and accountability to supervisee development. Any relational breaches must be addressed immediately and model cultural humility.

## Legal and Ethical Considerations

This anti-oppressive approach underscores every individual's intrinsic dignity and worth, emphasizing equity, access to services, and fair treatment as integral components of counseling and supervision. Mental health workers, in upholding nonmaleficence, actively confront social inequities and recognize how oppression influences clinical practice.

1. Talking about justice issues with clients and supervisees can be challenging. How do you manage your own feelings when things become challenging?
2. It is not uncommon for people to retreat from justice work when it becomes emotionally challenging or feels hard. How will you challenge yourself from retreating in your own work?
3. Using the appropriate IDM stage, identify your stage of development. What areas are strong for you? Which needs more development?

## Intervention Title: Unveiling Dominant Culture

## Author(s) and Affiliation(s)

Tina R. Paone, PhD, LPC, ACS, RPT-S
Monmouth University

Krista M. Malott, PhD, LPC
Villanova University

## Supervision Format and Modality

This intervention was developed for use within an in-person or virtual group of up to 15 supervisees.

## Supervisee Development

The intervention is relevant across all supervised developmental levels. This is an introductory-level supervision intervention.

## Supervisory Goals and Learning Objectives

1. Supervisees will develop a critical understanding of the impacts of dominant societal norms (often dubbed *Whiteness norms*), and name at least three examples, on self and others.
2. Supervisees will develop a critical lens and describe two examples of how it will foster ongoing recognition and analysis of dominant norms as they relate to multiple systems.

## Time Required

This intervention requires 50-60 minutes.

## Materials

Supervisors will need to familiarize themselves with the Assumptions of White Culture (Katz, 1990, 2003) and additional resources about dominant culture and the historical creation of Whiteness in the United States and its connections to mental health and diagnosis (Banks-VanAllen et al., 2023; Kendall, 2006). Materials include copies of the *Aspects or Assumptions of White Culture* table (Google image search 'Assumption of White Culture chart, Judith Katz'), Copies of the *Exploration of Values Worksheet* (see appendix), whiteboard or butcher paper, and markers.

## Intervention Instructions

1. Provide a copy of the *Exploration of Values Worksheet* to each supervisee, asking them to complete it and set it aside. The worksheet should be completed during a previous supervision session or, conversely, from home.

2. Ask the supervisees to think about the phrase *American culture* and what traits, values, or norms reflect American culture, specifying that the phrase will be used to refer exclusively to the United States.

3. As supervisees brainstorm thoughts and ideas, have them shout out responses while the supervisor writes them on a whiteboard or butcher paper to provide a visual. Write down all responses, even if they do not apply to the dominant culture of Whiteness.

4. Following the naming of cultural traits/practices, review the *Assumptions of White Culture* handout and ask them to compare what is on the list versus what is on the board. Ask them to name the things that they see in both places, circling the traits that they identified that are also on the list for a visual of overlap.

5. Supervisors should briefly describe the historical creation of race in the United States and link it to the creation of the dominant culture of Whiteness. An example of such an explanation entails the country was colonized (e.g., "founded") by individuals who were largely WASPS—White Anglo Saxons, Protestants, and cisgender males. Cultural traits, behaviors, language, religion, values, and aesthetics reflect those WASP norms by which all other groups in the U.S. were expected to adapt/assimilate in order to receive access to resources, opportunities, and power or privilege. Only those who were legally deemed 'White' were fully included in that privileged group, and the determination of who was White differed across state lines and over time. In turn, full inclusion and access to such resources and privileges have been prohibited for certain groups to this day due to not aligning with "whiteness" traits (e.g., Black or Asian Americans) (Tinsley, 2022).

6. To deepen exploration of the impacts of dominant norms, continue to prompt supervisee discussion by asking questions such as:

   • Do these Whiteness norms apply to all Americans?
   • If not, to whom do they apply?

- How does Whiteness, as defined by Katz, reflect dominant culture from an intersectional lens?
- How are folks impacted when they fail to align with certain Whiteness norms or traits (to make it personal and therefore more meaningful, ask them to identify a norm they 'fail' to embody—and to explore how that has impacted them)?
- What compromises or sacrifices might you or others (such as your clients) have to make in order to assimilate into specific norms?
- Are there assumptions on this list that are inherently bad? Or good? Which?
- Are there assumptions on this list that you disagree exist?

7. Ask the supervisees to refer to and reflect on the *Exploration of Values* sheet. Prompt them to take a few minutes to examine how the assumptions of Whiteness correspond to the supervisee's personal/family values.
8. Ask supervisees to note how their values and beliefs align with the dominant normative culture. Discuss these norms and if or how they have been systematically integrated into their families. Examine thoughts such as when their family came to the United States (electively or forcefully). ★Note: supervisees of color can be triggered by this component of the activity, recognizing how much Whiteness has dominated their lives. Have supervisees dialogue with a peer around this for a few minutes.
9. Return to the larger group and ask supervisees to share their reactions and conclusions.

## Supervisory Alliance and Relationship

Supervisees can experience an increased sense of vulnerability as they examine their values and beliefs surrounding dominant cultural norms. *Whiteness* norms, which are intersectional in nature (e.g., christonormativity, heteronormativity, patriarchy, neurotypicality, White supremacy), can elicit reactions from the supervisee. Depending upon the supervisee's previous work surrounding this topic, feelings may emerge that can derail or prohibit learning, examples including anger, guilt, grief/loss, shame, frustration, and oppression-associated trauma responses. Thus, the supervisor can model authenticity by naming their own emotional reactions to such topics as well as processing supervisee reactions in a non-judgmental manner. The supervisor is encouraged to continually check in with the supervisee about their experiences within supervision and how being challenged may impact the supervisory relationship.

## Legal and Ethical Considerations

This activity can elicit strong emotional reactions for some supervisees for differing reasons. For instance, some may feel that their core values are being 'attacked.' Some may feel rage or trauma-based reactions due to the oppression they have experienced from Whiteness norms. Others may feel a sense of shame or guilt for accessing certain privileges while simultaneously feeling a sense of grief or betrayal over their family having to forsake their heritage/certain traits to gain access to those resources. Hence, it is important to assure supervisees that they are not wrong or bad for possessing certain norms and to recognize the pain or grief around loss and oppression caused by these norms (and to add that their clients may also be impacted in these ways).

In addition, because emotional reactions can inhibit learning, take time to acknowledge common emotional reactions and offer time and space for reflection of those reactions via multiple modalities, either within or outside of the class session (journaling, dialoguing with a peer, video reflections). The supervisor would ideally also model the ways that you have managed reactions to this phenomenon, as well as how you have learned to address those harms in your professional and personal settings to normalize this reality.

## Reflective Questions

1. What did you learn about yourself today?
2. What will you take from this activity?
3. How do you now view Whiteness (as it has been defined in an intersectional way), and how are you impacted by Whiteness?
4. How will anything we talked about today help you work with clients of color or with those who do not fit into the Whiteness paradigm?

# APPENDIX: EXPLORATION OF VALUES

*Instructions: Decide how this value shows up for you. Write your responses in the first column. Is it a personal value (mine), family value (not mine, but my family holds this value), both (both my family and I hold this value), or N/A (Not applicable, neither I nor my family hold this value)?*

| *Whose Value* | *Values* |
|---|---|
| | Be self-reliant |
| | Be independent |
| | Individuals are in control of their environment |
| | Be number one |
| | Winner-loser dichotomy |
| | Must always "do something" about a situation |
| | Aggressiveness |
| | Majority rules |
| | Avoid conflict |
| | Be polite (don't raise voice) |
| | Avoid intimacy and emotion |
| | Christian values |
| | Hard work is key to success |
| | Work before play |
| | Objective thoughts |
| | Rational linear thinking |
| | Cause and effect relationships |
| | Wealth = worth |
| | Heavy value on ownership of goods, space, and property |
| | Your job is who you are |
| | Respect authority |
| | Adhere to time schedules |
| | Plan for future |
| | Delayed gratification |
| | Progress is always for the best |
| | Tomorrow will be better |
| | Nuclear family is ideal (father, mother, 2.5 children) |

CHAPTER 4

# Centering the Margins Through Empowerment and Liberation

*Clark D. Ausloos, Cirleen DeBlaere, Kirsis A. Dipre, Diana Gallardo, Arpana G. Inman, Melissa Luke, Kelly Moore, Harvey Charles Peters, Stacy A. Pinto and David P. Rivera*

## CHAPTER 4 INTERVENTIONS

### Intervention Title: Gnat in the Chat: Centering Clients and Supervisees Through Empowerment and Liberation

### Author(s) and Affiliation(s)

Melissa Luke, Ph.D., NCC, ACS, LMHC
Syracuse University

Harvey Charles Peters, Ph.D., NCC
Montclair State University

### Supervision Format and Modality

This intervention was developed for anti-oppressive supervision, modernizing the traditional *Bug in the ear* (Gallant & Thyer, 1989) and *Bug in the eye* (Weck et al., 2016) supervision. The intervention can also be adapted for use in live individual supervision triadic and group supervision that is conducted in person or virtually.

DOI: 10.4324/9781003470656-4

## Supervisee Development

supervisory intervention requires both client and supervisee consent and can be implemented with master's and doctoral students in training contexts, as well as pre- and post-licensed professional counselors and supervision of supervision (Jencius & Baltrinic, 2016).

## Supervisory Goals and Learning Objectives

1.  Supervisees will demonstrate an ability to prioritize the voices, narratives, and experiences of minoritized populations and communities within both their counseling and supervision.
2.  Supervisees will be able to identify ways to counteract the dominant and majoritarian forces, structures, and systems related to their counseling and supervision.
3.  Supervisees will identify strategies and resources to center historically excluded persons and perspectives within their counseling and supervision.
4.  Supervisees will increase their ability to intervene towards emancipation and liberation within their counseling and supervision.

## Time Required

This intervention typically requires one hour.

## Materials

This supervision intervention requires informed consent from both the client and supervisee, as well as adherence to federal and state laws and disciplinary ethical standards, including but not limited to the use of a HIPAA-compliant video conferencing platform.

Supervisors are encouraged to review supervisee goals and progress notes, as well as client case notes, in preparation for the use of live supervision using *Gnat in the Chat*, a synchronous text and/or direct messaging intervention during live supervision. We recommend short, concrete feedback where possible, limiting the number and focus of messages, and avoiding directives unless absolutely necessary, as these can in be in opposition to some of the aims of anti-oppressive supervision. While it is impossible to provide examples of these types of chat messages out of context, the following questions are offered as potential areas of foci consistent with the objectives of the intervention.

1. Who is the minoritized population and/or community in this instance?
2. What is stopping you from naming the minoritized population and/or community?
3. How can you prioritize the voices, narratives, and experiences of this population or community?
4. Could X counteract the dominant and majoritarian forces, structures, and systems here?
5. Might you explore the client's understanding of and experiences with the dominant and majoritarian forces, structures, and systems?
6. How are the immediate processes reflecting the dominant and majoritarian forces, structures, and systems? What if you addressed this?
7. Who is being centered right now, and what does this reflect in terms of identities and social locations?
8. What shifts if you center historically excluded persons and perspectives in this moment?
9. How can you intervene toward emancipation and liberation with this client?
10. Where might I support your emancipation and liberation in supervision?

## Intervention Instructions

1. Computer-mediated technology has been incorporated into clinical supervision for more than three decades; however, the types of technology have continued to evolve (Jencius & Baltrinic, 2016). The supervisor may benefit from familiarizing themselves with contemporary research and practice literature related to live, behind the mirror, bug in the ear, and bug in the eye supervision.
2. The supervisor explains the *Gnat in the Chat* live supervision intervention as part of the formal informed consent procedures. We recommend that the supervisor center input from the supervisee in the decision-making related to the procedures, such as whether or not the supervision will be recorded and whether or not they wish to share the content of the chat messages with the client.
3. The supervisor supports the supervisee in seeking consent from their client for participation in the live supervision. This begins with the supervisee developing an explanation of live supervision that includes

the anti-oppressive supervision intervention Gnat in the chat and also provides the client an opportunity to provide input.

4. Once the live supervision is scheduled, the counselor supervisee distributes log-on information to both their client and the supervisor.

5. The supervisor prepares for the live *Gnat in the Chat* supervision intervention by reviewing supervision and counseling case notes, the goals of the supervision intervention, and the sample questions.

6. Once logged on to the video conferencing platform, the supervisor reviews the purpose and procedures related to live supervision using the *Gnat in the Chat* intervention in an attempt to normalize potential anxiety and demystify the process. The supervisor intentionally invites the supervisee to assume a lead role in the discussion about the counselor and client's goals for the live supervision.

7. The supervisor shares their observations and enlists questions and comments from the client and the supervisee. We recommend that the supervisor invites the client and the counselor supervisee to recommend potential areas of foci for the supervisor's feedback.

8. The supervisor then turns off their video and audio functions while the counselor supervisee and client engage in the counseling session.

9. During the counseling session, the supervisor watches, listens, and may take notes on session content. The supervisor may wish to track session content and process related to the anti-oppressive goals of this intervention using a pre-developed form aligned with their supervisory model or framework.

10. The supervisor decides when and how to provide feedback and ask questions in the chat function. We recommend the supervisor be intentional when selecting what messages to send and in what form.

11. The supervisor sends a message to both the supervisee and the client when there are about ten minutes before the counseling session is scheduled to end, at which time the supervisor will rejoin with their audio and video to process the live supervision and reflect for about five minutes, and then leave the session so that the counselor and client have time to process and wrap up.

12. Once the counselor supervisee and client end the session and the supervisor is invited back, the supervisor rejoins with their audio and video on. The supervisor centers the client and counselor supervisee, taking cues from them about how to proceed, particularly in relation to principles of anti-oppression.

13. When appropriate, the supervisor provides brief, non-evaluative process observation that includes disclosure of some of the ways they were impacted by the content and process of this live supervision.

14. The supervisor then returns the process to the counselor supervisee and client, engaging in discussion as invited and appropriate.

15. The supervisor logs off of the live supervision, allowing the counselor and client to end the counseling session themselves. The supervisor will then prepare any written feedback for the counselor supervisee as previously determined and continue the discussion of the live supervision within the next scheduled supervision session.

## Supervisory Alliance and Relationship

We have found that having the supervisor meet with both the counselor and client at the start of the session and then again at the end of the session can be helpful to reinforce procedure and responsibilities, lower anxiety, and enhance alliance, as well as address any unresolved matters (Weck et al., 2016). Relatedly, when meeting with the counselor and client at the start and end of the session, the supervisor should consider both the supervisory working alliance and the therapeutic working alliance.

## Legal and Ethical Considerations

Supervisors must ensure that the use of HIPAA-compliant video conferencing platforms and session records, as well as informed consent documentation, adhere to both federal and state laws and ethical standards. This includes whether or not the counseling and supervision can occur across state lines, factors that may be discipline and/or state-specific. Supervisors are cautioned that not all supervisory techniques translate equally across online modalities. Therefore, we encourage future research into the use of *Gnat in the Chat*.

## Reflective Questions

1. How were the voices, narratives, and experiences of minoritized populations and communities attended to in your counseling and supervision, and what will you do to redress and prioritize moving forward?

2. Where did you counteract the dominant and majoritarian forces, structures, and systems related to their counseling and supervision, and how will you respond to what interfered?

3. What are two specific strategies and/or resources you will utilize to center historically excluded persons and perspectives within their counseling and supervision?

4. At which point in supervision were your skills to intervene towards emancipation and liberation within their counseling and supervision expanded, how so, and what can you take from this into your future anti-oppressive counseling and supervision?

5. Which aspects of your experience with live supervision matched your understanding of and expectations for anti-oppressive work, and what took you by surprise? How do you understand this?

### Intervention Title: Reflective Supervision: Centering Clients and Supervisees Through Empowerment and Liberation

### Author(s) and Affiliation(s)

Kelly Moore, PsyD
Rutgers University

Arpana G. Inman, PhD
Rutgers University

### Supervision Format and Modality

The anti-oppressive individual clinical supervision incorporates an adapted Reflective Local Practice (RLP) model by Sandeen et al. (2018), proving effective for both live and in-person reflective supervision and easily adaptable for triadic/group supervision settings.

### Supervisee Development

This supervisory intervention can be implemented with master's or doctoral-level clinicians, as well as licensed professionals seeking advanced study in culturally responsive approaches to clinical work.

### Supervisory Goals and Learning Objectives

1. Supervisees will increase their ability to recognize how their implicit biases may result in potential hidden spots (*language changed from "blind" to "hidden" to avoid language related to visual impairment*) that may impact the supervisory and/or therapeutic relationship.
2. Supervisees will be able to identify a minimum of three ways to counteract the dominant and majoritarian forces, structures, and systems related to their counseling and supervision.
3. Supervisees will identify at least one strategy and resource to center historically excluded persons and perspectives within their counseling and supervision.
4. Supervisees will increase their ability to intervene towards emancipation and liberation within their counseling and supervision through exploration of their areas of privilege and intersecting identities.

## Time Required

This intervention would require 60–90-minute supervision meetings for Parts 1, 2, and 3, respectively (a total of 3–4.5 hours total), with a subsequent hour to complete the optional Part 4.

## Materials

1. The Adapted Reflective Local Practice Model Form (see Table 4.1).
2. The Adapted ADDRESSING Framework Identity Handout (see Table 4.2) (Hays, 2001).

## Intervention Instructions

This anti-oppressive supervision intervention requires informed consent from both the client and supervisee, as well as adherence to federal and state laws and disciplinary ethical standards, including but not limited to the use of a HIPAA-compliant video conferencing platform.

## Part 1: Reflective Exercise to Facilitate Dialogue About Marginalized Aspects of the Supervisor and Supervisees' Identities

a. The supervisor first reviews the RLP model (Sandeen et al., 2018), their discipline's respective professional standard guidelines for Multicultural Supervision (the references in this chapter reflect the American Psychological Association Guidelines for Multicultural Supervision (APA, 2017), and the ADDRESSING Framework, which aims to increase a clinician's recognition of the multiple dimensions of identity (Hays, 2001).

b. The supervisor reviews the concepts of *bias spots* as outlined in the RLP model. These are hot, hidden, and soft spots that may indicate biases held by the supervisee or client and may also help to highlight potential areas of power, privilege, and neutrality (Sandeen, et al., 2018). For example, the supervisor might note if a supervisee shares an identity with a client. This may reflect a "soft" spot to be aware of in treatment.

## Part 2: Role-Play and Relational Perspective-Taking

a. The supervisor and supervisees then complete the adapted RLP Identity/Privilege form (see Table 4.1) and, using a self-in-relation approach, reflect on their various identities, identifying privilege/power or otherwise.

b.   The supervisor and supervisee share their completed forms, discussing areas of difference and similarity, including unexpected outcomes. The supervisor explains how the experience serves as a parallel process to the supervisee's client approach, emphasizing that supervisor self-disclosures can enhance supervisee self-disclosures.

c.   While completing the exercise, the supervisor or supervisee may complete the RLP Identity form as the client, noting potential identity privilege to enhance the supervisee's understanding of the impact of any marginalized identity on the social and emotional health of their client. By adopting this perspective, the supervisor aids the supervisee in examining their client relationship and enhancing the supervisee's comfort in providing space for the client's voice.

d.   During the activity, the supervisor and supervisee explore the following questions in consideration of how they can prioritize the voices, narratives, and experiences of the population or community with whom they are working. Guiding questions to help with this relational perspective-taking in this role-play are:

- What parts of your identity are marginalized? How do we (supervisor—supervisee) differ, and how might you (therapist) differ from your client?
- In what way are these identities visible to the world, and how does that impact how you might engage with me and with your clients?
- How does my/your experience reflect the impact of dominant and majoritarian forces, structures, and systems? Let's explore . . .
- How do your client's experiences reflect the impact of dominant and majoritarian forces, structures, and systems? Let's explore . . .
- How might you explore the client's understanding of and experiences with the dominant and majoritarian forces, structures, and systems?
- How can you center the aspect of identity that is least privileged in the therapy sessions with your client?
- What shifts if you center historically excluded persons and perspectives at this moment?
- How can you intervene toward emancipation and liberation with this client, while still recognizing the systemic forces that impact their experiences?
- What was it like to engage in this role-play? How might your client react to engaging in this activity?

## Part 3: Deeper Exploration of How to Engage a Client in this Exercise

The supervisor then reviews how the supervisee can approach this exercise with their client and discusses potential areas of implicit bias that may impact their therapeutic work, using Socratic questioning akin to the questions listed previously. Other discussion questions may include:

- After reflecting on your identities and areas of privilege, in what ways do you feel empowered in your identity? In what ways do you feel disempowered?
- What are your expectations of yourself that may be rooted in your various identities?
- How might these reflections relate to your ability to address your client's emotional health?

## Part 4 *(optional)*: Live Supervision to Assist Supervisee with Client

a.  If live supervision is an option, the supervisor (with written consent from the client) can log into a HIPAA-compliant video conferencing platform and help facilitate the completion of the RLP Identity/Bias form and follow-up with a discussion (reflection in action). The chat feature can be utilized to provide support for the supervisee in the follow-up question process.

b.  If live video supervision is not an option, then the supervisee should review the form with the supervisor at the subsequent supervision meeting and reflect on the experience of completing the exercise with the client (reflection on action).

## Supervisory Alliance and Relationship

The relationship between a supervisor and supervisee is vital to the development of competent clinicians in the behavioral health field. Supervisees who encounter supervisors who minimize or dismiss the role of cultural identity are less likely to share important information in supervision, impacting treatment outcomes (Ashley & Lipscomb, 2018; Burkard et.al., 2006; Constantine & Sue, 2007; Inman et al., 2014). Supervisors implementing the anti-oppressive practice outlined previously should engage in the intervention *with* their supervisees to establish their willingness to be vulnerable, an aspect that is critical to minimizing power and developing a strong supervisory relationship (Inman et al., 2014).

## Legal and Ethical Considerations

Supervisors must use HIPAA-compliant video conferencing platforms, maintain session records, and ensure informed consent documentation, adhering to federal and state laws and ethical standards. Note that the adapted intervention has been primarily applied to the clinician–client dyad but not the supervisor–supervisee dyad. Future research about its effectiveness and utility is needed.

## Reflective Questions

1.  What were some areas of similarities/differences related to power and privilege between you and the client(s) you served? In what ways did you help the client reflect on areas where they have power, if any?
2.  For identities where you, as the provider, had power and the client did not, how did you acknowledge that to the client? What strategies are helpful to empower the client to be the expert in the therapy room with a clinician who may not understand their lived experience?
3.  At which point in supervision were your skills to intervene towards emancipation and liberation within their counseling and supervision expanded? How so? What can you take from this into your future anti-oppressive counseling and supervision?

# APPENDIX

*Table 4.1* Adapted Reflective Local Practice Identity/Privilege Form

| Commonly identified dimensions of culture | Power/Privilege? (+) | Powerlessness? (-) | Neutral? (/) | Mixed Power? (+/-) | Unsure? (?) |
|---|---|---|---|---|---|
| Socioeconomic Status | | | | | |
| Sexual Orientation | | | | | |
| Gender Identity | | | | | |
| Education Level | | | | | |
| Gender Expression | | | | | |
| Body Type | | | | | |
| Geographic Location | | | | | |
| Veteran Status | | | | | |
| Race | | | | | |
| Ethnicity | | | | | |
| Religion | | | | | |
| Spirituality | | | | | |
| Professional Status | | | | | |
| Nationality | | | | | |

*Table 4.2* Adapted ADDRESSING Framework (Hays, 2001) Handout

| Cultural Influences | Examples of Minority Groups |
| --- | --- |
| **A**ge/generational | Children, elders, millennials, Gen-Z, etc. |
| **D**evelopmental disabilities, acquired disabilities | People born with Disabilities or those who acquired Disabilities later in life |
| **R**eligion & Spirituality | Religious minority groups |
| **E**thnic & Racial Identity | Ethnic and Racial minority groups |
| **S**ocioeconomic Status | People of lower income, with less education, living in areas that are disproportionality impacted by poverty and traumatically stressful situation |
| **S**exual Orientation | Gay, Lesbian, and Bisexual people, and also includes Gender Expansive Diverse Groups |
| **I**ndigenous Heritage | Indigenous, Aboriginal, and Native people |
| **N**ational origin | Refugees, Immigrants, and International students |
| **G**ender | Women, Transgender, and Gender Expansive persons |

## Intervention Title: Powerlines: Elucidating Dynamics of Privilege and Oppression to Inform Empowerment and Liberation

### Author(s) and Affiliation(s)

Cirleen DeBlaere, PhD
Georgia State University

David P. Rivera, PhD
Queens College, City University of New York

### Supervision Format and Modality

The *Powerlines* supervision intervention was developed for a group modality and can also be utilized in individual or triadic supervision. It was adapted from a *Powerlines* activity created to promote clinician self-awareness (Hook et al., 2017) and is intended for live in-person or virtual supervision.

### Supervisee Development

This intervention is ideal for students early in their training but can be utilized at any training level, from Master's practicum to postgraduate and post-licensed professionals, when a clinician would benefit from an increased awareness of the intersectional realities and privilege implications of their identity. The *Powerlines* intervention is an advanced introductory intervention. To increase the level of complexity, add more explicit exploration of the implications of one's positionalities within the context of broader systems (e.g., their organization or institution, policy, historical narratives).

### Supervisory Goals and Learning Objectives

1. Supervisees will demonstrate an understanding of intersectionality theory and the interplay, impact, and potential influence of their unique constellation of identities on their development and ways of engaging as people, clinicians, and supervisees.
2. Supervisees will develop a more nuanced understanding of the ways that oppression and privilege operate through their exploration of the interplay of their more privileged and oppressed identities.

3.  Supervisees will be able to identify at least two ways that their identities can be sources of empowerment and liberation of self and others.

## Time Required

This intervention typically requires one hour.

## Materials

Each supervisee should be provided a handout with the *Powerlines* figure (see Hook et al., 2017 for image), a writing utensil, and the following text:

## Intervention Instructions

*Directions*

*Pick six aspects of your cultural identity* and write down these identities in the rectangles—one identity in each box. Then, spend some time thinking and reflecting on each cultural identity. Does this particular identity afford you a high, medium, or low amount of power? Make a mark on the "power line" that connects the box to the large power oval at the top of the page. If the identity affords you a large amount of power, make a mark near the top of the line, close to the power oval. If the identity affords you a low amount of power, make a mark near the bottom of the line, far away from the power oval. If the identity affords you a medium amount of power, make a mark near the middle of the line.

1.  The supervisor first provides a discussion of intersectionality theory (Crenshaw, 2013; Hill-Collins, 2015) and its key tenets to orient the supervisees to their identities, the social locations and intersections of those identities, and the impact of their intersectional positionalities on their development and interactions.
2.  The supervisor presents a completed *Powerlines* handout example (ideally on a projected slide or other medium that allows for easy viewing and guided discussion) to illustrate where various identities (e.g., race/ethnicity, sexual orientation, ability, social class, neurodiversity) may be located. The supervisor can prepare a *Powerlines* handout of their identities to illustrate and allow for a subsequent discussion of the interaction of the supervisor's and supervisees' identities.

3.  In discussing the example, the supervisor should note the following:

    a.  Supervisees should select identities that are salient to them within the context of their current clinical work.
    b.  Although including sociocultural identities is common and important, salient identities can also include roles of importance to the supervisee that impact their experience as supervisees (e.g., student, caretaker, parent).

4.  Once supervisees have been oriented to the intervention, supervisees are instructed to complete their handout.
5.  After all supervisees have completed their handout, the supervisor poses the following questions in this general order. These can be projected on a slide or read aloud. Supervisees should note their responses on their handouts.

    a.  What surprised you about the identities that you listed?
    b.  Where did you note areas of more or less privilege?
    c.  How have those identities informed your understanding of how privilege and oppression operate in our society? Therapy? Supervision?

6.  After responding to these questions, supervisees discuss their responses in pairs.
7.  Subsequent to the dyadic discussion, the supervisor invites the group back to a larger group discussion; asking that they share an insight that they had about how their identities impact their orientations to power.
8.  The supervisor is encouraged to utilize what is shared by the supervisees to deepen the discussion of power, oppression, and liberation. For example, a few points to discuss would highlight that:

    a.  The identities that supervisees listed today would likely change if they were prompted to consider a different context (e.g., dinner with their family of origin). This is one illustration of how identity is fluid and how the salience of identities can change by context and circumstance despite society's tendency to enforce that identities are easily defined and immutable.
    b.  We largely lack a language of intersectionality as a society. Even this exercise asked supervisees to separate salient identities into boxes. The lack of language to represent inherently intersectional identities (with few exceptions, e.g., Latina) illustrates our society's

tendency to consider identity in singular and circumscribed ways, which does not reflect people's lived experiences.

    i.   When the responses are considered, complexity should be explored. For example, how do the intersections of marginalized identities (e.g., women of Color with a disability) impact experiences for different social identities (e.g., Asian women, Black women, Indigenous women, Latina women)? Do the supervisees note how intersectional invisibility (Purdie-Vaughns & Eibach, 2008) may operate and the implications for society and the supervisees' own understandings if these identities are centered?

    c.   In reflecting on our identities, we often have an easier time identifying our areas of less privilege than more, but we all have areas of privilege (e.g., obtaining a graduate degree reflects educational privilege); this is a tool of privilege to keep it unnamed and unchallenged. The group can consider other ways privilege operates based on this exercise.

9.   To emphasize empowerment and liberation, the intervention concludes with a discussion of strength and coping strategies that originated from the ways of being, intergenerational histories, and strengths cultivated within cultures that have been overlooked, understudied, and devalued in models of mental health care. To put this knowledge into action, the supervisee can discuss ways of applying intersectional and systems-level concepts to their therapeutic and supervisory experiences.

## Supervisory Alliance and Relationship

Literature indicates that explicit inclusion of cultural topics is critical to positive working alliances and supervisee disclosure in supervision (Zhang et al., 2022). Supervisors should endeavor to model a multicultural orientation (Hook et al., 2017). In this way, supervisors engage lifelong cultural learning, are attuned to the impact of their own intersectional cultural identity on the supervisory relationship, and avoid making assumptions about their supervisee's salient cultural identities (Hook et al., 2016).

## Legal and Ethical Considerations

The professional ethics codes, standards, and guidelines of your discipline and/or specialty should be followed.

## Reflective Questions

1. How can you use your awareness of your sociocultural identities and positionalities as a source of empowerment in your therapeutic work with clients?
2. How do your privileged identities and positionalities interact and impact your therapeutic work with clients? How do your identities and positionalities support oppression in your work?
3. Considering what liberation means for you, how does your understanding of your privileged and oppressed identities and positionalities influence what it means to be liberated?
4. What is something you can do to maintain awareness of how your privileged and oppressed identities and positionalities impact the therapeutic process?

## Intervention Title: Queering Socratic Questioning: Using Language for Exploration and Liberation

### Author(s) and Affiliation(s)

Clark D. Ausloos, PhD
Oakland University

Stacy A. Pinto, PhD
University of Denver

### Supervision Format and Modality

A queered version of Socratic questioning can be used to augment supervision within and between a broad range of identities. By destabilizing the assumption of normality in experience, the supervisory relationship is poised to support the unique identities of both the supervisee and the client. For the purpose of *this* intervention, it is conceptualized with lesbian, gay, bisexual, transgender, two-spirit, gender-expansive, queer, questioning, intersex, agender, asexual, aromantic, and/or pan/poly communities (LGBTGEQIAP+). Due to the dialogic nature of the intervention, synchronous (in-person or virtual) supervision settings are recommended. This flexible approach is inclusive of and beneficial to non-dominant and marginalized supervisees and clients with varied identities (e.g., race/ethnicity, social class, dis/ability), underscoring the intervention's potential to address intersectionality.

### Supervisee Development

This intervention can be used with LGBTGEQIAP+ identified pre-or post-licensed counselors and/or counselors-in-training (e.g., master's/doctoral students in field experience courses such as practicum/internship). The intervention is applicable across counseling specialties. This is an intermediate to advanced supervisory intervention.

### Supervisory Goals and Learning Objectives

1. Supervisees will reflect on their identities, articulating how these intersect with corresponding client identities, increasing self-awareness and ability to manage biases and dual relationships.

2.  Supervisees will use queered Socratic questioning to explore and strengthen the therapeutic alliance, enhance the therapeutic benefits for clients, and promote emancipation and liberation.

## Time Required

This intervention may be implemented regularly, as needed, and may take between 20 to 60 minutes each time.

## Materials

No physical materials are required.

## Intervention Instructions: Supervision Categories and Examples of Queering Socratic Questioning

A.  **Exploring Personal Identity, Professional Practice, and Power** (Goodrich et al., 2016)

- How do your own LGBTGEQIAP+ identities inform your approach to counseling and influence your interactions with LGBTGEQIAP+ clients?
- How do your personal identity and experience of disempowerment as an LGBTGEQIAP+ individual inform your critique of traditional counseling models, and how do you integrate this into affirming and liberatory counseling approaches for LGBTGEQIAP+ clients?

B.  **Challenging Societal Norms** (Chan et al., 2018)

- What actions can you take to dismantle societal perceptions and stereotypes about the LGBTGEQIAP+ community within your practice, creating a more supportive space for your LGBTGEQIAP+ clients?
- How does your understanding and personal experience of being marginalized within the LGBTGEQIAP+ community influence your approach to challenging societal norms in your therapeutic practice, and how do you use this understanding to advocate for broader change?

C.  **Reflecting on Intersectionality** (Frank & Cannon, 2010)

- How do your clients' non-LGBTGEQIAP+ identity factors (e.g., race, ethnicity, disability, social class) intersect with their

LGBTGEQIAP+ identities, and how are these factors similar or dissimilar to your identities/experiences?

- How do your identity intersections influence your perception and response to the diverse intersections present in your clients, and how do you integrate this awareness into a nuanced and empathetic counseling practice?

D.  **Understanding Oppression and Privilege** (Capobianco, 2020)

- As an LGBTGEQIAP+ identified counselor, how do you recognize and address the dynamics of oppression and privilege in your counseling practice, especially concerning LGBTGEQIAP+ clients who hold multiple marginalized identities?
- How do you navigate and reflect upon your multiple forms of marginalization within the therapeutic setting, and how does this awareness influence your approach to counseling and advocacy for and with clients?

E.  **Promoting Critical Discourse** (Frank & Cannon, 2010)

- As an LGBTGEQIAP+-identified counselor, what strategies do you use to foster critical discourse around LGBTGEQIAP+ issues in your sessions, and how do you ensure these discussions are empowering for your clients?
- Considering the unique perspectives/challenges that your LGBTGEQIAP+ identity brings, how do you incorporate these into critical discussions about intersectionality and diversity in your counseling sessions?

F.  **Fostering Empowerment, Emancipation, and Liberation** (Goodrich et al., 2016)

- How does your journey as an LGBTGEQIAP+ individual inform your approach to facilitating the empowerment, emancipation, and liberation of your LGBTGEQIAP+ clients, particularly in navigating and challenging societal norms/expectations?
- What actions do you take to promote the emancipation and liberation of LGBTGEQIAP+ clients within the counseling process, and how do you measure progress in this area?

1.  **Introduce** the intervention to your supervisee so that you are positioned to integrate it into (a) regular supervision and (b) individual reflection, as appropriate.

2. **Engage** in active listening throughout supervisee case presentations, with attention to identifying *Supervision Categories* that may be relevant to the supervisee's growth (e.g., hidden spots) that span various identities and experiences and emphasize the importance of empowerment and liberation.

3. **Collaborate** to identify aspects of your supervisee's work that may benefit from deeper analysis (whether individual cases or thematic discussion involving multiple clients). Guide supervisees to explore cases involving diverse identities, highlighting the importance of intersectionality and the unique challenges and needs of different client groups.

4. **Identify** a relevant *Supervision Category* (i.e., A through F). Examples are articulated in what follows.

    a. If a supervisee's conceptualizations seem overly aligned with their own experiences, failing to account for significant client differences (e.g., social class, educational background), supervisors may direct the conversation towards intersectionality (*Supervision Category C*) to help illuminate the diverse experiences within the LGBTGEQIAP+ community.

    b. If a supervisee faces challenges with a client's hesitancy toward public advocacy, applying empowerment concepts (*Supervision Category F*) can help them navigate similarities and differences in empowerment and advocacy strategies. This process involves posing questions that connect supervisees' personal experiences with their counseling sessions.

5. **Adapt**, as needed, an appropriate question within the identified *Supervision Category* to fit your supervisee's circumstances. Direct discussions to consider clients' multifaceted identities, using diverse examples to illustrate the intersection of sexuality, gender, race, ethnicity, and more.

6. **Prompt** your supervisee to engage in non-defensive reflection of potentially overlooked aspects of their case conceptualization(s) and/ or preconceived notions by responding to the question. Encourage supervisees to critically reflect on their biases and the complex layers of identity that affect their clients.

7. **Reflect** and **summarize** the information provided by your supervisee's response.

8. **Prompt** your supervisees to continue exploring their original thoughts related to the chosen question by asking questions focused

on *clarification, assumptions, evidence, perspective-taking,* and *consequences.* This process may support your supervisee in developing a richer understanding and empathy toward their client(s). Examples are articulated in what follows.

    a.   Encourage your supervisee to articulate *evidence* for their understanding of how their client's various identities intersect to inform their experience in the world.

    b.   Challenge your supervisee to identify potential *consequences* to engagement in public advocacy that their client may or may not have faced.

**9.**  **Share** details of this intervention with supervisees and encourage ongoing engagement with these queered Socratic questions outside of supervision sessions.

**Provide** opportunities during supervision sessions for discussion of additional reflections, insights, and challenges encountered during the intervention's application. This discussion fosters ongoing learning, enabling the adaptation of strategies to better address the needs of both supervisees and their clients.

## Supervisory Alliance and Relationship

This intervention aims to empower supervisees by integrating intersectional personal identity with professional practice through self-reflection, challenging societal norms, understanding oppression and privilege, and adapting counseling to clients' diverse experiences. The goal is to foster a therapeutic/supervisory environment that is affirming and empathetic to the unique needs of diverse supervisees and clients, promoting their emancipation and liberation.

## Legal and Ethical Considerations

This intervention requires compliance with relevant federal and state legislation and adherence to relevant professional ethical standards, including informed consent from both the supervisee and their client(s), confidentiality, and the use of HIPAA-compliant tools (e.g., video conferencing platform). It stresses the importance of self-awareness regarding biases and ethical practice. Supervisors are tasked with guiding supervisees to balance client autonomy with challenging systemic oppression, ensuring a supportive and brave space for all clients.

## Reflective Questions

1. How can I challenge my own assumptions and biases related to sex, sexuality, and gender and how they relate to interactions with my supervisees?
2. How am I fostering a brave space for critical discourse, and how can I better facilitate discussions that encourage my supervisees to critically examine their own assumptions about societal norms?
3. How am I skillfully integrating queered Socratic questioning to guide my supervisees to critically reflect on their own experiences and how this intersects with those of their clients?

**Intervention Title: Play, Pause, Rewind: Centering the Margins Through Empowerment and Liberation**

**Author(s) and Affiliation(s)**

Diana Gallardo, PhD
Northeastern Illinois University

Kirsis A. Dipre, PhD
Northeastern Illinois University

**Supervision Format and Modality**

This anti-oppressive supervision intervention is tailored for individual and triadic supervisory contexts, accommodating both virtual and in-person settings.

**Supervisee Development**

This supervisory intervention can be implemented with master's and doctoral students in training contexts and postgraduate pre-licensed professional counselors within their new professional contexts. In line with the Integrated Development Model (IDM) of supervision (Stoltenberg, 1981), this anti-oppressive supervision intervention focuses on level-one supervisees and can be implemented at different levels. Level-one supervisees are generally high in motivation yet high in anxiety and fear of evaluation (Kuo et al., 2016). However, supervisors can add additional questions depending on the supervisee's level.

**Supervisory Goals and Learning Objectives**

*Supervisees Will*

1. Identify at least two ways to respond to and challenge dominant systems and structures to create more inclusive and equitable counseling practices.
2. Increase their self-efficacy in applying counseling interventions that foster empowerment and liberation for both clients and supervisees.
3. Demonstrate an increased awareness and understanding of counseling and supervisory practices that promote emancipation and liberation.

## Time Required

This intervention typically requires 60 to 90 minutes, depending on the supervision format and modality.

## Materials

Although no materials are required for this intervention, supervisors must follow the following steps in preparation for the supervision session.

## Intervention Instructions

*Pre-session Preparation*

1. The supervisor familiarizes themselves with the technology involved in recording client sessions and the procedures for utilizing *the Play, pause, and rewind* intervention.
2. The supervisee obtains the client's (s) consent to record the session and explain the purpose of recording, emphasizing the focus on the development and enhancement of counselor skills and their development of growth and awareness.
3. Supervisors review the identified recording, paying attention to strengths, growth areas, and content related to culture and oppressive systems.
4. Supervisors review client goals, session progress notes, and relevant documentation.
5. Obtain a computer through which the sessions can be reviewed.

*Session Instructions*

The *Play, pause, rewind* intervention was developed specifically for anti-oppressive supervision, reforming the traditional *audio and video recordings* pioneered by Rogers and Covner (Bernard & Goodyear, 2019). The *Play, pause, rewind* intervention allows the supervisor and supervisee to review specific session sections individually (play and pause) and together (rewind).

1. During the first supervision session, the supervisor discusses the purpose of supervision and explains the *Play, pause, and rewind* intervention to the supervisee(s), emphasizing the importance of selecting appropriate video segments of the counseling session to share in supervision. Consistent with the aims of anti-oppressive supervision,

we recommend that the supervisor center the supervisee's input in the decision-making process around equipment selection. Special attention should be paid to accessibility (e.g., captions, accessibility to recording space, etc.) in terms of use and cost for the supervisee.

2.  Relatedly, the supervisor thoughtfully and intentionally teaches the supervisee how to select three 5-minute segments. Next, the supervisor adopts a directive approach, teaching and illustrating the concepts of strengths, growth, and cultural and oppressive systems to the supervisee. For example, the supervisor might say, "Areas of growth are the instances where you think you could have done better; strengths are where you feel confident in your abilities, while cultural and oppressive systems refer to the instances where you are addressing or failing to address systemic influences."

3.  The supervisor provides the supervisee(s) with the opportunity to ask questions to ensure expectations are clear and achievable before agreeing to start the intervention during the following supervisory meeting. Once scheduled, this intervention becomes integrated into their upcoming supervision session. The supervisee will share their selections with their supervisor prior to the supervision (based on the agreed-upon timeline).

4.  The supervisor continues to engage their preparation for the *Play, pause, and rewind* intervention in accordance with steps 3 and 4 in the pre-session preparation.

5.  Once in the supervision session, the supervisor is encouraged to emphasize the relational aspect of the supervisory process by centering mutuality and connection. Utilizing critical theories (e.g., Relational cultural theory) to build a strong alliance while simultaneously modeling how they may engage with their client.

6.  Depending on the supervisee's needs, the supervisor works with the supervisee to develop a clear structure and process to foster a supervisee's sense of agency and empowerment. It may be beneficial for the supervisee to show the segments as they occur and have them attempt to identify which of the three areas they fall in (i.e., strengths, growth areas, and/or content related to culture and oppressive systems). While watching each segment, the supervisor takes notes of the recording and the supervisee's reactions and actions while in session and supervision. The supervisor ideally pays close attention to whether there is acknowledgment or disregard of the potential impact of personal beliefs held by the client, supervisor, and supervisee and its impact on therapeutic and supervisory alliances.

7.  After watching the first segment fully, the supervisor encourages the supervisees to share their perceptions of the segment, inviting

reflection and critical consciousness. The supervisor provides feedback that responds to the supervisee's questions and incorporates additional insights from their notes and observations. It is essential the supervisor is intentional in their delivery of feedback, focusing on a combination of the following: (a) achievement of realistic goals for the supervised session (e.g., highlighting missed opportunities and offering examples of how to intervene effectively), (b) internal processes across contexts encouraging storytelling and valuing of diverse narratives (e.g., inviting supervisee to notice their internal experience while in session and in supervision, potentially highlighting parallel processes), and (c) moderate discrepancies between supervisee performance and target performance (e.g., noting discrepancies in supervisee perception of effectiveness and accuracy of effectiveness). The supervisor then repeats this process for the remaining two areas.

8.  After feedback is provided on each of the three areas, for approximately 15 minutes each, the supervisor proceeds to the final stage of the supervision session by checking in with the supervisee and how they experienced the supervision and counseling session went, asking if they had questions, reflecting on what they found to be helpful during the session. Explicitly acknowledging power dynamics, biases, and socialization within the supervisory relationship. During this time, the supervisor and supervisee can intentionally challenge and deconstruct potential factors and biases that may arise during their session while fostering an inclusive and affirming environment. For example, the supervisor might say, "When the client disclosed their challenges on campus related to their identities, what happened here (use video to show the exchange happening) for you as I noticed you froze to respond?"

9.  Lastly, the supervisor and supervisee conclude the session by collaboratively establishing realistic goals (e.g., SMART) for the upcoming client session.

## Supervisory Alliance and Relationship

Supervisors prioritize mutual empowerment, recognizing that both parties contribute to the growth and development of the other. Open communication where power dynamics are acknowledged based on roles and responsibilities should be maintained. Additionally, supervisors should promote critical consciousness, wherein supervisors and supervisees reflect on their biases, privileges, and socialization and their impact on the therapeutic and supervisory alliances.

## Legal and Ethical Considerations

Supervisors must ensure the use of HIPAA-compliant video conferencing platforms and session records, as well as informed consent documentation, and adhere to both federal and state laws and ethical standards. Specific attention is paid to whether counseling and supervision can occur across state lines and factors that may be discipline-and/or state-specific. As an anti-oppressive supervisory intervention, *Play, pause, and rewind* is transtheoretical and can be integrated across theory-based, developmental, process model, and second-generation supervisory frameworks (Bernard & Goodyear, 2019).

## Reflective Questions

1.  In what ways have I embraced a transformative learning approach, actively engaging in critical reflection and growth as a supervisor?
2.  How do I encourage and model critical consciousness among supervisees, facilitating reflection on biases, privileges, and socialization?
3.  In what specific ways have I actively worked towards addressing systemic inequalities and promoting social justice within the supervisory context?
4.  How have I prioritized mutual empowerment, and how have these efforts contributed to the growth and development of both myself and my supervisees?

# Wellness and Self-Care Through Acts of Compassion and Vigilance

*Katie Gamby, Melissa Luke, Jeff Moe, Dilani Perera, Harvey Charles Peters, and Laura Wood*

## CHAPTER FIVE INTERVENTIONS

### Intervention Title: Wellness and Self-Care Plan: A Practice of Accountability and Anti-Oppression

### Author(s) and Affiliation(s)

Harvey Charles Peters, Ph.D., NCC
Montclair State University

Melissa Luke, Ph.D., NCC, ACS, LMHC
Syracuse University

### Supervision Format and Modality

This anti-oppressive supervision intervention was developed for group supervision with a maximum group size of 12 members conducted virtually or in person. With minor modifications, this supervision intervention can be implemented in individual, triadic, or peer supervision. It can also be adapted to use with clients.

DOI: 10.4324/9781003470656-5

## Supervisee Development

While supervisees' exposure to wellness, self-care, anti-oppression, and trauma-informed care may vary, supervisors should tailor interventions to their development level, whether they are in a master's or doctoral practicum, internship, professional development, or post-graduate stage.

## Supervisory Goals and Learning Objectives

1. Discuss and review each supervisee's understanding of and experience with self-care and wellness.
2. Discuss and review each supervisee's understanding of and experience with burnout, compassion fatigue, vicarious trauma, secondary traumatic stress, and/or socio-cultural battle fatigue.
3. Facilitate the development of wellness and self-care plans grounded in accountability and anti-oppression.

## Time Required

Depending upon group size, level of discussion, and review of key concepts, the intervention can range from 45 to 75 minutes. Based on the allotted time, supervisors can make adjustments as they see necessary.

## Materials

Before using this intervention, which is adapted from the work of Myers and Sweeney (2004), the supervisor should review the materials and create their own wellness and self-care plan to understand the content and process. They can prepare handouts on wellness, self-care, and related issues (e.g., burnout, compassion fatigue) and use process questions to facilitate the intervention. Additionally, the supervisor should ensure the workspace accommodates both in-person and virtual participants, providing necessary writing tools and digital resources to support various needs and abilities.

## Instructions

1. To begin, the supervisor will facilitate a discussion on wellness and self-care. The supervisor should begin by exploring the supervisees' understanding and experiences with wellness and self-care. The supervisor can ask questions such as (a) What does self-care and

wellness mean to you personally and professionally? (b) What have you been taught about wellness and self-care? (c) Why is wellness and self-care important for mental health professionals? (d) How do oppression and discrimination (e.g., racism, genderism, heterosexism, ableism, transmisia, and nationalism) impact wellness and self-care? (e) What do wellness and self-care look like, and how can we practice without engaging in cultural appropriation and socio-cultural harm? The supervisor should create a brave space to address the influence of dominant socio-cultural values, privilege, and oppression (Gamby et al., 2021).

2. Next, the supervisor should provide a little background information and psychoeducation on key concepts from self-care and wellness (e.g., wellness, self-care, compassion fatigue, burnout). The supervisor might also introduce related concepts, including but not limited to vicarious trauma (i.e., emotional and psychological stress experienced by individuals who are exposed to the traumatic experiences of others, such as clients), secondary traumatic stress (i.e., emotional and psychological symptoms that develop in individuals who have experienced vicarious trauma), and socio-cultural battle fatigue (i.e., physical and emotional exhaustion experienced by individuals exposed to oppression, discrimination, interpersonal violence, and high-stress situations for prolonged periods; Mack, 2021). The supervisor can discuss the impact of oppressive structures and the importance of addressing them as mental health professionals.

3. After contextualizing and introducing key concepts, the supervisor can introduce the intervention. The Supervisors can assign key articles (see references) pre- or post-supervision to aid in their ongoing personal and professional development (Graham & Pehrsson, 2009).

4. Using a sheet of paper and writing utensils, dry-erase board and pen, or electronic documentation (e.g., Google Docs), each supervisee will be asked to develop a wellness and self-care plan that can be revisited and continually adapted throughout supervision. The coping plan will consist of six domains (i.e., essential self, creative self, coping self, social self, physical self, and anti-oppressive self). The first five domains are from Myers and Sweeney (2004), and the sixth is an adaption of the authors. The *essential self* is comprised of social-cultural identities, a sense of spirituality, and self-care. The *creative self* is comprised of a combination of personal characteristics and human experiences that inform one's social interactions, including thinking, emotions, control, humor, and work. The *coping self* is comprised of elements

that regulate one's responses to life events and provide a means for transcending their negative events, including realistic beliefs, stress management, self-worth, and leisure. The social self is comprised of friendship, love, and intimacy. The physical self is comprised of exercise and nutrition (Gibson et al., 2021; Myers & Sweeney, 2004). The *anti-oppressive self* is comprised of elements that support individuals in their development and liberation related to advocacy, civil disobedience, anti-oppression, and liberation.

5.    Following, each supervisee will develop a wellness and self-care plan, which will outline how they will intentionally and critically engage in various wellness and self-care practices throughout the identified period of time. Each supervisee should begin by defining what wellness and self-care mean to them.

6.    Next, the supervisee can identify and list some of their key personal, professional, and oppressive stressors. After they have independently identified key stressors, they can check in with their body (e.g., body scan) and identify how this stress shows up for them emotionally and psychologically. After this, each supervisee will list all six wellness and self-care domains (i.e., essential self, creative self, coping self, social self, physical self, and anti-oppressive self).

7.    Beneath each domain, they will list: (a) two to three specific, intentional actions they will enact, (b) identify how they will check in with themselves (e.g., emotionally and physiologically) to assess for stress, burnout, compassion fatigue, etc., (c) identify the frequency in which the intentional actions will be completed (e.g., once a day or weekly), (d) the general time the intentional action will be completed (e.g., morning, before bed), (e) identify positional barriers to their wellness and self-care plan and actions (e.g., intrapersonal, interpersonal, community, and societal), (f) identify needed supports and an accountability partner, whether that be within or external to the group, and (g) identify how they ensure they are not appropriating or harming minoritized communities.

8.    After each supervisee has completed their initial wellness and self-care plan, the supervisor can have the group reflect on their experience and invite participants to share their plan. Such questions can include: (a) What was this process like? (b) What did you learn about yourself? (c) How can we promote culturally attuned and critical practices of wellness and self-care individually and collectively? (d) What considerations or needs are present for this group?

9.    This discussion will allow other members to visualize and be introduced to various practices and considerations. It is essential that the supervisor frame this as a dynamic process. Each supervisee will need

to continuously revisit and revise their plan. Lastly, the group can close by reflecting upon how they can support and be accountable for their self-care, wellness, and roles and responsibilities as anti-oppressive professionals.

## Supervisory Alliance and Relationship

When discussing wellness, self-care, trauma, and anti-oppression in a group context, the supervisor should address social-cultural and anti-oppressive issues within the group process. Attending to intrapersonal, interpersonal, and group dynamics is crucial in addressing oppression and harmful rhetoric. Supervisors must also acknowledge and navigate power dynamics, social locations, and roles, ensuring a focus on disrupting domination and harm. By doing so, the supervisor creates a braver space for critically examining these constructs while addressing potential ruptures within the group.

## Legal and Ethical Considerations

When exploring issues related to vicarious trauma, secondary traumatic stress, and socio-cultural battle fatigue in clinical supervision (Mack, 2021), it is essential that supervisors balance their roles and responsibilities to integrate trauma-informed supervision and the distinction and boundary between supervision and counseling (Borders et al., 2022). Supervisors can consult the relevant competencies, professional standards, and professional ethics in their field to ascertain the separation of supervision and counseling.

## Reflective Questions

1. How can you practice wellness and self-care using a framework of accountability and liberation?
2. How can you use wellness and self-care to continue your growth and journey toward anti-oppression?
3. How can wellness and self-care informed by anti-oppression be used within your clinical praxis?

## Intervention Title: Compassion Building Toward Self and Other: IFS and Drama Therapy in Action

### Author(s) and Affiliation(s)

Laura Wood, PhD, LMHC, LPC, RDT/BCT
Lesley University

### Supervision Format and Modality

This intervention is designed for triadic or group supervision and can be used in live, in-person supervision.

### Supervisee Development

This intervention can be used within master's and doctoral practicum/internship, as well as with post-graduate pre/post licensed professionals. This intervention is designed for intermediate and advanced levels of supervision.

### Supervisory Goals and Learning Objectives

1. Supervisees will articulate at least one previously unvoiced aspect of their own internal responses to clients.
2. Supervisees will build insight in service of fostering self-compassion and increased clarity and connectedness in the clinical dynamic in service of growing as an anti-oppression clinician.
3. Using sculpting and dramatic reality, supervisees will demonstrate the ability to externalize and embody the internal parts of themselves that surface in clinical settings in service of separating out from the client.

### Time Required

This intervention will take 30–60 minutes, depending on the size of the group and the number of people working.

### Materials

Participants should be in clothing that you can move in, as well as have access to extra chairs.

## Intervention Instructions

This exercise, grounded in Internal Family Systems (IFS) and Drama Therapy, aims to help clinicians and trainees identify both obvious and hidden reactions within clinical interactions, emphasizing hands-on learning. At the heart of IFS is the 'Self,' which is defined by eight qualities: compassion, curiosity, connection, creativity, courage, clarity, calmness, and confidence. Schwartz argues that everyone is born with a 'Self,' and one thrives through positive engagements with others exhibiting similar 'Self energy' (Schwartz & Sweezy, 2019; Wood, 2015).

Challenges occur when individuals face emotionally or physically distressing situations. These situations can result in the creation of 'exiled' parts that carry this emotional weight. To ensure exiled parts never have to feel the pain of the past again, people form protective strategies, namely 'managers' for everyday protection and 'firefighters' for emergency protection. In the IFS model, all parts are welcome, and all parts are understood as having important functions (Schwartz & Sweezy, 2019). IFS therapy's main goal is to nurture relationships between the 'Self' and the parts (managers, firefighters, and exiles), encouraging healing and integration.

In the context of diversity, equity, and anti-oppression, Schwartz's model challenges practitioners to examine the protective parts that may have formed due to societal messages or personal experiences concerning identities different from our own. The model advocates for an approach of curiosity and compassion towards these protective parts, encouraging a deeper understanding of the beliefs and biases they may carry in service of meeting our clients from a place of Self, rather than bias and enhancing solidarity through highlighting the value of difference (Schwartz, 2016).

Complementing IFS, Drama Therapy utilizes the dynamic and transformative power of drama and theatre processes to facilitate mental, emotional, behavioral, or psychological change. Core processes in Drama Therapy include embodiment, play, dramatic reality, role-playing, storytelling, metaphor creation, and the use of aesthetic distance. These processes are instrumental in creating a safe yet evocative space for exploration and change (Johnson & Emunah, 2009).

This supervision intervention is both reflective and interactive and combines an IFS lens with drama therapy tools. To implement, the supervisor does the following:

1. Selects a supervisee and asks them to recall a specific moment where they felt stuck or had a reactive response to a client's behavior, a

particular clinical interaction, an aspect of the client's intersecting identities, or explore a culturally dominant narrative of one's feelings.

2. Asks the supervisee to verbally or non-verbally identify and share this scenario with the supervisor and group.

3. Supports the supervisee in asking a peer supervisee to 'play' the role of the client. The supervisee chooses a line that encapsulates the essence of the moment and a corresponding physical posture or 'sculpt' that represents their perception of the client in that instance. For example, if the supervisee is working with a client who expressed feeling 'resentful of being a mother,' the chosen peer supervisee would embody this sentiment through a physical posture that the supervisee determined to represent this emotion (a slumped over, annoyed-looking posture, for example) and would utter the line that encapsulates the client's sentiment "I'm so sick of being a mother, this isn't the life I wanted."

4. Facilitates the supervisee's observation of the enacted scenario, paying close attention to their emotional responses and encourages the supervisee to identify the most prominent emotion or 'part' that surfaces during this observation. For instance, if the supervisee identifies a feeling of disgust, the supervisor may suggest they engage another group member to embody this specific emotion. This embodiment involves adopting a physical posture (or 'sculpt') that represents the feeling of disgust and vocalizing a line that encapsulates this emotion. For example, the supervisee has the 'disgusting' part sculpted by wrinkling its nose and pulling its body away in relationship to the client and provides a line such as: "I feel disgusted by this mother; some people are so desperate for children, and here she is being ungrateful." By exploring the root of this disgust in relation to identity and oppression, the supervisee can uncover underlying biases and societal constructs that shape their emotional responses, fostering a deeper understanding of how personal and systemic prejudices influence their clinical practice.

5. Invites the supervision triad/group collectively to examine both the sculpt of the client and the embodiment of the supervisee's emotional response to try to foster feelings of curiosity or compassion towards the supervisee's own emotional part (in this example, their disgust). The supervisor helps the supervisee engage with their reaction with curiosity and supports them to understand the underlying reasons for this response. The supervisor can also encourage the triad/group to assist the supervisee by asking questions from a place of Self. For example: "I'm curious how your experience of disgust might be influenced by

personal encounters with identity and oppression?" Other supervisees should not interpret, guess, or offer leading questions.

6.  Asks the person embodying the part to 'shake off' this role and sit down and then invites the supervisee to sit across from the person enacting their client and reassess their feelings. If the supervisee can now relate to the client with one of the 'C' words from the IFS model, move on to step 7. If, however, the supervisee experiences a different emotion towards the client, the exercise is repeated, this time focusing on this new emotion.

7.  Instructs the supervisee to create a new 'sculpt' of the relationship between the supervisee and client that represents how they wish to engage in their next session with the client. The supervisor encourages the supervisee to incorporate the metaphor into a plan or approach. This step enables the supervisees to translate their insights and emotional shifts into a concrete plan of action and encourages them to consciously integrate tangible anti-oppressive and identity-affirming strategies.

8.  Engages everyone in the triad/group in a physical activity to 'shake out' their bodies, symbolically returning to their own selves and concluding the exercise.

## Supervisory Alliance and Relationship

This exercise enhances supervisees' understanding of internal dynamics and biases, offering tools for improved anti-oppressive clinical practice. It's especially valuable for addressing 'parts' related to clients with diverse identities, requiring vulnerability and trust. Supervisors must model risk-taking and embody Self energy, with a focus on embodied techniques for success. Drama Therapy can rapidly evoke emotions; hence, preparing supervisees and ensuring cultural sensitivity without stereotypes is essential for a respectful and effective process.

## Legal and Ethical Considerations

As is the case with all experiential learning, supervisors should attend to informed consent and consider the scope of practice with embodied work. Supervisors should have some familiarity with and practice in embodied or chair-type work or should seek supervision from someone who has that training before trying this intervention for the first time.

## Reflective Questions

1. What did you learn about yourself in supervision today (e.g., through the sculpting)?
2. Describe how you will transfer what you witnessed today into future triadic/group supervision.
3. How can identity, culture, and privilege promote and hinder compassion, connectedness, and curiosity?

## Intervention Title: Uncovering the Depths: Enhancing Compassion and Vigilance Through Guided Imagery

## Author(s) Name, Credentials, and Affiliation(s)

Katie Gamby, PhD, LPCC-S
The Wellife, LLC

## Supervision Format and Modality

This supervisory intervention can be completed in individual, triadic, or group supervision and can be experienced in person or virtually.

## Supervisee Development

Supervisors should tailor this intervention to fit the supervisee's developmental stage. For beginners, some pre-reading on wellness, self-care, anti-oppression, bias, intersectionality, or other themes that show up in the guided imagery can be helpful. This is an intermediate exercise, but supervisors can adjust prompts for a higher intervention level.

## Supervisory Goals and Learning Objectives

After the intervention, supervisees will be able to:

1.  Define guided imagery, grounding, embodiment, self-care, and wellness.
2.  Explain how guided imagery deepens awareness, specifically toward marginalized groups.
3.  Evaluate their self-care and wellness strategies to increase vigilance toward anti-oppressive practices.

## Time Required

The supervisory intervention takes 30–45 minutes, followed by at least 15 minutes of processing. Discussion time depends on group size, requiring more time for larger groups.

## Materials

Supervisors should observe their own physical and mental responses while experiencing the intervention themselves, seeking support if needed before guiding others. Journaling during and after the guided imagery is recommended. Paper and pens, computers, or other technological devices can be used to capture information.

## Intervention Instructions

1.  Before delving into the guided imagery, supervisors should discuss the impact of oppression on wellness practices (see Gamby et al., 2021) and the vigilance it takes to be anti-oppressive. Next, the supervisor should facilitate conversations about the purposes of guided imagery (Owen, 2010) and share the reasons for incorporating this guided imagery in supervision, such as opening the mind to new and novel ideas or experiences (Utay & Miller, 2006).

2.  The guided imagery is trauma-informed, but it might still evoke challenging content. Since supervisees may use guided imagery with clients, it is crucial for the supervisor to discuss how guided imagery can bring up unprocessed material and help supervisees learn grounding and anchoring techniques before proceeding (Van Der Winjgaart, 2021).

3.  The supervisor shares the following guided imagery, pausing for 15–20 seconds when seeing an ellipsis (. . .):

    a.  Take a moment to notice your body. Maybe you notice your back up against the chair you are sitting in, or your feet planted firmly on the floor . . . now, close your eyes or keep them open and move your gaze to something still . . . turn your attention to your breath and notice it. If you notice any judgment, allow your breath to release the judgment with the next exhale . . . perhaps you start to deepen your breath if that feels good, or you continue to notice your breath as is . . .

    b.  I invite you now to remember a recent time when you felt defensive or felt the need to protect yourself in your physical body. This may have been a time when you felt particularly protective of your own identities, culture, values, or beliefs. The invitation is to bring up a memory that is recent and mild, something that isn't too far in the past or completely unprocessed . . . (30-second pause).

    c.  Once you have that memory in mind, note the physical sensations you felt in your body . . .

    d.  Maybe you felt nauseous, muscle tension, or increased heart rate . . . maybe you noticed your face flushing, your hands getting clammy, or trembling. Whatever you experienced, notice that now . . .

e.  Now notice what your body wanted to do in this experience. Perhaps you wanted to or decided to defend yourself by talking back . . . perhaps your tone became elevated, or your voice increased in volume . . . perhaps you numbed out or disassociated . . . perhaps you blamed others without taking responsibility, or something else. Become aware of your go-to behaviors or the urges you had in this particular situation . . .

f.  As best you can, notice who you were engaging with . . . what was going on in the image that caused this kind of reaction?

g.  Now, take a few breaths, and with each exhalation, allow yourself to move from the past situation back to the present moment. To do this, you might touch your fingers together or slowly tap on your knees or thighs.

h.  Notice your body now . . . with each breath, allow yourself to come back to the present moment and let the past image get fuzzy as it moves to the background and your body in this present moment moves to the foreground.

i.  Now, notice any body reactions, specifically body reactions you may just have had in the last image toward the following groups. You may have a body reaction or an image, an emotion, or something else. These might be positive or negative. After each group, I will give you about 30 seconds to notice what comes up in your physical body and about 30 seconds to jot down any reactions you had. You will have time to process it in more detail later.

   i.  Supervisor: use a list of intersections to invite participants to explore and uncover body responses and reactions to various groups and determine these ahead of time. For example, Asian women, disabled people, gay men, cisgender White men, etc. After each group is read, invite breath before moving on to the next group.

j.  Now, take a breath, remembering what you need for this experience.

k.  One more breath, becoming present in this moment, noticing your feet on the floor or your back up against the chair.

l.  Last breath, waking up your body in the way that feels best, perhaps fluttering your eyes open, wiggling your fingers or toes, or something else.

m.  Now, take 15 minutes to journal, type, or process the experience. The following questions might help:

   i.  How did your body feel when you were defensive or disgusted? What, if anything, surprised you about this? How might knowing this information be helpful when working with clients?

ii.    What physical reactions did you notice toward certain groups? Were you already aware of this? If so, how do you usually handle these reactions? Are there any additional things you want to add to increase your awareness? If you were unaware, how do you plan to address such reactions in the future to promote an anti-oppressive worldview?

iii.   How can you notice and manage these bodily reactions with clients? How might your supervisor assist you in navigating these sensations, emotions, and experiences?

iv.    What other self-care or wellness practices can you adopt without culturally appropriating or causing cultural harm (Gamby et al., 2021)?

n.    Supervisors should allow supervisees time to verbally process the experience after the journal exercise, paying attention to exploring how the guided imagery experience can be a jumping-off point for supervisees to be aware of their internal biases and use this information to encourage vigilance toward anti-oppressive commitments. For example, the supervisor may query/suggest cultural responsivity training, community involvement, reading and education, collaborative projects, etc. Elicit ideas from the supervisee(s) in the discussion to allow for idea generation as well.

## Supervisory Alliance and Relationship

Discussions on anti-oppression can lack focus on embodiment (i.e., somatic or body-centered) levels, which may cause confusion and distress for students experiencing unexpected bodily responses. As supervisees are in different developmental stages (Bernard & Goodyear, 2019) regarding anti-oppression, some may feel shame, disgust, or guilt about their body reactions. The supervisor should help supervisees distinguish between intentional harm and a willingness to address internal biases. Encouraging sharing while challenging intentionally harmful behaviors is essential.

## Legal and Ethical Considerations

This exercise may evoke strong feelings towards oneself and others. It is vital to recognize the limits of supervision and suggest therapy or specialized groups if the material requires deeper exploration (Bernard & Goodyear,

2019). As part of informed consent, supervisors should acknowledge these possibilities beforehand and ensure they have available resources to share with supervisees as they are needed or requested.

## Reflective Questions

1. How did this guided imagery intervention decrease anti-oppression, and what might facilitate this further?
2. How does this intervention assist the exploration of feelings, body sensations, and images toward oppressed groups?
3. How did this guided imagery intervention boost compassion and self-awareness?

### Intervention Title: Reclaiming Wellness: Centering Intersectional Identities and Coping in Self-Care

### Author(s) and Affiliation(s)

Jeff Moe, Ph.D., LPC, NCC, CCMHC
Old Dominion University

Dilani Perera, Ph.D., LPCC-S, LICDC-S, NCC, MAC, BC-TMH
Fairfield University

### Supervision Format and Modality

This wellness activity is best suited for individual or triadic supervision, as Principle 4 involves re-appropriating and re-contextualizing concepts that have been misappropriated by exploitive systems. This activity could be adapted for application with clients by supervisees who have engaged in critical conversations and reflections on wellness.

### Supervisee Development

Based on the principle of critical reflexivity, supervisors can adapt the reclaiming wellness intervention for master's and doctoral students as well as pre- and post-licensed counselors. When working on supervisee developmental and remediation plans, it will be helpful to discuss wellness as a component of the plan to facilitate healthy coping and development. The reclaiming wellness intervention is best suited for intermediate or advanced levels but can be calibrated to meet introductory supervisory needs as well.

### Supervisory Goals and Learning Objectives

*Supervisees Will*

1. Review the Indivisible Self Model of holistic wellness (Myers & Sweeney, 2008) with an emphasis on the Essential Self and Coping Self domains.
2. Critically evaluate at least one wellness concept based on an intersecting identities framework, identifying at least two items for discussion (Moe et al., 2023).
3. Foster evaluation of authentic wellness and identify two self-care practices based on the relational-cultural theory principle of affirming and enhancing connection (Hammer et al., 2021).

4.  Identify at least two social and systemic barriers to wellness and self-care informed by experiences of marginalization, as well as strategies for personal and group advocacy to overcome barriers (Perera-Diltz & Moe, 2020).

## Time Required

This activity requires approximately 20 minutes for each of the two supervisory sessions and five to ten minutes for future sessions as needed.

## Materials

Supervisors should be familiar with the Indivisible Self Model of Holistic Wellness (IS-WEL) and the 5 Good Things from relational-cultural theory (RCT). We recommend using a graphic handout to summarize both concepts for supervisees, which can continue to serve as a reminder of how to integrate IS-WEL and RCT concepts. Instructions for the reclaiming wellness activity should be shared with supervisees, including the process and reflection questions that should guide the critique of wellness concepts and the identification of meaningful, connection-enhancing wellness activities.

## Intervention Instructions

1.  **Orient:** First, discuss feminist and RCT principles that emphasize mutuality and power-with vs. hierarchy and power-over dynamics. Then, invite supervisees to reflect on the power dynamics and oppressive systems present in the supervisory relationship, including what could be improved and how power can be shared mutually. Assessing supervisee comfort level, inviting constructive feedback from supervisors. Invite shared decision-making to emphasize collaboration. Here, supervisors also attend to their own personal biases and possible supervisory counter-transference with supervisees. For instance, it is helpful to identify, own, and change your own defensive behaviors so this exercise can be fruitful.
2.  **Broach:** Introduce the subject of social identities and oppression employing a trauma-informed approach, recognizing that minoritized supervisees may have encountered bullying, subjugation, and other traumatic events linked to their intersectional identities. Engage in listening practices with empathy (not sympathy) and without interruption to allow the supervisee to share their traumatic and unpleasant experiences. Use appropriate self-disclosure about aspects of personal

identity associated with privilege, marginalization, and complicated experiences. For example, briefly share an instance where you have experienced bullying or microaggressions and how it affected you.

3.  **Evaluate:** Using a strength-based, anti-oppressive perspective, assess the supervisee's familiarity with wellness and self-care. Self-disclose as appropriate, especially struggles to engage in wellness as a professional counselor to humanize the experience. Provide an overview of the principles of holism and the IS-WEL model, including Myers and Sweeney's (2008) 4-step process for applying wellness (assessment, goal setting, intervention, and evaluation).

4.  **Reflect and Recontextualize:** Prompt critical reflection on the 5 IS-WEL domains and intersecting dimensions of personal identity. Re-contextualize attempts to engage in wellness practices by discussing how being members of a minoritized group can impact wellness. Invite supervisees to share how marginalization has impacted their engagement with wellness. Facilitate supervisees' identification of barriers to wellness and self-care, such as locating safe places to exercise, experiencing discrimination in the healthcare system, and the emphasis on individualism vs. collectivism prevalent in certain spaces. Prompt supervisees to reflect on how wellness relates to their salient and intersecting sources of personal identity and oppressive systems. Prompt supervisees to consider what groups seem most associated with a given wellness activity or space and whether that group represents a dominant culture or marginalized culture.

5.  **Center and Integrate**: Utilize centering techniques such as mindful breathing or body scanning to address areas of wellness that are impacted by minoritized intersectional identities. Facilitate the supervisee to focus on the here and now, removing the power of the outside world that does not accept the intersectional identities and even invalidate their experience. Be cognizant of microaggressions, oppressive ideology, and disrespectful expressions or actions on the part of the supervisor, and be intentional in word and action choices. For instance, ask the supervisee to focus on their current needs and reclaim wellness, compartmentalizing the oppression that limits the supervisee's wellness.

6.  **Reclaim and Discuss:** Invite consideration of the 5 Good Things from RCT: zest, clarity, worth, productivity, and a desire for more connection. Ask supervisees to consider: 1) if an activity promotes a sense of zest or fun, 2) comes with clarity about the meaning or worth of the activity, 3) enhances feelings of self-worth, 4) helps supervisees be more productive both at work and other areas of life, and

5) fosters a desire to see and spend time with other people. As each of the 5 Good Things is explored, ask supervisees to consider how their intersecting identities affect experiences in each domain. For example, ask whether their gender, ethno-racial, or sexual identity impacts their ability to experience fun or zest when engaging in a particular wellness behavior such as exercise. Facilitate identification of wellness-promoting activities that account for multiple minority stress factors, such as overcoming barriers to wellness. Reframe engagement in newly identified activities as reclaiming wellness.

7. **Connect and Establish:** Close with extended reflection on the activity, encouraging the enactment of the supervisee's wellness plan. Focus on the processes within the reclaiming wellness intervention, such as what was difficult or confusing, how power shifted and was engaged, etc. Together, determine ways to extend the activity to further mobilize wellness from an anti-oppressive lens with clients, colleagues, and supervisee and supervisor personal lives, also should be included.

8. **Revisit:** In the future, revisit the wellness plan and its effectiveness for supervisee wellness as necessary.

## Supervisory Alliance and Relationship

Relationships, whether they are between counselor-client or supervisor-supervisee, are transformative tools for personal and professional development. Addressing and exploring identity, power dynamics, oppression, and collaboration within these relationships is essential to building an environment of bravery, empathy, humility, attunement, and non-defensiveness. Collectively, these dispositions and practices support relationships that support authenticity, wellness, and anti-oppression.

## Legal and Ethical Considerations

Legal statutes protect the consumer, in this case, the supervisee. Therefore, supervisor competence in providing anti-oppressive and culturally attuned supervision that does not harm or discriminate against the supervisee is necessary. Similarly, mental health provider self-care and non-impairment are mandated for effective client service. Barriers to wellness that stem from social factors related to ethnicity/race, sexual and gender identities, among others, cannot be changed by the individual. Therefore, it is both ethical and legal for wellness to be taught, monitored, and supported by supervisors to provide appropriate and effective care to clients.

## Reflective Questions

1. When should the wellness of a supervisee/client be addressed in supervision?

2. How do you, as a counselor/supervisor, address your own biases? Do you give permission for your supervisee/client to challenge those biases, such as calling out unintentional micro-aggressions and disrespectful expressions or actions?

3. What intersectional identities do you find uncomfortable or less knowledgeable to address related to wellness with your supervisee/client?

4. What types of supervisees/clients make you uncomfortable, and how does that impact your engagement in wellness discussions with the supervisee?

5. How do you repair relationship breaches with a supervisee/client as you work to deepen their wellness?

## Intervention Title: Radical Healing and Hope Within Clinical Supervision

## Author(s) and Affiliation(s)

Harvey Charles Peters, Ph.D., NCC
Montclair State University

Melissa Luke, Ph.D., NCC, ACS, LMHC
Syracuse University

## Supervision Format and Modality

This anti-oppressive supervision intervention was developed for individual supervision being conducted virtually or in person. With minor modifications, this supervision intervention can be implemented through triadic, peer, or group supervision. It can also be adapted to use with clients.

## Supervisee Development

While supervisees' exposure to wellness, self-care, anti-oppression, and radical healing may vary, supervisors should tailor interventions to their development level, whether they are in a master's or doctoral practicum, internship, professional development, or post-graduate stage.

## Supervisory Goals and Learning Objectives

*Supervisee's Will*

1. Summarize key concepts from readings on radical healing and radical hope.
2. Explain the components of radical healing, including their applicability to themselves and clients.
3. Reflect on their experiences of oppression, radical healing, and radical hope and connect them to their clinical practice.
4. Create a personalized model and identify actions to promote radical healing and hope.

## Time Required

The intervention initially requires 60 minutes, with supervisors adjusting the necessary time based on the supervisee. Supervisors should allocate additional time across supervision sessions.

## Materials

Before using this intervention, which is adapted from the work of French et al. (2020), the supervisor should review the materials and develop their own model of radical healing and hope. The supervisor can ensure access to articles, prepare handouts, and prepare materials to help guide the discussion and development of a radical healing model (e.g., pencils, paper, tablet, etc.).

## Intervention Instructions

1. To begin, the supervisor should familiarize themselves with the interdisciplinary scholarship on radical healing and radical hope (see French et al., 2020; Mosley et al., 2020, 2021).
2. Following the review, the supervisor should engage with the model, scholarship, and be able to have a working understanding of the concepts, constructs, model, and application in counseling and supervision.
3. Next, the supervisor will have the supervisee read French et al. (2020) prior to the start of supervision.
4. The supervisor will provide a brief overview of the psychological framework of radical healing that integrates liberation psychology, Intersectionality theory, Black psychology, and ethnopolitical psychology. Although not required, a brief handout may be of use to the supervisor and supervisee. Additionally, based on the writings of French et al. (2020) and Mosley et al. (2020), the supervisor can operationalize radical healing as navigating the space between resisting oppression and striving for hope, freedom, and wellness. It requires individuals to engage and be present with the dialectic tension by acknowledging current realities while envisioning and committing to possibilities for change. By balancing the despair of oppression with hope for a better future, people can avoid the pitfalls of disempowerment and detachment. This process emphasizes the importance of recognizing systemic injustices and actively pursuing wellness and liberation. Engaging in this continual dialectical process can ultimately foster healing, enabling individuals and communities to cultivate

resilience and agency amid adversity and oppression (French et al., 2020; Mosley et al., 2020).

5.  After this, the supervisor and supervisee can begin by discussing the contexts of racism and White supremacy in relation to racial, historical, and intergenerational trauma. Some questions include: (a) How have your personal experiences or observations shaped your understanding of racial trauma and oppression in your personal and professional environments? (b) In what ways do you see the impact of historical trauma and oppression manifesting in the lives of individuals from marginalized communities today? (c) How do you see racial trauma and oppression impacting people's health, wellness, and liberation? (d) What role do racial trauma and oppression play in the social determinants of mental health?

6.  The follow up the previous component is to include other marginalized social locations, whether they be individual or multiplistic in nature, and discuss the role and impact of oppressive, historical, and intergenerational trauma on the health, wellness, and hope of these marginalized communities. The supervisor can adapt the aforementioned question to apply to these communities.

7.  Next, the supervisor and supervisee review and discuss each competent of the psychology of radical healing model. The model (see French et al., 2020) includes: (a) critical consciousness (i.e., a person's ability to critically and consciously examine, reflect, and act within their privileged to marginalized socio-cultural-political environments), (b) cultural authenticity and self-knowledge (i.e., an evolving self-definition and socio-cultural authenticity not defined by or centering oppressive ontology and epistemology), (c) radical hope (i.e., developing and restoring wholeness despite historical and persistent experiences of oppression that negatively affect individuals from marginalized communities, such as race, ethnicity, and other socio-cultural identities), (d) emotional and social support (i.e., power of and the necessity for connection, community, belonging, and balance, and (e) strength and resistance (i.e., cultivating joy and well-being while actively resisting systemic oppression and trauma by drawing on collective experiences and the potential for transformative change). In addition, they are informed by the dialectic tension between interlocking systems of oppression and hate and envisioning justice and liberation.

8.  The next aspect of this intervention is to have a discussion to further explore the supervisee's experiences of and desires to promote their radical healing and hope within the supervisory and clinical contexts. Some guiding prompts include: (a) How do you see or experience the difference between surviving and coping with the symptoms of

oppressive and hate-based trauma and healing? (b) How can you shift toward radical healing and hope in your personal and professional practice? (c) In what ways can you actively challenge the oppressive systems that contribute to oppressive trauma that impact your health, wellness, and sense of belonging and authenticity? What might radical healing and hope look like in terms of anti-oppressive self-care and wellness?

9. After the review and discussion, the supervisory dyad should work towards developing a model using each component of the previously referenced model to develop the supervisee's model for radical healing and hope. The supervisor and supervisee should collaboratively begin working on this model to aid the supervisee in doing this work. The supervisor can encourage, empower, and be in community with the supervisee. If the supervisee needs more time, it can be completed and brought to the subsequent supervision session.

10. Next, the supervisor should process and reflect on the supervisee's emotional, cognitive, behavioral, relational, and systemic experiences.

11. Last, the supervisor and supervisee should explore and discuss the applicability of this within the supervisee's clinical work with marginalized communities, especially people of the global majority (e.g., Black, Indigenous, and People of Color). Some guiding questions include: (a) How can you integrate the concept of collective resistance into your work with clients? (b) How can you promote cultural authenticity and self-knowledge in your therapeutic relationships with clients? (c) How can you shift your focus from merely helping clients cope with symptoms of oppressive trauma to fostering their capacity for healing and resistance?

## Supervisory Alliance and Relationship

When discussing radical healing, radical hope, and anti-oppression, the supervisor should address social-cultural and anti-oppressive issues within the supervisory relationship. In addition, when discussing or facilitating personal and professional reflection related to anti-oppression, the supervisor should not decenter racial, ethnic, and other marginalized community knowledge, identity, experiences, or praxis or recenter dominant and oppressive perspectives of radical healing and hope or anti-oppression.

## Legal and Ethical Considerations

Before engaging in such work, the supervisor must ensure informed consent, maintain confidentiality, and be aware of potential vicarious trauma among supervisees. They should create a brave, trauma-informed environment that encourages open dialogue about racial trauma and oppression while adhering to ethical guidelines. Additionally, supervisors must promote cultural humility and respect supervisee boundaries without discussing their experiences of racism and interlocking systems of oppression, especially if the supervisor holds predominantly dominant social locations.

## Reflective Questions

1. What ways can you actively challenge the oppressive systems that contribute to oppressive and racial trauma in your clinical practice and within the broader community?
2. How can you navigate the tension between recognizing systemic oppression and fostering hope for healing in your clients?
3. How can we prioritize and center radical healing and hope within sessions to promote our health, wellness, and self-care?

CHAPTER 6

# Co-Constructing a Brave Space Through Relationships and Community

*Jane E. Atieno Okech, Mina Attia,
Kenya G. Bledsoe, Bagmi Das,
Mary DeRaedt, Melissa Luke,
Harvey Charles Peters, Deborah Rubel,
and Jaimie Stickl Haugen*

## CHAPTER 6 INTERVENTIONS

### Intervention Title: Props in the Brave Space Box

### Author(s) and Affiliation(s)

Melissa Luke, Ph.D., NCC, ACS, LMHC
Syracuse University

Harvey Charles Peters, Ph.D., NCC
Montclair State University

### Supervision Format and Modality

This supervision intervention was developed for use within in-person group supervision with 6–12 supervisees. The intervention could be adapted for individual and/or triadic supervision as well.

DOI: 10.4324/9781003470656-6

## Supervisee Development

This supervision intervention can be used across all levels of supervisee development, and it is particularly beneficial in introducing the concepts of multiple perspectives, cultural empathy, and brave spaces.

## Supervisory Goals and Learning Objectives

1. Supervisees will actively engage in the co-construction of a brave space.
2. Supervisees will explore and demonstrate empathy for multiple perspectives as related to client and supervisee experiences.
3. Supervisees will increase their skills to explore and equitably respond to the needs of others across counseling and supervisory relationships (i.e., clients, peer supervisees).
4. Supervisees will examine and acknowledge their impact in counseling and supervision.
5. Supervisees will expand their ability to foster difficult dialogues, courage, and compassion within counseling and supervision.

## Time Required

This intervention is designed for a 60 to 75-minute supervisory session.

## Materials

The supervisor prepares the brave space box with at least 30–40 objects that can be used as props, including props that evoke or represent facilitative and detracting brave space opportunities and processes. Luke (2008a) suggested including small toys, sand tray figures, and household objects such as "keys, large paperclip, bottle cap, human figures, pinecone, credit card, play dishes, bar of soap, roll of masking tape, matchbox car, wrench, floppy disc, bird nest, envelope, plastic animals, seashells, and eraser" (p. 111).

## Intervention Instructions

The communication within supervision has largely taken place through verbal means (Mullen et al., 2007); however, there has been increased recognition of the role of experiential techniques and symbolic expression within supervision (Luke, 2008a). Before the intervention begins, the supervisor introduces the role of a brave space in anti-oppressive supervision, identifies the goals of Props in the Brave Space Box, and reviews the concepts of experiential interventions, symbolic communication, and physical metaphor.

1.  The supervisor illustrates how the props will help the supervisees communicate their unique needs and perspectives as well as co-construct group expectations and norms for a brave space. To do so, the supervisor displays two objects (.i.e., light bulb, lock), and models that the light bulb can convey that supervisees will contribute their ideas and authentic reactions throughout the intervention, and the lock could symbolize supervisees appropriately guarding the information that is shared in supervision.

2.  The supervisor displays the Brave Space Box and places the props on a table or the floor in the middle of the room, allowing the supervisees to see and have good access to them.

3.  The supervisor differentiates a brave space from a safe space and invites supervisees to explore how so. The supervisor indicates that a brave space looks and feels differently to people and that to begin, each member of the supervisory group will select a prop to represent their perspective about what constitutes a brave space. During this time, the supervisor provides process observations such as "You knew exactly what you wanted," "Sometimes it's hard to find just the right thing," "You seem disappointed that the one you wanted was already selected," or "Maybe it's familiar to you to observe first before you engage."

4.  Once the supervisees have each selected an object, the supervisor facilitates the supervisees in sharing what they selected, what it represents about a brave space, and how this might operate in group supervision. Throughout this, the supervisor identifies opportunities to follow up with supervisees about their experiences and expectations for the benefits and challenges with difficult dialogues, as well as how the group can engage in empathy, courage, and compassion for others' experiences.

5.  The supervisor uses basic group work skills to draw out and block supervisees as appropriate, to link supervisees to one another through content and process, and to make "clear points of divergent opinion" (Goodrich & Luke, 2016, p. 43) across supervisees.

6.  The supervisor asks the supervisees to select another prop from those remaining that will represent their in-the-moment reaction to understanding the multiple differing perspectives and needs within the supervision group, specifically with respect to how they as a supervisee may respond to the potential intra-and inter-personal difficulties

that can be associated (e.g., embarrassment, vulnerability, judgment, invalidation, conflict, microaggression).

7. The supervisor invites the supervisees to share their props and what they represent, encouraging supervisees to explore their prior and current life experiences that inform their perspective and help them examine how this may have an impact on others in the supervision group. For example, the supervisor may say, "What from your past informs what's happening now," "Tell us more about the connection between this and an anti-oppressive brave space," or "How could your perspective impact others in this supervision group?"

8. The supervisor identifies opportunities to respond to the group as a whole and can use process observation and feedback about the group dynamics, looking for opportunities to validate, provide a psychoeducational context, and utilize reframing when appropriate. For example, the supervisor could note, "It's common for people to have received overt and covert messages about what is appropriate or acceptable to share in a group. I wonder how this supervision group will take that up in a brave space?" or "I'm noticing that many of you are looking to me as you speak. This makes sense to me on the one hand, as I am the supervisor facilitating the intervention, and at the same time, I invite you to consider how this could interfere with your learning needs in terms of the brave space we are co-constructing" or "Although we have a wide range of experiences and perspectives in this room and a variety of props in our brave space box, it seems the group remains undecided about if or how it will engage difficult dialogues."

9. The supervisor may choose to engage supervisees in brainstorming varied strategies to foster difficult dialogues, courageously address relational ruptures, and compassionately be accountable for impacting others and the supervisory working alliance. To do so, the supervisor can ask supervisees to swap their previously selected props with two other supervisees in the supervision group and then select one of these props or another that has not yet been used (still in the middle of the room) to represent their response.

10. As the supervisor solicits supervisees' input, they will continue to shift focus between the content of the responses and the intra-and inter-personal processes taking place in the group. The supervisor can also encourage supervisees to deepen their reflection and begin to transfer their supervisory experiences to counseling. For example, the supervisor could note, "Thank you for sharing. How might we recognize this is happening at the moment," "This is helpful to understand. What could interfere with this happening and what might assist," "When

you think about your experiences, what might you need from the group to reach your brave space goals," or "How do you think what you've identified could similarly apply to your counseling work?"

11. The supervisor asks the supervisees if there is anything additional they wish to add to the brave space box that has not yet been addressed and what type of prop would symbolize this, inviting the other supervisees to improvise using the remaining props. This becomes an opportunity for the supervisor to highlight and normalize not only differing perspectives but also alternative ways of thinking. The supervisor then asks the supervisees to place all of the props used in the supervision session in one place and can take a photo of the Props in Brave Space Box that can be used in the future.

## Supervisory Alliance and Relationship

Although originally developed as a group counseling intervention to assist in establishing ground rules and expectations (Luke, 2008b), Goodrich and Luke (2016) adapted the Props in a Box intervention to focus on the working alliance, noting the impact of working alliance on both group counseling process and outcome. Extending Baltrinic and Luke's (2022) conceptualization of multidimensional empathy (e.g., cultural, cognitive, affective, behavioral), the supervisor can use this intervention to model cultural empathy and strengthen the working alliance by affirming supervisees' identities, social locations, and cultural experiences. Supervisors address instances of mis-attunement, wherein the supervisor or peer supervisees may have overlooked opportunities for cultural empathy and/ or mistook or mis-identified the cultural experiences of a supervisee. Failing to redress such instances risks a rupture in the supervisory relationship and damage to the ongoing working alliance.

## Legal and Ethical Considerations

The supervisor intentionally determines the amount of structure to impose within this Props in the Brave Space Box intervention, continually assessing the individual supervisees and the group as a whole's needs, experiences, and development, as well the intra, inter, and systemic dynamics that are processed. The supervisor should also ensure that their professional disclosure statement, syllabi, and/or supervisory contract include information about the use of experiential and symbolic supervisory interventions and how these relate to the learning within supervision (Goodyear, 2014).

## Reflective Questions

1.  What stood out to you about your experience during this intervention, and what did you notice happening in the group?
2.  Where did you observe yourself impacting the group?
3.  When did you feel most accountable to someone else in the group?
4.  How would you have ranked the bravery in this space at the start of supervision today compared to right now, at the end?
5.  How can you envision using something you learned today with your future clients?

### Intervention Title: Using Anonymous Polling to Co-Construct Brave Spaces in Anti-Oppressive Online Group Supervision

### Author(s) and Affiliation(s)

Deborah Rubel, PhD
Oregon State University

Jane E. Atieno Okech, PhD
University of Vermont

### Supervision Format and Modality

This supervision intervention is designed for online supervision groups with 6–8 supervisees and can also be adapted for in-person supervision.

### Supervisee Development

This intervention is designed primarily for master's students (Practicum/ Internship) but can be adapted for all supervisee developmental levels, including doctoral and pre-licensure groups.

### Supervisory Goals and Learning Objectives

After the use of this intervention, the group and supervisees may:

1. Feel safer and be more willing to take risks related to engaging in anti-oppressive processes and learning.
2. Be better at assessing their comfort with disclosing challenging experiences and feedback related to anti-oppressive processes.
3. Gain more awareness of others' experiences in learning anti-oppressive processes and practices.
4. Identify at least two personal and systemic factors influencing brave space creation in relationships, groups, and communities.

### Time Required

This intervention is designed to be used as needed during a 90-minute group supervision session and may take from 5–20 minutes.

## Materials

For this intervention, the required resources are essential technology (i.e., computers, phones, other handheld devices), access to the internet, and supervisor proficiency with online polls.

Essential technology

The technology must enable three functions: 1) creation of polls, 2) easy supervisee participation, and 3) anonymous sharing of results. This intervention was created for group supervision conducted via Zoom and Microsoft Teams, which have polling features. Online group supervision platforms without a polling feature necessitate using a tool like Mentimeter, Kahoot, or Slido that allows anonymous results sharing. Adaption for face-to-face group supervision requires that the three functions be present and useable in a physical space.

Polls that uncover issues impacting the creation of brave spaces

Supervision groups are psychoeducational groups that facilitate clinical learning. Anonymous polls meant to co-construct brave spaces should 1) foster a group culture that is both safe and stimulating, 2) involve supervisees in each other's learning, 3) allow supervisees to explore their authentic reactions to the content of their learning (Champe & Rubel, 2012). The following are examples of polls that address various needs. Processing the results is necessary, and suggestions are offered in the instructions.

Early group development poll designed to foster a safe and stimulating group culture:

How safe do you feel disclosing your social locations in this supervision group? I feel:

a.  Unsafe.
b.  Safe disclosing a few of my social locations.
c.  Safe disclosing most of my social locations.
d.  Safe disclosing all my social locations.

Later group development poll designed to involve supervisees in each other's learning:

I am confident I can provide challenging feedback about peers' anti-oppressive personalization, conceptualization, or intervention skills in this group.

a.  True
b.  False

Poll designed to open space for supervisees to explore their reactions to anti-oppressive content:

To what degree do you agree with the concept of "*Centering the margins through empowerment and liberation*"?

a.   I mostly disagree with it.
b.   I partly agree and disagree with it.
c.   I mostly agree with it.
d.   I do not understand the concept well enough to agree or disagree.

## Intervention Instructions

The group therapeutic factors of acceptance, cohesion, self-disclosure, and interpersonal learning parallel the characteristics of brave spaces that promote anti-oppressive learning (Okech et al., 2023b). Group supervision enables anti-oppressive learning when supervisors encourage supervisees to actively co-construct brave spaces (Okech et al., 2023a). Research indicates that online anonymity may correlate positively with self-disclosure (Clark-Gordon et al., 2019). This intervention uses anonymous polling to broach and process questions critical to creating brave spaces.

1.   The supervisor introduces the idea of anonymous polls, explains their purpose, and demonstrates by launching a poll. In this introduction, the supervisor discusses the importance of participation, honesty, and the right to pass during group processing.
2.   The supervisor can schedule or initiate polls when issues arise in creating a brave space. The supervisor may initiate polling by announcing a check-in poll whenever they sense the group may benefit from one (e.g., group stage change, impasse in conflict resolution, peer feedback is superficial or missing anti-racist perspective).
3.   The supervisor launches the poll, instructs the supervisees to respond honestly, and provides a clear timeline for a response.
4.   After polling, the supervisor shares the results, asks supervisees to reflect on their reactions, and communicates a clear timeline for reflection.
5.   Then, the supervisor leads processing to facilitate individual, interpersonal, and group-as-a-whole meaning-making. The following represents a processing progression for the first example poll:

   a.   What do you notice about the results of this poll and the safety of disclosing social locations?
   b.   What feelings come up for you about these results?

    c.   How do you make sense of the results in the context of this group being a supportive environment for growth as an anti-oppressive clinician?

    d.   What actions would you like to take based on these results?

6.   While processing, the supervisor may ask for voluntary supervisee self-disclosure about their poll response. In this case, a processing progression related to the second poll may look like this:

    a.   What do you notice about the results of this poll on broaching ability status?

    b.   Would anyone like to share how they responded and why?

    c.   Would someone with a different response like to share?

    d.   How do you make sense of the results and what has been shared about this supervision group being a brave space?

    e.   What actions to build compassion and connection would you like to take based on the results?

## Supervisory Alliance and Relationship

The anonymous poll intervention is designed to broach issues in the multilayered relationships of online group supervision. Conducting an anonymous poll and processing the results as a group can positively or negatively affect these relationships. The polls should attend to all these relationships and enable feedback exchange among the group members and from supervisees to the supervisor. The supervisor is likely the most powerful individual in the group and needs to be aware of their impact on the process and learning environment. Thus, anonymous polls inviting feedback for the supervisor should be included early and regularly.

The polls should be tailored to the group's readiness and the supervisor's confidence in managing intercultural conflict (Okech et al., 2016). For a supervision group early in its development, an overly intense poll might be, "I feel judged for my values by someone in the supervision group." This type of query might raise anxiety enough to stall processing or uncover conflict when trust is low. A better choice for a poll might be, "I hope this group can delve into our different identities and values," or "I would like to delve into my identity and values."

## Legal and Ethical Considerations

Supervisors must adhere to the ethical requirement of adequately preparing supervisees for the process of group supervision, providing informed consent for anti-oppressive content and processes, and the anonymous polling intervention. This group intervention's primary legal and ethical concern is maintaining anonymity in polling methods. Supervisors must ensure anonymity is preserved. If self-disclosure about the polls is encouraged, supervisors must counsel supervisees not to self-disclose if they feel vulnerable or coerced. To prevent harm, the supervisor must be cognizant of the poll's potential to initiate conflict and consider the group's diversity, supervisees' potential trauma histories, past cohort or supervision group dynamics, and sociopolitical current events when selecting the topic and wording of a poll. The supervisor should be confident and skilled at effectively managing and addressing conflicts within supervision groups.

### Reflective Questions

These reflective questions may help supervisees make sense of their learning experience with anonymous polls:

1.  What issues related to creating a brave space continue in this group?
2.  What have you learned about yourself as a clinician through the anonymous polls?
3.  What differences have you observed in your behavior and disclosures when interacting anonymously in the group and when your identity is known?
4.  How does anonymity, or the absence of it, relate to the work of being an anti-oppressive clinician?

## Intervention Title: The Brave Space Zine

## Author(s) and Affiliation(s)

Bagmi Das, PhD, LMFT
The George Washington University

Mina Attia, PhD, NCC
The George Washington University

## Supervision Format and Modality

This anti-oppressive supervision intervention is designed for live group supervision. It can be used both in-person and via virtual supervision. This supervision intervention can be used in Masters' or Doctoral level practica or internships and includes an initial and more dynamic version. This intervention is designed for intermediate anti-oppressive development; it works best when the group of supervisees has formed a working relationship.

## Supervisory Goals and Learning Objectives

*The Supervisee Will*

- Engage in reflective practice to identify salient social locations.
- Identify values they ascribe to their social locations.
- Build awareness of at least two situations in which they find comfort and safety in sharing their thoughts.
- Share and identify one or more things they have learned from others' experiences in the supervisory environment.

## Time Required

The initial Zine intervention and related reflexive exercises require ~90 minutes. The more dynamic Zine requires additional time, one or two subsequent supervision sessions (30–60 minutes each). Please see the detailed instructions to add these options.

## Materials

There are two approaches to this Zine, and both have different benefits. The initial option is to create a paper Zine, which allows people to use their hands and own words to create the product. This Zine would be a one-time intervention that can be returned to the supervisee in later supervision groups. To create this Zine, the supervisor provides plain 8.5"x11" paper, coloring and writing implements (e.g., markers and colored pencils), and scissors (at least one for the group). The supervisor also provides or encourages supervisees to bring in magazines, stamps, and stickers that they are drawn to. For this Zine exercise, the supervisor will want to learn the Zine folding technique (www.readbrightly.com/how-to-make-zine/) or provide the video during supervision.

The second option is to create a dynamic Zine, which can be revisited and adjusted during the course of supervision. This allows supervisees to reflect on their own anti-oppressive development over time, specifically as regards their changes in salient social locations due to historical events and the related care they need from themselves and others. The supervisor might consider: How do current world events place emphasis on or endanger particular social locations? Altogether, this encourages both the development of critical consciousness through critical reflexivity and the potential centering of wellness and self-care through acts of compassion in addition to the co-construction of this brave space. In order to engage in the dynamic Zine, the supervisees will need their own laptops loaded with Microsoft PowerPoint or Presi. They will also need access to the internet in order to download pictures.

### Intervention Instructions

1.  Introduce Zine before group supervision. A Zine, derived from "magazine," is an artifact of a point in time. Just as a magazine has a focused theme but has different ways of engaging with that theme, a Zine, too, has a central idea and uses art and text to reflect on that theme in different ways. To encourage students to think about the Zine prior to the group supervision, ask students to bring anything salient to them regarding their social locations, such as religious artifacts (e.g., symbols) or ethnocultural artifacts (e.g., textiles, flags, words in different languages). The supervisor can create their own Zine, deciding whether to share it based on AO Principle 3, which emphasizes centering marginalized voices. Supervisors should also engage in a separate consulting group for personal reflexivity, distinct from the group supervision setting.

2.  In group supervision, provide pieces of paper and use a Zine folding guide to direct supervisees in creating the initial Zine. If completed in an online setting, ask supervisees to come prepared with materials. If completing a dynamic Zine, the supervisor should ask supervisees to come with their computers or tablets to create an eight-page PowerPoint (no pre-loaded layouts) or eight-section Presi presentation. This should take two to three minutes.

3.  In progression, the supervisor utilizes the following prompts per page. It is also advised that the supervisor engage in tracking, reflecting, linking, and use of immediacy while the supervisees work. For example, the supervisor might note, "I see that several of you are behaviorally engaged and intently focused, and others look as if they are carefully contemplating their next steps. Approaching this type of work comes in many forms." The supervisor should encourage supervisees to consider their needs while completing their Zine. They may observe shifts in verbal and nonverbal behaviors. Allocate five to ten minutes per interior page, allowing flexibility, and two to three minutes for the cover and back pages to guide this reflective process effectively.

|  | *Guided prompt* |
|---|---|
| #1/Cover | Create a title page for your Brave Space Zine (e.g. [insert name here]'s Brave Space Zine). You are welcome to spend some time decorating this as you see fit. |
| #2 | Turn the cover to the first, left-side page. Before putting anything on the page, consider what social locations (e.g., faith, country/culture of origin, peer groups, etc.) inform your value systems. You can use text, art, or items you have brought to fill in this page with your salient social locations. Please stay on this left side. |
| #3 | On the right hand of this page, use text, art, and items to show 3–5 of your core values. |
| #4 | Flip to the next two blank pages. On the left side only, reflect on the prompt "How do you take care of yourself?" Use whatever means to convey your response on this page. |
| #5 | On the right-hand side, reflect on the prompt, "How do you take care of yourself as a counselor?" You might consider how the former two pages' contents (social locations and values) impact your understanding of care. Continue using art, text, and other objects to show these. |
| #6 | Now flip to the final two blank pages that are side by side. On the left, reflect on "How do you take care of yourself as an anti-oppressive advocate/activist?" and convey this through whatever means you would like. |
| #7 | On this last right-hand page, please list, draw, or otherwise convey your wishes for this group space as it relates to anti-oppression. You might want to reflect on your goals for engaging in advocacy and critical discussion in class, how you like to be held accountable, how you plan to hold others accountable, and how you want to care for yourself and others when engaging in this work? |
| #8/Back | Flip over that page, and you should be looking at a back "cover." Here, I encourage you to put quotes, words, or images that motivate you toward being brave. |

4. After completing Zines, allow supervisees unstructured time to embellish their Zines.
5. In small groups of 3–4, ask supervisees to share their Zines with each other. They share how they processed each prompt and what they have depicted on each page. We recommend that one supervisee goes over their full Zine before moving on to the next supervisee. The supervisor should plan to allot five minutes of sharing per group member (e.g., a group of three should be given 15 minutes).
6. Use the reflective questions listed later on to guide a larger group discussion. It is recommended that the supervisor be aware of group dynamics so as to not have one supervisee bear the load of responding to each question. As folks process at different speeds, it may also be helpful for the supervisor to provide reflective questions to the supervisees and guide the discussion in the next supervision meeting.
7. To end this intervention, the supervisor will thank the students for their involvement and end with a group share of their back cover.
8. For supervisors interested in a dynamic Zine: The supervisor will remind supervisees that they will revisit their Zines and walk them through the guided prompts 2–7 once again, using "Reflect on what has changed" to the end of each prompt. Instead of a small group share, the supervisees will focus on a group reflection of reflective question #3 below. It is recommended that the supervisor wait at least 7–10 supervision sessions to allow time for development before coming back to the Zine. Supervisors may also use current events to guide the revisit to the Zine. For instance, in times of conflict, the Zine may be a way to identify salience for supervisees and reorient self-care and group supervision to facilitate brave space.

### Supervisory Alliance and Relationship

This Zine is focused on building awareness of how social locations and coping methods inform each supervisee's approach and affiliation with anti-racist and anti-oppressive movements. Given this, we would recommend that this Zine project be introduced well after the students have formed a group identity and become comfortable discussing self-care/well-being and have also gone through the process of video presentations for group critique.

### Legal and Ethical Considerations

The supervisor should secure informed consent from supervisees by clearly outlining the activity's purpose, potential risks, and benefits in clinical or academic settings. Supervisors must explain confidentiality limits, emphasizing ethical standards like the ACA Code of Ethics (2014). To minimize risks, supervisors should foster a supportive environment, offer resources for those in distress, and provide opportunities to debrief. Encouraging cultural humility and self-reflection on beliefs, biases, and privileges is essential. Supervisors should offer consistent guidance and support to supervisees throughout the activity, ensuring a respectful and ethical learning experience.

## Reflective Questions

1. What have you learned from this activity as you reflected on your anti-oppressive identity as a supervisor/supervisee?
2. What prompts were challenging as you completed the Zine? Which ones were particularly facilitative and why?
3. How can we all create guidelines on our anti-oppressive group supervision based on what you all have added to page 7?
4. What did you learn from your peers in the small group sharing?
5. Please title your Zine and offer a brief rationale.

## Intervention Title: Co-Creation Supervision in the Sand

## Author(s) and Affiliation(s)

Mary DeRaedt, PhD, LPC
The George Washington University

## Supervision Format and Modality

Originally created for in-person individual supervision, this intervention is adaptable for triadic settings and can also be effectively used virtually with an online sand tray.

**Supervisee Development:** (i.e., master's practicum or internship, doctoral practicum or internship, professional development plans/remediation plans, post-graduate and pre-licensed professionals, post-graduate and post-licensed professionals). This supervision intervention is appropriate across the developmental spectrum of supervision. The purpose and depth of exploration will differ across the developmental spectrum, but it offers non-hierarchical, culturally empathic, and brave opportunities for all clinicians and supervisors.

## Supervisory Goals and Learning Objectives

1. Supervisees will examine their impact on the supervision relationship.
2. Supervisees will increase their skill in processing sand tray content.
3. Supervisees will expand their ability to participate in a co-creation of the supervisory experience with their supervisor in a non-hierarchical manner.
4. Supervisees will increase their ability to participate in a brave space with their supervisor.
5. Supervisees will expand their understanding of the impact of creating a brave space for clients and in supervision.

## Time Required

The timing, ranging from 45–60 minutes, will depend on the supervisee's comfort level and the depth of processing involved in the intervention.

## Materials

A sandtray includes a variety of miniatures, or it can be adapted as an online sand tray, making it essential to have miniatures from key categories to support full expression. These categories include fantasy, dangerous, scary, foliage, animals from various ecosystems, vehicles, construction materials, buildings, diverse people, food items, household items, and religious items across diverse social locations.

## Intervention Instructions

Sandtray is an intervention appropriate for all populations in anti-oppressive supervision as it is founded on the principle of unconscious meaning-making where self-created metaphors inherently place the participant in the non-hierarchical space of being the expert on their own experience while inviting them to be brave by embracing the vulnerability of the process (Homeyer & Sweeney, 2023, Anekstein et al., 2014). "Co-creation of Experience" invites the supervisor and supervisee to engage in this brave space mutually, exploring egalitarian vulnerability. By allowing room for the co-created metaphor, both participants share their own experiences and then bravely allow for adaptation of their own experience in service of a mutual understanding and metaphor. Before beginning, the supervisor reviews the power of metaphor and the value of unconscious content, followed by an explanation of the vulnerability of exposing unconscious experience. This should include an exploration of the value of a brave space in anti-oppressive and anti-racist supervision.

1. The supervisor begins the session by introducing the sandtray materials and checking in with the supervisee about their previous experience with sandtray. It is recommended that this activity not be the introduction to the sandtray technique. Supervisees who have no previous experience with the intervention may rely too heavily on observing and copying the supervisor's sandtray as a way of learning about the approach, as opposed to feeling brave enough to create their own unique half of the tray. If the supervisee has no previous understanding of sandtray as an intervention, it is recommended to begin with an individual sandtray intervention such as "put counseling in the sandtray." After determining that the intern has some understanding of the approach, the supervisor will describe that they will be co-creating a sandtray today. Explain that supervision is a unique combination of the supervisees' experience and the supervisor's experience, and by creating a sandtray with both experiences and then combining the two halves, the dyad bravely engages in the act of co-creation.
2. The supervisor then invites the supervisee to discuss how they will agree to divide the sandtray space. This discussion should include exploring multiple ways the tray could be divided, the role of power

and anti-oppression within the relationship, and then mutually agree on the dividing line. It is recommended that the dyad try drawing lines in the sand to represent the many options for dividing the space and discuss how their visceral responses to each possibility. This begins the dual process of bravely sharing individual experiences and beginning to tap into the unconscious experience. It could be referred to as the "warm up" prior to beginning.

3. Once the dividing line is agreed upon and drawn in the sand, either by the supervisee or the supervisor (both options have implications, and the decision could also be processed for affective and somatic experience)

4. The supervisor then begins the building stage by first inviting the supervisee to participate in two or three deep cleansing breaths together and then prompting with "Put your experience of our supervision in the tray." This allows both participants to begin choosing miniatures to represent their experience. It can be helpful to have duplicates of some miniatures so that both participants have equal opportunity to utilize a miniature, but it is not required. Once the trays are combined, the mutual desire for the same miniature can be a valuable part of the final co-created tray and indicate a place of mutuality. Allow as much time as each participant needs to complete their tray. Once the pair sit down and appear to be done, the supervisor invites them to view what they have created and check in with themselves about whether or not the tray feels "finished." Once both individuals feel that their trays are done, processing can begin.

5. The supervisor starts with the prompt to the supervisee, "Tell me about your tray." After the supervisee discusses their tray, they will provide the supervisor with the same prompt. This will open up further process-oriented questions as both participants explore and expand on their understanding of their trays. Some process-oriented questions could be: What do you notice about your tray? How do you feel when you view your tray? Does this figure evoke any memories or strong reactions? If this figure could speak, what would it say? How is power, hierarchy, oppression, or anti-oppression captured within your tray?

6. The supervisor will then begin the process of co-creating a mutual metaphor by introducing the idea of commonalities in the two trays. If a second sand tray is available, the two participants will move complimentary elements and common-themed miniatures to the second brave space tray. If there is only one tray, they can agree to "erase" the line drawn in the sand and begin moving miniatures around to create a common brave space in the center of the tray. The negotiation of

what will be placed in the center will be led by the supervisor inviting the supervisee to participate in moving and reorienting the figures in the tray to represent a mutual experience of supervision.

7.  Closure involves a final discussion around the experience of co-creating the brave space tray of supervision. Process questions to be asked: What was the experience like to shift from a self-created tray to a co-created tray? How does it feel to view the new co-created tray? What do you notice about the co-created tray? Which miniatures in the co-created tray evoke a strong reaction? Do we feel there is anything missing from the co-created tray? And if yes, what elements would we add? How did power, hierarchy, and anti-oppression shift in the co-created tray?

8.  The final step is for the supervisor and supervisee to process how it felt to participate in this intervention together. Opening the discussion up to include potentially uncomfortable feelings or hesitation allows further opportunities for the supervisee to engage in the space with bravery. The supervisor should also offer their experience. The intervention can conclude by relating back to their identity, roles, and responsibility as anti-oppressive agents for change.

## Supervisory Alliance and Relationship

The use of sandtray in clinical supervision is established as an effective tool for enhancing counseling outcomes and fostering trust. Perryman et al. (2021) highlight the value of modeling sandtray techniques in supervision, especially for offering creative approaches. However, using sandtray early in a master's practicum may challenge the supervisory alliance, given supervisees' heightened vulnerability. Supervisors trained in sandtray should only employ this technique with supervisees who have prior experience. Before implementation, supervisors must assess the strength of the supervisory relationship. By acknowledging supervisees' social identities, sandtray can build trust and help externalize internal experiences, providing a safe space to explore emerging identities and biases (Carnes-Holt et al., 2014). Given the vulnerable nature of sandtray work, this approach can lead to ruptures in the supervisory relationship if cultural disconnections within trays are not processed with empathy. Supervisors should model self-awareness and non-reactionary responses when addressing conflicting tray elements (Cormier et al., 2023). Recognizing systemic power dynamics, supervisors can mitigate authority-based cultural responses by reframing these differences as opportunities to strengthen the supervisory alliance. Directly acknowledging misaligned elements within the trays can model a strengths-based, culturally responsive approach. Embracing these differences helps supervisees view diversity as valuable, fostering a supportive and growth-oriented environment.

## Legal and Ethical Considerations

When establishing any supervisory relationship, it is the responsibility of the supervisor to provide the supervisee with the scope of practice of the supervisor. Having a supervision contract that includes the use of expressive techniques as well as a description of the potential added vulnerability of these interventions will provide the supervisee with informed consent.

Furthermore, the supervisor should make sure they have appropriate training and supervision in sandtray as a way of ensuring that the intervention is being used skillfully. It is unethical for supervisors to practice outside the scope of their expertise.

## Reflective Questions

Please note that process questions are provided in the instructions for this intervention. The following questions can be used post-intervention. It is recommended to do follow-up reflection in the follow-up session.

1.  How did you experience the time after the session ended? Somatic and cognitive responses?
2.  As you review the experience of co-creating supervision in the sand, what are some thoughts or reactions you have had in the time since the sandtray experience?
3.  Take a moment to review the metaphors identified in the sandtray. Which metaphors are still in your mind, and how are you thinking of them now?

## Intervention Title: Framing Brave Spaces Through Collage Art: A Perspective on Counseling Supervision

### Author(s) and Affiliation(s)

Kenya G. Bledsoe, PhD, LPC-S NCC, NCSC, BC-TMH
The University of Mississippi

Jaimie Stickl Haugen, PhD, LPC, NCC, ACS
William & Mary

### Supervision Format and Modality

This supervision intervention is in-person group supervision with three or more supervisees, a maximum of 12. Supervisors can adapt this intervention for triadic supervision and peer supervision. This supervision intervention is applicable across all levels of supervisee development and intervention levels (e.g., introductory, advanced).

### Supervisory Goals and Learning Objectives

1.  Engage supervisees in a dialogue about the nuances between brave and safe spaces, encouraging them to take risks in discussing controversial topics related to anti-oppression, justice, and equity.
2.  Guide supervisees in visually representing their diverse experiences via a communal collage to foster communication, engagement, and relationship-building within a brave space.
3.  Facilitate group discussion among supervisees around the completed collage, exploring common themes and personal and professional challenges and identifying areas for growth within a brave space.

### Time Required

This 90-minute group supervision session is split into two 45-minute parts. Part one establishes a foundation for co-constructing a brave space through collage art, encouraging reflection on cultural identities. In part two, supervisees explore how their identities impact others, fostering dialogue to co-create a brave space within the group.

## Materials

The supervisor is responsible for securing an open space so supervisees can spread out. Also, the supervisor should supply as many creative art materials and supplies as possible to execute the collage activity. The supervisor should assimilate all the required items for the collage, including magazines, a blank canvas or mural paper, a poster board cut into pie-shaped pieces (see Figure 6.1), scissors, glue sticks, or adhesive. Art supplies such as magic markers and colored pencils are needed.

## Intervention Instructions

### Session Preparation

1.  Before group supervision, the supervisor should draw a large circle on a poster board and dissect the circle into pie-shaped pieces according to the number of supervisees in the group (see Figure 6.1). The supervisor will cut pie-shaped pieces, one for each supervisee and one for themselves.
2.  The supervisor should arrange collage materials in an accessible space, considering the number of supervisees, available time, and supervisees' abilities to facilitate engagement and reduce resistance to art-based strategies.
3.  Before the session, supervisees should bring magazines with diverse cultures and perspectives, looking for images, texts, and colors that reflect diversity. They are also encouraged to bring cultural artifacts, like flags or family crests, representing their values, identities, and heritage.

### Session Intervention

Counseling supervisors can use weekly group supervision to tackle racism and oppression via a brave space where supervisees can actively reflect, identify biases and areas of uncertainty, and participate in conversations with respect and civility. Collages have frequently been used for individual and family counseling. The visual arts (e.g., photographs, clay work, drawing) empower clients to address issues symbolically, serving as a catalyst and conduit for self-exploration in a broader context (Gladding, 2016). Considering the benefits of visual art and creative expression in counseling, art-based approaches have also been incorporated into group supervision to elevate the supervision experience by fostering new learning and self-confidence (Liberati & Agbisit, 2017). Hence, the present intervention employs a collage to cultivate supervisee awareness and reflection. It encourages supervisees to capture and express emotions and thoughts through visual and symbolic means (Gladding, 2016).

### Part One—Approximately 45 minutes

To begin, the supervisor provides an overview of creative arts and expressive techniques in counseling and the benefits of incorporating art-based strategies in clinical supervision. Creative supervision techniques provide supervisees with an opportunity for deep reflection while decreasing defensiveness and enhancing self-awareness and openness (Graham et al., 2014). The supervisor can share visuals of collages as art therapy with clients using magazines and other materials. The supervisor explains their supervisory role during the process, who will facilitate the group and contribute to the collage. Before the intervention, the supervisor should identify the goals of the collage and discuss the role of creative arts interventions to enhance communication and awareness. The supervisor can normalize that art-based activities may cause anxiety or discomfort for some individuals based on prior experiences or preconceived notions of personal art skills or abilities. We have found it helpful to reiterate that creative interventions are about the *process* rather than the *outcome*.

1. The supervisor starts by asking supervisees to define "cultural identity" and leads a discussion on how intersecting social identities (e.g., gender, age, religion, affectional orientation, and race) shape our interactions with others and the world. Supervisees are encouraged to explore how these intersections form their unique perspectives and consider how images can help reflect and communicate their identities and life experiences to others.
2. The supervisor then gives each supervisee a pie-shaped poster board (see Figure 6.1) and invites them to create a collage reflecting their cultural identity. Supervisees are encouraged to sit around a table with magazines and art materials placed in the center for easy access and engage in conversation with each other during this activity.
3. The supervisor provides 20 minutes for supervisees to reflect on their life experiences while exploring the art materials. Supervisees are encouraged to cut out images, text, and patterns from magazines, sorting them by color or theme, and glue them to their pie-shaped piece to create a collage. They can also use additional art

materials to add elements not found in the magazines. The supervisor, as part of the group process, also creates their own collage. Soft background music can be played during this time, and the supervisor should provide time updates at the five-minute and one-minute mark.

4. When time is up, the supervisor invites each supervisee to share their collage and explain the meanings behind their chosen images and symbols. The supervisor facilitates deeper reflection by encouraging supervisees to consider how their identities and experiences may impact others in the group. They might note similarities and differences among the collages and ask questions like, "How do your experiences shape your perceptions of others in this group?" or "How do your intersecting identities influence how you present yourself to others?"

5. After each supervisee shares, they place their pie piece onto a large canvas or mural paper. The supervisor arranges the pieces to form a complete circle of identities (see Figure 6.1). They then prompt reflection by asking, "What do you notice about our collection of identities as a group?" and encourage consideration of the strengths and challenges associated with the diverse identities represented.

### Part 2—Approximately 45 Minutes

In part two, the supervisor introduces the concept of a brave space and its role in anti-oppressive supervision. Integrating the discussions during the first session is vital as supervisees consider how their unique identities and prior experiences influence their co-creation of a brave space.

1. The supervisor begins by discussing brave spaces versus safe spaces in supervision, emphasizing that brave spaces foster accountability and shared learning.

2. Next, the supervisor displays the identity collage from Session 1, placing it in view. They draw a square around the collage to symbolize framing a brave space and remind supervisees how unique experiences shape interactions by saying (see Figure 6.2), "It's important to intentionally frame a brave space around all of our identities within the context of our shared space."

3. The supervisor invites supervisees to reflect on what a brave space means to them, considering the group's unique identities. They have 15 minutes to gather words and images from magazines that represent their vision, then glue these around the identity collage but

within the square, symbolizing the "framing of a brave space" (see Figure 6.2).

4. After supervisees glue their images to the paper, the supervisor leads a discussion on their selections, exploring what each image represents and how these ideas might shape group supervision. The supervisor may ask, "How might this show up when we encounter challenging discussions, different perspectives, or diverse opinions," "How might this help us respond to conflict, controversy, or relational challenges we encounter in our group," or "How will our creation of this brave space help us own our intentions and impact on others?"

5. The supervisor uses facilitation skills to observe the process of creating the brave space collage. For example, they might say, "Some of you took longer to find images for a brave space than for your identity. Why do you think that is?" The supervisor also notes common themes and differences, emphasizing that a brave space may look different for each person.

6. To conclude, the supervisor invites supervisees to share any final thoughts on brave spaces. As they complete the collage, they can also add more images, words, or ideas using the available art materials.

7. Once the collage is complete, allow it to dry fully. If desired, the supervisor can then apply a protective covering to preserve it. When dry, consider framing or mounting the collage to serve as a visual reminder of the group's brave space for future sessions.

## Supervisory Alliance and Relationship

Supervision is an ongoing process that requires attention, care, and mutual respect for the supervisee's ideas and alternative perspectives (Bernard & Goodyear, 2019). The supervisory alliance is a collaborative partnership that supports the supervisee's growth and development while ensuring clients' well-being (Ganske et al., 2015). A foundation of a solid supervisory alliance inclusive of trust and respect is crucial to creating a safe space for supervisees to be vulnerable (Perryman et al., 2021). Constructing a brave space needs to be considered within a trusting supervisory alliance to allow supervisees to tackle topics they may find difficult to broach. Incorporating creative interventions into supervision can provide structure and guidance to scaffold the development of the supervisory alliance (Perryman et al., 2021). Expanding on previous multicultural and social justice counseling research, the supervisor can use this intervention to cultivate a brave space that respects and accepts supervisees' interests, values, and feelings while tackling anti-racism and oppression. A good supervisor provides ongoing guidance and support within a trusting relationship while encouraging supervisees to self-reflect and use critical thinking to improve their counseling skills. The group supervision setting for constructing a brave space is ideal for peer engagement in an environment where supervisees can recognize and respect diverse cultural backgrounds, beliefs, and values crucial for effective counseling, ongoing cultural competence, and anti-oppressive counseling.

## Legal and Ethical Considerations

Supervisors must model legal and ethical behavior, guide supervisees in navigating ethical dilemmas, and allow the ethical codes to serve as the moral compass to influence supervisees' work within the art collage intervention. Additionally, the supervisor should explicitly communicate informed consent and adequate discussion of the purpose, rationale, and intention of using creative interventions in supervision, as evidenced in the professional disclosure statement, course syllabi, supervisory contract, and state board counseling paperwork. Also, the supervisors should carefully consider how to store the collage and protect the supervisees' confidentiality and privacy in a way that replaces supervisees' vulnerability with affirmation and representation. Creating brave spaces may be a new concept for some supervisors and supervisees. Consider the supervisor's comfort level with integrating creative intervention techniques and obtain additional training or consultation as needed. Supervisors need to consider the "use of creativity within the context of the developmental level of the supervisee, the nature of the supervisory alliance, and their skill level" (Graham et al., 2014, p. 424).

## Reflective Questions

1. Describe the importance of a brave space when engaging in anti-oppressive work with a client. During supervision?
2. How impactful was it to hear the reactions or experiences of colleagues in group supervision? What emotions emerged?
3. As you reflect on this brave space experience and recognize this is an ongoing process, what areas can you identify for professional growth?
4. Describe one takeaway that you can apply with your future clients.

# APPENDIX: COLLAGE CIRCLE OF IDENTITIES

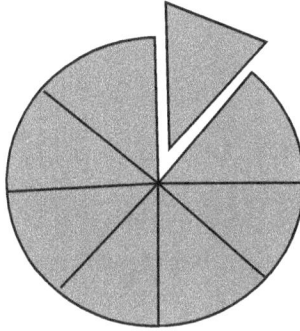

*Figure 6.1* Collage Circle of Identities

*Note:* The number of pie pieces should correspond with the number of supervisees in the group, with the addition of the supervisor.

## Framing a Brave Space Around Our Identities

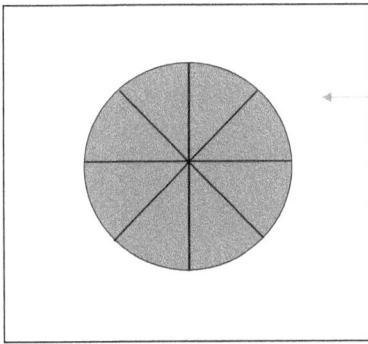

*Supervisees will add images and words inside the square to represent their depiction of a brave space around the identity mosaic*

*Figure 6.2* Framing a Brave Space Around Our Identities

CHAPTER 7

# Developing Goals and Assessing Outcomes Through Stakeholder Investment

*Casey Barrio Minton, Lindsey M. Bell, Theodore R. Burnes, Kristopher Goodrich, Dan Li, Yanhong Liu, Melissa Luke, Harvey Charles Peters, and Maria Reyna*

## CHAPTER 7 INTERVENTIONS

### Intervention Title: A Deliberate Practice Intervention to Develop Authoritative and Facilitative Skills

### Author(s) and Affiliation(s)

Melissa Luke, Ph.D., NCC, ACS, LMHC
Syracuse University

Harvey Charles Peters, Ph.D., NCC
Montclair State University

### Supervision Format and Modality

This supervision intervention was developed for use within triadic supervision conducted in in-person supervision.

### Supervisee Development

This supervision intervention can be used across all levels of supervisee development; however, it is specifically designed to develop the supervisee's

DOI: 10.4324/9781003470656-7

understanding and application of authoritative and facilitative intervention skills. We find the intervention particularly helpful for supervisees who are newly exposed to principles of anti-oppression and/or the development and assessment of community stakeholder engagement.

## Supervisory Goals and Learning Objectives

1. Supervisees will be able to distinguish between and demonstrate all six intervention types within Heron's framework (e.g., prescriptive, informative, confronting, cathartic, catalytic, and supportive).
2. Supervisees will be able to identify short and long-term anti-oppressive goals related to their counseling and supervision work.
3. Supervisees will demonstrate the ability to connect the six intervention skill types to the development, facilitation, and assessment of anti-oppressive counseling goals.

## Time Required

This intervention is designed for a 75-minute supervisory session.

## Materials

The supervisor can use the handout provided or prepare other visual aids to support the supervisees in their learning and practice, the implementation of the six types of skills.

## Intervention Instructions

Prior to supervision, the supervisor reviews Heron's (2001) framework consisting of two primary types of interventions, authoritative and facilitative, each with three sub-categories. The three sub-categories of authoritative interventions include prescriptive, informative, and confronting, whereas facilitative interventions include cathartic, catalytic, and supportive interventions.

1. The supervisor explains the purpose of the intervention, reviewing the learning objectives and engaging the supervisees in a discussion about how these fit within their overall supervisory development thus far.
2. The supervisor introduces Heron's (2001) framework for helping interventions (a handout may be helpful), noting that they observed

the supervisees implementing many of these types of interventions in their prior work, even if they had not been named.

3. After familiarizing the supervisees with the definitions of authoritative and facilitative interventions, the supervisor invites the supervisees to consider when they have used authoritative and facilitative interventions in counseling or when they have observed their triadic peer supervisee having done so. For example, the supervisor can suggest that "an intervention is authoritative when it provides information, challenge, structure, or suggestion, whereas an intervention is facilitative when it draws out, explores, or enables increased insight, understanding, or action."

4. The supervisor asks the supervisees to identify the ways in which these two intervention types converge and diverge in terms of their purpose and impact. The supervisor might ask, "What is similar about authoritative and facilitative interventions, and what is different?" As the supervisor facilitates the examination, they can offer examples of when they have used or witnessed the supervisees using authoritative and facilitative interventions in supervision. The supervisor can inquire about the supervisees' reactions by asking, "Which type of intervention skill are you more comfortable using," "How might your identity and social locations contribute to the likelihood or frequency of you using this type of intervention skill," or "What else might you consider when deciding whether or not to implement this type of intervention skill?"

5. The supervisor directs the supervisees to take turns reading the information about each of the six intervention types within Heron's framework (e.g., prescriptive, informative, confronting, cathartic, catalytic, supportive), pausing after each for clarification and processing. The supervisor might ask, "What in the example offered makes this a _____ type intervention skill," "How could the example offered be changed to turn it into a _____ type intervention skill," or "What kind of impact/response does this type of intervention skill tend to elicit?" The supervisor repeats the clarification and processing until all six intervention types have been covered.

6. The supervisor helps the supervisees connect their previously identified supervisory goals and development to Heron's (2001) framework. The supervisor supports the supervisees in extending this into concrete (and ideally measurable) short- and long-term anti-oppressive goals for their counseling and/or supervision work. The supervisor might ask, "Where can you envision the six intervention skill types assisting you in reaching your goals," "How might _____ intervention skill type be integrated into short- or long-term anti-oppressive goals related to your counseling," or "What about our triadic supervision; what can we apply from Heron to our anti-oppressive supervision?"

7.  The supervisor asks the supervisees to take turns developing their own examples of each type of the six intervention skills that can be implemented with stakeholders to elicit input and evaluation of the anti-oppressive goals. The supervisor can facilitate the supervisees in providing feedback to one another by saying, "What did you notice about developing an example for use with stakeholders," "How did this compare to use with clients or fellow supervisee," or "Which of these are you drawn to using and where do you still have questions?

8.  The supervisor models intervention skill types as they begin to consolidate the supervision intervention. For example, the supervisor might say, "Supervisee A, please tell Supervisee B one connection that you see between authoritative intervention skills and the development of anti-oppressive counseling goals?" followed by "Supervisee B, what type of intervention skill type did I just use?" Alternatively, the supervisor can suggest, "Supervisee B, perhaps you can select one facilitative intervention skill type and use it with Supervisee A to assess their progress today related to anti-oppressive counseling or supervision goals" followed by "Supervisee A, what intervention skill type did I use and how did you observe it to function?"

9.  The supervisor uses the reflective questions that follow to support supervisees in transferring the learning from the supervision intervention into their future work.

## Supervisory Alliance and Relationship

Given that the prior literature centers the alliance and relationship within stakeholder engagement across community projects (Häberlein & Hövel, 2023), as well specifically within counselor community engagement across needs assessments, interventions (Storlie et al., 2016), and evaluation processes (Sheperis & Bayles, 2022), the supervisor should be attentive to the supervisory working alliance and the impact of both the intervention content and processes on the relationships.

## Legal and Ethical Considerations

Although supervisors are familiar with and intervene in multicultural, social justice, and advocacy content, they may lack substantial prior experience with anti-oppressive practices and stakeholder engagement and thus could find themselves unwittingly in a regressive pairing with their supervisee. As such, we encourage supervisors finding themselves in this situation to develop their own community engagement intervention to address this gap.

## Reflective Questions

1. What stood out to you about your experience during this anti-oppressive supervision intervention, and what did you notice happening between you and your co-supervisee and/or you and your supervisor?

2. Where did you observe yourself struggling today, and how do you understand this?

3. When did you feel most competent today, and how might this impact your future anti-oppressive goals as well as stakeholder engagement?

4. In what ways might you apply Heron's (2001) six types of interventions in your in-session counseling and/or our future supervision session?

5. How do you envision clients and/or stakeholders responding to authoritative and facilitative interventions?

**Intervention Title: The Small Experiment Framework (SEF)**

**Author(s) and Affiliation(s)**

Maria Reyna, PhD, LPC-S (TX)
Seminary of the Southwest

Casey Barrio Minton, PhD, NCC
The University of Tennessee, Knoxville

**Supervision Format and Modality**

This supervision intervention was developed for use within individual, in-person supervision. However, the intervention may be adapted to a variety of formats and modalities.

**Supervisee Development**

This supervision intervention can be used across all levels of supervisee development; however, the intervention is designed to support supervisees in identifying their internalized oppressive beliefs and behaviors with the goal of promoting awareness and transformation. We find the intervention to be most useful with supervisees who have a working knowledge of the principles of anti-oppression. This is an intermediate or advanced intervention.

**Supervisory Goals and Learning Objectives**

1. Supervisees will identify, process, and explore at least two internalized oppressive beliefs, attitudes, and behaviors that impact their counseling work.
2. Supervisees will develop at least one anti-oppressive goal related to their counseling and supervision work.
3. Supervisees will assess and evaluate progress towards their anti-oppressive goals, adjusting as they deem necessary.

**Time Required**

This intervention is designed to be implemented as a conversation across at least three successive 60-minute supervision sessions.

## Materials

The supervisor may use the provided Small Experiment Bento Box handout, the 10 principles of anti-oppression, and any additional resources to support the supervisee in developing awareness and goals.

## Intervention Instructions

The Small Experiment Framework (SEF) is a constructivist intervention based on monastic traditions and behavioral science. The supervisee and supervisor collaborate to develop, implement, and assess at least one anti-oppressive goal, which moves the learning process from intellectual exercise to embodied action in counseling and supervision.

1.  The supervisor begins by introducing the SEF intervention, reviewing learning goals (e.g., increasing the use of immediacy), and processing how the intervention may be useful in the supervisee's professional development. We suggest the supervisor provide the supervisee with the included Small Experiment Bento Box handout.
2.  The supervisor invites exploration regarding how the supervisee's learning goals link to the 10 principles of anti-oppression, including what an anti-oppressive goal might mean to the supervisee. Based on the discussion with the supervisee, the supervisor may provide relevant anti-oppression-related materials, such as the MSJCCs (Ratts et al., 2016) or an identity development model responsive to the learning goals. Supervisors are encouraged to review the supplemental materials with the supervisee, collaboratively noting the supervisee's areas of strength and growth.
3.  After a thorough review of supplemental materials, the supervisor encourages the supervisees to explore their areas of growth with the aim of identifying one area of focus for the SEF. The supervisor asks open-ended questions to support the supervisee's reflective process, such as: *Which area of growth seems to be the most pressing to you at this time? When have you noticed this area of growth impacting your work with clients? What have you done in the past to support your growth in this area?*
4.  The supervisor asks the supervisee to reflect on beliefs and attitudes that are limiting their growth in the identified area. At this point, the supervisor asks the supervisee to engage in a reflective process outside of the supervision session. The supervisor provides the supervisee with prompts corresponding to the four quadrants on the SEF worksheet. Such prompts can include: *What are my current behaviors in this*

*area of growth? To what ideal behaviors do I aspire? What do I believe about myself, others, and the world regarding this area of growth? What would I need to believe in order to move towards my ideal behavior?*

5.  In the following supervision session, the supervisor and supervisee debrief the reflective assignment, including the supervisee's experience of the process (*What was this process like for you?*), the content of their reflections (*Tell me what came up for you in your reflection.*), and their reactions to the debriefing (*How are you feeling at this moment? What is sitting with you?*). If the supervisee struggles to identify beliefs or behaviors with depth or brings reflections inconsistent with the supervisor's observations, the supervisor may facilitate a deeper exploration in the session.

6.  Next, the supervisor and supervisee collaboratively develop a small experiment based on the supervisee's aspirational behavior. The supervisor may use a goal development framework, such as S.M.A.R.T. goals (Doran, 1981), to support the supervisee in the creation of a goal that is specific, measurable, attainable, realistic, and time-bound. The supervisor may use the following preface to support the goal development process:

    *Many of us set large, unrealistic goals, and we forget that we are all human and in process. This often sets us up to fail; we feel shame, guilt, and discouragement, and then we often are harshly self-critical, give up on the goal, and/ or become apathetic. To interrupt this human tendency, let's create a goal that is the smallest experiment of your overall aspirational behavior. For example, right now, you have noticed yourself avoiding any recognition of your client's physical disability, and you wonder if it is a barrier in your relationship. You want to believe that disability can be an asset and that your clients can bring their whole selves to work with you. At this time, your behavior is to not address disability with your client out of fear of offending them, and your aspirational behavior is to humbly but comfortably invite your clients to explore how they experience their physical disability related to their presenting concern and your work together. A small experiment could be you making an audio recording of how you might open the conversation with your client, listening back, reflecting on what you hear, and bringing your reflections back to supervision.*

7.  After the supervisee decides on their small experiment, the supervisee and supervisor identify a timeframe during which the supervisee will conduct the experiment. At the conclusion of the timeframe, the supervisor invites the supervisees to debrief their implementation of the experiment. The supervisor may use the debriefing questions

suggested previously. Additionally, the supervisor invites the supervisee to identify adjustments to the experiment that would support their growth. The supervisor may choose to conclude the intervention or encourage the supervisee to continue with the experimentation process until they are ready to address another area of growth.

## Supervisory Alliance and Relationship Considerations

When utilizing this intervention, it is important that the supervisor have a clear understanding of the supervisee's level of development (e.g., within anti-oppressive principles, identity related to the area of focus) to inform expectations of the supervisee's ability and capacity for honest self-reflection, vulnerability, and openness. The supervisor is encouraged to gauge the level of rapport, trust, and safety established in the relationship to establish their expectations of the level of supervisee's engagement with the intervention. The utility of the intervention is quite flexible. The supervisor could use it at the beginning of the supervisory relationship to facilitate a deeper exploration of supervisees' personalized goals. The supervisor could also initiate the SEF in response to observations of supervisee skill or engagement in supervision as the supervision relationship gains solidity over time.

## Legal and Ethical Considerations

Supervisors must uphold an ethical obligation to protect the profession and the public and adhere to legal requirements while also supporting supervisee development and matriculation into their professions. In the recent past, there have been several legal challenges from remediated trainees who claim that professional standards and ethical codes are discriminatory against their religious beliefs and threaten their First Amendment rights (Hutchens et al., 2013). Given the sociopolitical climate and rise of divisive concepts and laws, it is important to center professional work behavior, rather than harmful beliefs and attitudes, as the target of the intervention. Should supervisors become concerned about supervisees' competency, clinical performance, or harmful beliefs and attitudes, they are responsible for developing and implementing professional development plans that uphold their ethical and legal responsibilities.

**Reflective Questions**

1.  Consider the mutual experience of the supervision relationship. What is a small experiment you might design to support your forward progress in the principles of anti-oppression?
2.  In your own process of growth in anti-oppression principles, what has been helpful, supportive, and facilitative? How do you know that you have made progress?
3.  What expectations do you have of yourself and those around you regarding growth and change? How might this be influencing your supervision relationships, specifically regarding growth in anti-oppression principles?

# Appendix: Worksheet for Small Experiments

|  | The Present | The Possibility |
|---|---|---|
| Behavior |  |  |
| Belief |  |  |
| Experiment: |  |  |

### Intervention Title: Developing and Assessing Anti-Oppressive Goals: A Supervision of Group Work Intervention

### Author(s) and Affiliation(s)

Lindsey M. Bell, MS,
The University of New Mexico

Kristopher Goodrich, Ph.D.,
The University of New Mexico

### Supervision Format and Modality

This intervention is intended for in-person group supervision of group work.

### Supervisee Development

This intervention was developed to assist supervisees in their master's practicum or internship. This intervention can be applied across all levels of supervisee development.

### Supervisory Goals and Learning Objectives

*Supervisees Will*

1. Identify and assess at least one short- and long-term anti-oppressive goal related to their group counseling and supervision work.
2. Demonstrate the ability to connect their goals to the three areas of multicultural competence foci (i.e., knowledge, awareness, and skills).
3. Describe the impact of the development and assessment of anti-oppressive goals and outcomes on each of the following: stakeholders, including the supervisee, supervisory group, group members, and the broader community.

### Time Required

This intervention is designed to be utilized throughout one academic semester during 60-minute supervisory sessions and may be repeated more than once.

**Materials:** Materials are optional; however, the supervisor can develop a handout for this intervention to aid the supervisees in their learning and application of the anti-oppressive intervention and development of 360 goals (i.e., connect proposed anti-oppressive intervention goals across the multicultural foci).

## Intervention Instructions

This anti-oppressive supervision intervention expands upon Goodrich and Luke's (2011) LGBTQ Responsive Model for Supervision of Group Work (RMSGW) to enhance supervisees' skills related to *Principle 6: Developing Goals and Assessing Outcomes Through Stakeholder Investment.* While Goodrich and Luke's LGBTQ RMSGW is a atheoretical model of group supervision developed to address the unique needs of LGBTQ individuals, the model's concepts can be adapted to provide culturally responsive group supervision for members from various social locations and intersectional identities. Stage-by-stage instructions are provided in what follows.

1.  The supervisor introduces the objectives of the intervention and discusses with the supervisees how these might fit within their overall supervisory development. In doing so, the supervisees and supervisor define and discuss 360 goals for the application of the intervention and how it will best aid the supervisees' development. If the supervisor prepared the suggested handouts or resources given previously, they should be provided to supervisees at this time.
2.  The supervisor introduces the areas of multicultural competence foci from Goodrich and Luke's (2011) LGBTQ RMSGW. Approaching the conversation from the consultant or teacher role, the supervisor might ask, "What motivates you to continually develop and assess your knowledge, awareness, and skills when working with individuals from marginalized groups in a group setting?" or "As you select interventions, what kind of impact/response do you wish to elicit from your group members?" The supervisor continues to ask reflective questions and clarify as needed related to the multicultural competence foci.
3.  The supervisor adopts the counselor role and intervenes at the intrapersonal level by inviting the supervisees to reflect on their current knowledge, awareness, and skills related to group work with members who experience intersectional oppression. For example, the supervisor can ask supervisees to identify challenges they have faced in addressing intersectional oppression within group settings and how they have approached these challenges thus far.

To help facilitate reflection, the supervisor transitions to the teacher role and offers examples of knowledge, awareness, and skills related to multicultural competence at interpersonal, intrapersonal, group-as-whole, and supra-group levels. The supervisor and supervisees also offer instances in which they have witnessed peers demonstrating any of these competencies in supervision. The supervisor can inquire about the supervisees' reflections by asking questions such as "What would be an example of an anti-oppressive group intervention that applies to your group work?" or "How might your cultural identities and social locations contribute to your present-day knowledge, awareness, and skills?"

4. The supervisor briefly proceeds into a didactic teacher role and introduces the concept of establishing and evaluating anti-oppressive 360 goals. The 360-degree goal evaluation model emphasizes the viewpoint of all relevant stakeholders (e.g., including but not limited to supervisees, supervisors, group members, and the broader community) that are closely associated with the intended goal outcomes (McCombs, 2014). Focusing on the intrapersonal point of entry, the supervisor directs supervisees to reflect individually and then as a group on short- and long-term 360 goals that will improve their knowledge, awareness, and skills in working with group members from diverse social locations and intersectional identities. The supervisor then transitions into the consultant role and supports the supervisees' goal setting by asking questions such as "What immediate actions will you take to expand your knowledge and awareness regarding your group members' lived experiences and cultural identities," or "How can you improve your knowledge, awareness, and skills to contribute to an inclusive, anti-oppressive group environment over time," or "How can reflecting on your own cultural identities, beliefs, and biases as well as your anti-oppressive responsibilities be integrated into short- or long-term anti-oppressive goals related to your group work?"

5. Returning to the teacher role, the supervisor explains who the stakeholders are and describes the importance of stakeholder investment. The supervisor asks the supervisees to identify stakeholders in their group work and reflect on the importance of stakeholder evaluation methods related to their short- and long-term anti-oppressive goals. After the supervisees share their reflections with the larger group, the supervisor facilitates the supervisees in discussing their observations. For example, the supervisor, acting as a consultant, might say, "What did you observe about including stakeholders using an anti-oppressive

approach? How did this change your ideas of short-and long-term anti-oppressive goals?" or "How might we involve input and evaluation from stakeholders given the short-and long-term goals developed today?"

6. Lastly, the supervisor assumes the role of the teacher and assists supervisees in refining their anti-oppressive 360 goals as needed by collaborating with the supervisees to create evaluation plans for their goals. Evaluation plans are personalized for each supervisee and include assessment methods tailored to the supervisees' anti-oppressive goals. For example, evaluation could occur at the intrapersonal level through mid-term and end-of-the-semester evaluations by the supervisor and self-assessments by the supervisees, as well as the group-as-whole level through anonymously surveying group members' perceptions of the supervisees' cultural responsiveness and anti-oppressiveness as group leaders at the conclusion of the group. The supervisor assumes the counselor role and uses the reflective questions that follow to support supervisees in integrating their learning from the intervention into their overall professional identity and future work.

## Supervisory Alliance and Relationship

Discussing anti-oppressive issues and attending to areas of recognized (or not) prejudice, bias, discrimination, and oppression can be cognitively, emotionally, and professionally challenging, both for the supervisor and supervisee. It is important to create a shared brave space where there is honesty, trust, open communication, and shared understanding. Setting initial ground rules/expectations may be helpful to review periodically. It is also important to explore the different identities that both the supervisor and supervisees bring to the work, how these influence perspectives and understandings, the relationships to group work, and how they impact the supervisory work and relationship.

## Legal and Ethical Considerations

Not all supervisors or supervisees are aware of anti-oppressive principles, although they may be more familiar with multicultural and social justice principles in counseling. As such, they should familiarize themselves with current literature in anti-oppression as well as the relevant ethical code and field-based ethical decision-making models.

## Reflective Questions

1. What motivates you to continually develop and assess your knowledge, awareness, and skills when working with individuals from marginalized groups in a group setting?
2. How might your cultural identities and social locations contribute to your present-day knowledge, awareness, and skills?
3. In what ways can you improve your knowledge, awareness, and skills to contribute to an inclusive, anti-oppressive group environment over time?
4. How might reflecting on your own cultural identities, beliefs, and biases be integrated into short- or long-term anti-oppressive goals related to your group work?
5. Moving forward, in what ways will you continue to involve input and evaluation from stakeholders in your short-and long-term anti-oppressive goal setting?

## Intervention Title: Supervisor Assessment from an Anti-Oppression Framework

## Author(s) Name, Credentials, and Affiliation(s)

Theodore R. Burnes, Ph.D.
University of Southern California

## Supervision Format and Modality

This supervision intervention was developed for use with individual supervisees conducted in-person.

## Supervisee Development

This intervention can be used across all levels of supervisee development; however, it is specifically designed to develop supervisee's understanding after at least six months of work. In addition, supervisees who have some introductory engagement with anti-oppression would be ideal for this intervention. This is an introductory level intervention.

## Supervisory Goals and Learning Objectives

1. Supervisees will be able to self-assess their initial development and articulate at least two areas of their own growth as clinicians.
2. Supervisees will be able to identify strategies for ongoing self-assessment and implement one new assessment strategy (co-constructed with supervisor).
3. Supervisees will be able to increase their own resilience and community care and implement one new strategy (co-constructed with supervisor) for increasing their resilience at an individual or community level.

## Time Required

This intervention is designed for a 60-minute supervisory session. The follow-up process may occur intermittently, taking 15 minutes of subsequent supervision sessions.

## Materials

The supervisor can use the attached handout or take notes throughout the process (a tablet and/or pen and paper are required for this alternative).

## Intervention Instructions

Consistent with strategies for clinical supervision grounded in cultural humility (Burnes & Manese, 2019) and anti-oppression (Peters & Luke, 2022), this supervision intervention assists the supervisee to self-assess skills related to Principle 6: *Developing Goals and Assessing Outcomes Through Stakeholder Investment.* As existing methods of assessment of supervisee skills are often problematic due to their grounding in oppressive ideologies, it is imperative that principles of anti-oppression be used in the assessment of supervisees' development.

1. The supervisor begins by explaining the importance of skills assessment as part of the supervision process, reviewing the learning objectives, and engaging the supervisee in a discussion about how these fit within both the overall supervisory relationship and the supervisee's overall learning goals.
2. As supervisees from various backgrounds may have experiences with assessment and evaluation rooted in oppression (del Mar Fariña & O'Neill, 2022), the supervisor invites the supervisee to consider how the assessment has felt unhelpful or biased. The supervisor can invite the supervisee to consider any experience throughout their history.
3. The supervisor then reviews any initial goals formed at the beginning of the supervisory relationship. The supervisor asks, "What progress have you made on these initial goals for yourself?" The supervisor can model by naming examples of when the supervisor has witnessed progress on one or more goals.
4. Next, the supervisor should facilitate the supervisee's exploration of how the supervisee's social locations have impacted their meeting of goals. For example, if a white male-identifying supervisee has wanted to work more with silence in the room and has a caseload of eight Mexican female-identified clients, the supervisor and supervisee should explore how the supervisee's race and gender have impacted the exploration (or lack of exploration) of silence in the room.
5. The supervisor should reflect examples of growth and also examples of challenge. Writing these down on a piece of paper or tablet that both the supervisor and the supervisee can see will allow both to build upon collective thought.

6. Following the assessment of initial goals, the supervisor should articulate some competencies specific to supervisees in the clinical setting. These competencies can be clinical (e.g., skills related to intervention, diagnostic, outreach, documentation, etc.), professional (e.g., interpersonal skills, affective regulation, integration of supervisory feedback, etc.), and community-contextual (e.g., working with larger communities; Burnes & Manese, 2019). The supervisor might ask, "What progress have you made in developing one or more of these competencies for yourself?" As the supervisor facilitates the supervisee's self-examination for this second domain, the supervisor can model examples of witnessed progress on one or more goals.

7. Next, the supervisor should facilitate the supervisee's exploration of how the supervisee's social locations have impacted the growth of these competencies. For example, if a cisgender male-identifying supervisee wants to gain more competency in assessing gender dysphoria with gender-diverse clients, the supervisee and supervisee could explore how the supervisee's gender identity has impacted the exploration (or lack of exploration) of dysphoria with clients.

8. Next, the supervisor checks in with the supervisee about how the assessment is feeling so far ("Can I stop us? How is this feeling? What might be helpful to name or attend to in our process right now?"). The supervisor can model by naming their own feelings that have emerged. The supervisor may also equalize this process by self-disclosing some of their feelings during their own self-assessment process, as supervisory self-disclosure can be a vital tool in evaluation processes within clinical supervision (Ertl et al., 2023). The supervisor then summarizes the process thus far, naming specific competencies and goals and how the supervisee's social locations have impacted development.

9. The supervisor then asks the supervisee what specific areas need to still be addressed. As the supervisor and supervisee address areas of growth, the supervisor facilitates a co-construction of goals for the supervisee. For each goal, the supervisor should ask about assessment strategies ("How will you know if you're getting closer to that goal?"). These goals and competencies may be in terms of clinical skill development, impact of community advocacy and liberation efforts, professional development markers, or growth in the self-of-the-clinician.

10. With the supervisee, the supervisor then identifies and addresses barriers through resistance and opposition (Peters & Luke, 2022); the supervisor and supervisee address potential barriers to any of the formulated goals. Such barriers could be intrapersonal (including lack of

self-care and/or internalized oppression), interpersonal, relational, or systemic. The supervisor continues to offer support and brainstorm strategies to counteract these future obstacles.

11. The supervisor and supervisee also reflect on the supervisee's wellness, self-care, and community care through relationships and community (Peters & Luke, 2022). As self-care is mostly defined by what individuals do for themselves, community care is what people put into and receive from the community that they have built around themselves (Adkins-Jackson et al., 2023). Thus, an assessment of a supervisee's progress and outcomes must include their development of self-care and community care that is infused into their professional development. The supervisor completes the intervention by asking the supervisee to outline different self-care and community-care strategies.

## Supervisory Alliance and Relationship

As supervisors must deconstruct privilege and oppression within supervisory relationships and processes, the supervisor should be attentive to various aspects of the supervisory relationship and the impact of both the intervention content and processes on this relational dynamic. For example, differences in supervisor and supervisee social locations and cultural identities may result in the supervisee feeling shamed for some of their goals about which they have a source of pride. Further, the supervisor should attend to their own pitch and tone when suggesting certain growth edges or skills so as not to shame a supervisee, which could be exacerbated by cultural differences in the supervision relationship.

## Legal and Ethical Considerations

It is the supervisor's responsibility to remain informed of and adherent to the relevant laws and ethics impacting both their and their supervisee's work (sometimes, the license of the supervisee and supervisor may differ, and the supervisor should be aware of both). Although supervisors must reflect contemporary multicultural, social justice, and advocacy laws and ethics, they may be less familiar with the application of these laws and ethics to anti-oppressive principles (Peters & Luke, 2022). Such lack of familiarity may result in supervisors needing to consult with other supervisors about their supervisee's competencies. Such consultation is critical, especially if the supervisor may exhibit an unawareness of how a supervisee's cultural identity may impact their professional development.

## Reflective Questions

1.  What resonated for you during this anti-oppressive supervision intervention?
2.  How did it feel to name areas in which you have grown with your supervisor? How did it feel to name future areas of growth?
3.  When did you feel most connected today to your professional identity? How might this connection impact your future anti-oppressive goals?

## Intervention Title: The Gestalt Dialogue Between the "Old" and "New" Selves: An Expressive Arts-Based Anti-Oppressive Supervision Intervention

### Author(s) and Affiliation(s)

Dan Li, Ph.D., NCC, LSC (K-12, NC)
University of Oklahoma Health Sciences

Yanhong Liu, Ph.D., NCC
Syracuse University

### Supervision Format and Modality

This intervention was specifically developed for use in individual, in-person sessions due to the expressive arts nature of this intervention; however, it can be adapted for various formats, including triadic, group, and peer supervision.

### Supervisee Development

This intervention is applicable at all levels of supervisee development but is specifically tailored for international supervisees early in their training (master's or doctoral) who are navigating the dual process of acculturation on both personal and professional levels. This intervention is particularly helpful for international supervisees early in their training.

### Supervisory Goals and Learning Objectives

1. Supervisees will be able to explore the dual process of acculturation at both personal and professional levels.
2. Supervisees will be able to make their unheard voices heard by externalizing an internal dialogue between their old and new selves as related to counseling and supervision.
3. Supervisees will be able to identify at least one short-term and one long-term anti-oppressive goal related to their counseling and supervision work.

### Time Required

This intervention could be used during the first half of a one-hour-long supervision session (duration), on a weekly basis (frequency).

## Materials

The setup for this activity includes a visual board with markers or, alternatively, paper and pen for participants to use. Additionally, there is a collection of expressive arts supplies available, which includes two empty chairs and a variety of toys and materials that encourage creative expression. These materials are carefully chosen to offer a diverse representation of cultures and abilities, featuring small figurines of people, animals, and symbolic objects.

## Intervention Instructions

Informed by Principle 6, this intervention emphasizes the ongoing cycle of setting and evaluating anti-oppressive goals, reflecting the continuous evolution of our old and new selves. At the beginning of each session, supervisees reflect on a significant incident from their last supervision, exploring how an intersection of their identities (e.g., age, gender, sexual orientation, ability status), positionalities (e.g., English language proficiency, immigration status), and social locations (e.g., socioeconomic status, perceived prestige of affiliated institutions), both old and new, have influenced their decision-making. This intervention embodies the liberating spirit of anti-oppression by unveiling what is present, absent, and at the margins—a process of *deconstruction*. For instance, a supervisee becomes aware of explicit and implicit factors that inform their decision-making in ethical dilemmas through externalizing the internal dialogue. Additionally, this intervention involves constructing structures and traditions that prioritize the voices and needs of marginalized individuals—a form of *reconstruction*. For example, a supervisee acknowledges, embraces, and even celebrates their differences (e.g., cultural, linguistic), viewing them as strengths that ground them rather than deficits that constrain them. It aids in setting goals for the current session and provides supervisors with valuable context for deliberate feedback in the long term. The intervention serves as an action-based approach to enhance supervisees' technical, perceptual, interpersonal, reflective, and personal competencies (Pugh & Margetts, 2020). Notably, although this intervention is specifically illustrated through the experiences of international supervisees, it can be adapted to various socio-cultural contexts, especially for populations whose voices have historically been unheard or marginalized.

1.  The supervisor explains the purpose and process of this intervention, utilizing visual aids or writing tools to illustrate the acculturation process at personal and professional levels. Drawing on Berry's acculturation theory (1997), this approach identifies with two dimensions—origin culture and host culture—leading to four outcomes:

marginalization, separation, assimilation, and integration, representing varying degrees of cultural identification. In this context, "old" signifies personal values and beliefs, while "new" represents the counseling profession's history, philosophy, and ethics (Li & Ai, 2020).

2.  If the supervisee agrees to the intervention, the supervisor offers various options for proceeding, allowing supervisees to choose their preferred expressive means. This flexibility in expression could be especially beneficial for international students whose first language is not English and for those new to counselor training (Li et al., 2018; Li & Liu, 2020).

3.  Using empty chairs as an example, the supervisor arranges two chairs facing each other to symbolize the supervisee's current/new and old selves. Guided by the supervisor, the supervisee moves physically and psychologically between the chairs, adopting different perspectives. This method assists the supervisee in making abstract thoughts or feelings more concrete and in externalizing potential internal conflicts. Consequently, the supervisor can more effectively identify the supervisee's strengths (e.g., resilience and the ability to navigate various cultures and spaces) and pinpoint areas requiring support (e.g., enhancing clarity in communicating the cross-cultural impact on counseling). The supervisor can then provide targeted support and guidance and improve stakeholder engagement as needed (e.g., involving the supervisee in guest speaker events for other classes or highlighting available writing and speaking services on campus).

4.  The supervisor needs to foster a safe and inclusive environment, allowing the supervisees to explore various aspects of themselves and deepen their dialogue. For example, the supervisor may indicate the importance of dismantling oppressive narratives and power structures. Additionally, they focus on how the intersection of these aspects could potentially impact their therapeutic work with clients by noting the need for culturally responsive and equitable practices. The intervention aims to bring some resolution or closure to internal conflicts embedded within multilayered cultural, social, political, legal, and economic contexts.

5.  Here is a series of probing questions:

    a.  Can you identify one short-term anti-oppressive goal that we can establish to enhance your supervision experience?
    b.  Can you describe who the empty chair represents for you today?
    c.  What would you like to say to [the old/new self] represented in the chair?
    d.  What do you wish [the old/new self] understood about your thoughts or perspectives?

e.  Now that you are in the other chair, representing a different self, how does it feel to be [the old/new self]?

f.  What do you think [the old/new self] would say in response to what you have just expressed?

g.  What are you learning about yourself in this dialogue?

h.  What does each side of this conversation need in order to find a resolution?

i.  How does this dialogue inform your ethical decision-making in similar scenarios?

j.  In light of today's dialogue, can you identify one long-term anti-oppressive supervisory goal?

## Supervisory Alliance and Relationship

Building a strong supervisory alliance involves more than just establishing a bond; it requires a mutual understanding of the intervention's goals and methods in supervision. The supervisor should communicate to the supervisee the potential of this intervention as a powerful method for exploring internal conflicts between their old and new selves and for promoting self-awareness and personal growth. Importantly, supervisors should emphasize that participation in this intervention is entirely voluntary. The supervisee is assured that their preference for alternative interventions will in no way influence their evaluation or standing, underscoring the commitment to a supportive and non-coercive supervisory relationship.

## Legal and Ethical Considerations

Beyond regular supervision, this intervention could be particularly beneficial for international supervisees in navigating and processing ethical dilemmas that arise from conflicts between professional and personal values. Additionally, it serves as a powerful tool for exploring supervisees' internal conflicts, especially those related to socio-cultural, political, legal, and economic factors. Accordingly, supervisors must clearly explain the grounding of Gestalt theory and its empirical foundation, as well as outline the potential risks, benefits, and ethical considerations associated with using this intervention. In delivering this intervention, the supervisor remains acutely aware of their role and boundaries within the supervision context. The supervisee may exhibit intense emotional reactions during experiential activities, such as the empty-chair dialogue. It is imperative for the supervisor to exercise clinical judgment and make professional referrals if they identify any significant personal needs of the supervisee that cannot be adequately addressed within the supervision context.

### Reflective Questions

1.  What stood out to you during this anti-oppressive supervision intervention, and what did you notice happening between you and your supervisor?
2.  In what ways might you apply this intervention to your counseling and our future supervision?
3.  When did you feel most competent today, and how might this impact your future anti-oppressive goals as well as stakeholder engagement?
4.  Where did you notice yourself struggling today, and what is needed to address this struggle?

# Challenging and Disrupting Oppression Through Broaching and Accountability

*Susan Branco, Michael M. Gale, Connie T. Jones, Kelly M. King, Melissa Luke, Harvey Charles Peters, and Melanie M. Wilcox*

## CHAPTER 8 INTERVENTIONS

### Intervention Title: Oppression Impact and Redress Plan

### Author(s) and Affiliation(s)

Harvey Charles Peters, Ph.D., NCC
Montclair State University

Melissa Luke, Ph.D., NCC, ACS, LMHC
Syracuse University

### Supervision Format and Modality

This anti-oppressive supervision intervention was developed for individual supervision being conducted virtually or in-person. With minor modifications, this supervision intervention can be implemented in triadic, group, or peer supervision.

### Supervisee Development

The intervention can be applied across all development levels, from master's and doctoral practicums to post-graduate professionals. The supervisor

DOI: 10.4324/9781003470656-8

should tailor the intervention to each supervisee's development level, considering their training in anti-oppression.

## Supervisory Goals and Learning Objectives

### Supervisors will:

1. Explore the supervisee's understanding of how oppression influences their therapeutic space and relationships.
2. Facilitate the supervisee's development of an action plan with supervisees to address oppression in clinical work.
3. Aid the supervisee in reviewing and learning from the process of addressing oppression in therapeutic spaces and relationships.
4. Review supervisees' adherence to accountability measures and commitment to addressing harm through supervision notes and follow-up discussions.

## Time Required

The intervention requires approximately 60 minutes for the initial intervention and an additional 20–30 minutes for subsequent supervision check-ins, with supervisors adjusting the time based on the supervisee's needs and process. Supervisors should allocate additional time and consider the group's dynamics if adapted for triadic or group supervision.

## Materials

Prior to the supervision session, the supervisor should review materials related to oppression, accountability, and redressing harm (Heitz & Rappaport, 2023; Ramírez Stege et al., 2020). The supervisor may consider providing the supervisee with resources that can aid in the intervention. The supervisor and/or supervisee will also need access to writing utensils and paper or electronic documentation (e.g., Word, Google Docs, etc.) as well as space to conduct a role-play. Supervisors should ensure accessible spaces, whether in-person or virtual, allowing supervisees to develop interventions suited to diverse needs.

## Intervention Instructions

The aim of this intervention is to aid a supervisee in the difficult and important work associated with addressing and redressing the impact of oppression within the therapeutic space and relationship that is essential for fostering an equitable and liberatory environment (Ramírez Stege et al., 2020). The Oppression Impact and Redress Plan (OIRP) is a structured approach to identifying, addressing, and repairing harm caused by oppressive actions, policies, and systems. Below is a systematic guide for implementing the OIRP with the aim of supporting supervisees' abilities to apply this plan in their work with clients.

1. The supervisor will begin this intervention by discussing and exploring a supervisee's understanding of the various dimensions and forms of oppression that can manifest in clinical work, including microaggressions, cultural erasure, interpersonal violence, and systemic injustices. The supervisor and supervisee can discuss and unpack questions, such as: (a) What does oppression mean to you personally and professionally? (b) How does oppression show up in the therapeutic space and relationship? (c) Can you tell me about a time when you have observed oppression (or related terms/constructs) in your therapeutic space and relationship? and (d) Can you tell me about how you work to identify and address instances of oppression within the therapeutic space and relationship? During this exploration, it is vital that the supervisor model and assist the supervisee in broaching to build a foundation of reflexivity, transparency, and vulnerability.

2. The supervisor builds upon the examples and impact identified in the initial discussion to frame the importance of intentionality, proactivity, and reflexivity in addressing and attending to intersectional oppression. Without intentionality, proactivity, and reflexivity, it is easy to reproduce and uphold systems of oppression within the therapeutic space and relationship. The supervisor and supervisee should briefly discuss and define what intentionality, proactivity, and reflexivity look like in anti-oppressive clinical work.

3. In addition, the supervisory dyad can explore that despite such efforts, it is easy and common to reproduce systems and cycles of violence. Thus, it is essential to intentionally plan and utilize tools to address oppression and the interpersonal and systemic harm it reproduces in the therapeutic space and relationship. The discussion can explore questions such as: (a) How does being aware of your role in perpetuating oppression affect you cognitively, emotionally, and somatically? (b) Can you tell me of a time when you did and did not broach and redress oppression caused in a therapeutic space and relationship? (c) How have you redressed oppression in your therapeutic space and relationship?

4. Following the conversation, the supervisor invites the supervisee to begin the process and work associated with using intentionality, pro-activity, and reflexivity to redress oppression and harm that occurred within the therapeutic space and relationship. Using a writing utensil and paper or another form of documentation (e.g., Word, Google Docs, etc.), the supervisor will provide the supervisee with the OIRP and guide them through the process. Although it may make sense to move in a linear fashion, the supervisory dyad can identify and decide the best process and course of action. The OIRP should include:

1. Identifying the oppressive event(s).
2. Identifying the harm (i.e., impact) and associated social locations (e.g., identities and structural inequalities).
3. Completing a personal assessment of one's biases, privilege, subjectivities (e.g., socio-cultural-political positionality), and structural components (e.g., racism, ableism, nationalism, hetero-sexism) that influenced the oppression.
4. Exploring the supervisee's intrapersonal experiences of the oppressive event to inform their accountability and redress the oppression.
5. Naming of the type(s) of oppression and impact it had on the client(s) emotionally, somatically, cognitively, and culturally.
6. Identifying the potential implications for the client as well as the therapeutic space and relationship.
7. Co-creating guiding objectives used to guide the redressing of oppression.
8. Locating and reviewing relevant scholarship, resources, and tools to inform the redressing of oppression in the therapeutic space and relationship.
9. Reviewing and identifying potential actions and practices that can be used to redress the oppression based on the client's socio-cultural-political needs and values.
10. Solidifying a list of actions accompanied by intrapersonal (i.e., self-betterment-focused) and interpersonal (i.e., client-focused) objectives.
11. Engaging in supervisor-supervisee role play to support the super-visee in practicing accountability and to redress oppression.
12. Implementing the proposed sequence of actions outside of supervision.
13. Revisiting the implantation and assessing the effectiveness (and address plan as needed).

14. Engaging in continued reflexivity to commitment towards redressing the oppression and maintaining accountability moving forward.

5. The supervisor and supervisee can conclude this intervention by outlining how they will follow up on the intervention in the subsequent supervision session. Moreover, they can determine if and how they will integrate accountability for and address oppression within the supervisory space moving forward.

## Supervisory Alliance and Relationship

This intervention necessitates supervisors and supervisors to work towards a strong supervisory alliance. Supervisors must model and co-construct an open, brave, and liberatory environment where oppression can be discussed honestly. Given supervisees are being asked to demonstrate humility, vulnerability, and accountability to redress oppression within the therapeutic space and relationship, the use of empathy, mutuality, and humility is essential to ensure supervisees feel understood, supported, and challenged. Accordingly, supervisors must also remain receptive to feedback and uphold the characteristics, values, and practices being asked of the supervisee, which is important yet difficult work. By cultivating an inclusive and anti-oppressive environment, supervisors can effectively support supervisees in applying the OIRP, thereby improving client care and fostering a more equitable therapeutic environment.

## Legal and Ethical Considerations

The supervisor should ensure that the intervention and OIRP do no harm (non-maleficence) and actively promote the well-being (beneficence) of both clients and supervisees (Ivey et al., 2023). It is important for supervisors to respect the supervisee's professional autonomy and the parallel process within the supervisee–client relationship while guiding them in the implementation of the OIRP. Given the nature of the intervention, supervisors must discuss potential legal liabilities for both themselves and the supervisees when addressing oppression in clinical work, particularly considering the legal risks associated with challenging oppressive behaviors within clinical systems.

## Reflective Questions

1. How can this intervention be used to inform the continued practice of taking accountability for and redressing oppression within the therapeutic space and relationship?
2. How can I continuously and systematically assess my practice of taking accountability and redressing oppression within the therapeutic space and relationship?
3. How can I work toward proactively limiting my recreating or upholding oppression within the therapeutic space and relationship?
4. How am I at allowing others to take accountability and redress oppression within my personal and professional spaces and relationships?

## Intervention Title: Group Supervision Broaching Presentations and Critical Analysis

## Author(s) Name, Credentials, and Affiliation(s)

Kelly M. King, PhD, LPCC, LMHC, NCC
*California State University, Sacramento*

## Supervision Format and Modality

This exercise is tailored to either in-person or virtual group supervision. If assigned in individual or triadic supervision, the supervisor can pose additional reflective questions and provide broaching examples with different features (e.g., varied goals and identities of members in the dyad) to maintain the goal of appreciating the complexity of broaching conversations.

## Supervisee Development

Supervisees receiving this intervention could be at the master's internship, doctoral practicum, or internship level. The intervention should follow classroom-based instruction on socio-cultural issues in counseling to bridge into the application of a culturally responsive counseling skill. The intervention level is intermediate. Some introductory knowledge of broaching is assumed; however, the supervisee is relatively new to the counselor role and is beginning to encounter the complexities of applying multicultural counseling skills.

## Supervisory Goals and Learning Objectives

1. Reflect on an initial broaching conversation with a counseling client.
2. Compare and contrast at least two different approaches to broaching across supervisees/counselors in the context of interpersonal style, identities represented in the counseling dyad, and broaching goals.
3. Define various applications for broaching and anti-oppression skillsets.
4. Describe one relational and one situational factor to consider when broaching.

## Time Required

The length of time required will depend on the number of supervisees in the group (ideally 4–6 members) and the amount of space devoted to the critical analysis portion. Supervisee presentations should be 5–10 minutes long.

At the conclusion of all presentations, a minimum of 20 minutes should be allocated to critical analysis following the supervisor's discussion prompts.

## Materials

In the simplest version of this exercise, you will need your supervision platform (i.e., videoconferencing room) and supervisee notes with responses to presentation prompts (for their reference or distribution). In a more elaborate version, you might use recording playback equipment. Ensure the equipment is charged, turned on, and cued up to the portion of tape that supervisees will play to streamline presentations. Supervisors can refer to analysis and reflection questions as needed by bringing this book or recording questions elsewhere.

## Intervention Instructions

1. **Assess supervisees' existing knowledge:** Supervisors can assess supervisees' existing knowledge of broaching by asking supervisees to generate a definition of the skill and list recommendations for application (King, 2021). Supervisors should ensure that both individual-level (e.g., differences in worldview and the counseling relationship) and systems-level (e.g., social stratification and unjust conditions that are oppressive to the client) elements of broaching are included in the supervisees' description. This assessment could inform supplemental reading assignments (see Bayne & Branco, 2018; Day-Vines et al., 2020; King & Borders, 2019) and guide supervisor feedback during the analysis portion of the exercise.

2. **Assign the exercise:** Provide supervisees with the below prompts that encourage reflection on their approach to broaching conversations (Day-Vines et al., 2021; King, 2021) before the supervision session in which you will facilitate the intervention:

   a. Identify an initial broaching conversation (e.g., early in the counseling relationship, first one to three sessions, first explicit discussion addressing cultural and/or power dynamics) you have had with a client that you feel was effective.

   b. Select an approximately two-minute clip of this recorded conversation, beginning with your opening broaching statement. **OR** Summarize an outline of this conversation (e.g., How did you phrase your broaching statement? How did you address identity and experiences of privilege and/or oppression? How did the client respond? How did you conceptualize and follow-up on the client's response?)

c.  Share your reflections on the following questions: What considerations did you make when deciding when and how to broach with this client? What do you believe makes this broaching conversation effective? To what extent is anti-oppression infused in the conversation? What appeared to be the impact of broaching on the client? How did you feel before, during, and after the broaching conversation?

3.  **Facilitate supervisee presentations:** During the supervision session, determine the order in which supervisees will present. Frame the intervention around the goal to deepen understanding of the complexity of broaching and anti-oppression dialogues and factors that can shape them. Before beginning presentations, identify common hesitations to broaching and briefly process related supervisee worries. For example, supervisors can ask about possible barriers to broaching and sources of discomfort for supervisees, such as possible emotional reactions, fear of exposing personal biases, worry about harming the client or how the client could view the counselor's identities, and uncertainty about how to navigate cultural differences (Wei et al., 2011). Instruct supervisees to attend to critical analysis questions while listening to presentations and to hold group discussions until the conclusion of all presentations. Monitor time so that each supervisee's presentation is between 5–10 minutes.

4.  **Engage in critical analysis:** The supervisor will open discussion by posing each prompt to the group and soliciting specific examples from presentations. The supervisor will then moderate the discussion, linking skills to identify common strengths and struggles across supervisee broaching examples. For example, the supervisor may note an example when a supervisee addressed structural oppression impacting the client or they could indicate missed opportunities to further explore relevant power dynamics. The supervisor will balance providing supportive and constructive feedback and offering challenges to supervisees as needed.

a.  What are the common features of these early, effective broaching conversations? How do these features contrast from instances when broaching was ineffective or did not unfold as intended?

b.  Distinctions across broaching examples? With respect to:

  i.  Broaching goal (e.g., address privilege, gather background information, identify the impact of oppression, repair rupture following microaggression).

ii. Identities represented (consider intersectionality of both client and counselor).

iii. Interpersonal style (e.g., tone, disposition, body language, comfort, self-disclosure).

iv. Individual and systems-level aspects of broaching (how were issues of identity, power, privilege, and oppression addressed?).

## Supervisory Alliance and Relationship

This exercise allows supervisees to compare real-world broaching conversations with attention to the nuances of this skill. Supervisees will likely differ in their positionalities, cultural identity development, and multicultural and anti-oppressive orientation. Presenting an example broaching conversation could feel vulnerable. Supervisors can acknowledge this reality and encourage supervisees to view culturally responsive counseling as an ideal to strive toward with humility and acceptance of personal limitations, emphasizing these qualities of multicultural orientation (Jones & Branco, 2020). If they have not already done so during supervision, the supervisor might model broaching before initiating this intervention to address the multiple identities and experiences in the room and share about their own developmental process with this skillset (Wilcox et al., 2022a). Supervisor modeling and reflecting on their personal development could normalize supervisee insecurities and reduce the power differential. For example, a supervisor might note ways that gaining more cultural self-awareness has improved their authenticity in broaching.

## Legal and Ethical Considerations

Whenever using session recordings in clinical supervision, it is necessary to ensure HIPAA and/or FERPA compliance, including proper storage and handling of confidential material. Further, if other group members could be acquainted with the client in the session, the group will need to take care to identify these instances and excuse the group members in question. Additionally, self-disclosure and sharing information about cultural group memberships are often part of broaching interventions. The supervisor can take steps to ensure that this information is not shared beyond the group setting without the member's approval and should encourage members to reflect on which cultural identities and associated life experiences they feel comfortable speaking about in clinical and supervisory contexts.

## Reflective Questions

1. How do we define and/or understand broaching differently now?
2. What considerations seemed to influence how the broaching statements were worded (e.g., which identities were addressed or overlooked, more or less comfortable to approach)?
3. What relational and situational factors should we consider when broaching with clients?
4. How can we use this deeper understanding to improve our broaching efforts in the future?
5. What, if anything, might differ when considering broaching with clients, peer group supervisees, and with me as the supervisor?

## Intervention Title: The Broaching Cultural Genogram: An Equitable and Empowering Supervisory Intervention

### Author(s) and Affiliation(s)

Connie T. Jones, PhD, LCMHCA, LCAS, NCC, ACS,
The University of North Carolina at Greensboro

Susan Branco, PhD, LPC, NCC, ACS, BC-TMH,
Palo Alto University

### Supervision Format and Modality

This anti-oppressive supervision intervention was developed for individual, triadic, or group supervision conducted virtually or in person. In triadic and group supervision, the supervisor engages with the supervisees and encourages and facilitates discussion between supervisees.

### Supervisee Development

This intervention can be used across developmental levels for supervisees in master's or doctoral practicum or internship, those with professional development/remediation plans, and post-graduate pre- and post-licensed professionals. The intervention level can be applied at the introductory, intermediate, and advanced levels.

### Supervisory Goals and Learning Objectives

1. Create and facilitate an inclusive and belonging environment where important socio-cultural identities and socio-cultural aspects are broached and explored.
2. Model for and train supervisees on how to use a Broaching Cultural Genogram (BCG) with clients.
3. Utilize the BCG to discuss concepts of power, privilege, and oppression in the supervisory relationship, the counselor-client relationship, and sociopolitical issues in the global society.
4. Use the BCG as an accountability method to highlight supervisor and supervisee growth and strength areas.

## Time Required

The intervention is ~30 to 50 minutes, depending on the levels of awareness of the supervisor and supervisee. If used in a triadic or group setting, the allotted time may need to be increased.

## Materials

The supervisor should review genogram examples with the awareness that the history of genograms is rooted in patriarchal and white supremacist values. Therefore, the supervisor should prepare to offer recommendations for an expansive and equitable genogram, as described by Warde (2012). Paper, pencils, markers, crayons, and stickers may be utilized for in-person supervision. The whiteboard function on an electronic video platform can be used in tele-supervision. Tele-supervision can also create a paper genogram and share it on their screen. A wide variety of expressive strategies (e.g., photograph/photovoice, sand tray/virtual sand tray, mixed media) can also be utilized.

## Intervention Instructions

1. The supervisor provides a rationale for the Broaching Cultural Genogram (BCG) to build supervisory relationships, discover more about salient identities, and explore how identities influence supervisee work with clients. The cultural genogram visually supports supervisees' ongoing awareness of how their identities influence their growth as professionals (Warde, 2012). For the purposes of modeling broaching behavior, the supervisor discusses how the BCG aids in discussions of power, privilege, and oppression in the supervisory relationship, the counselor-client relationship, and sociopolitical issues in the global society. For example: *What are your initial thoughts and reactions on using the BCG in our supervisory relationship? How do you envision this intervention helping us understand and navigate our identities in the context of our work together?*
2. Both supervisor and supervisee(s) create a genogram with as many generations as desired with emphasis on family of origin. The supervisor notes that access to many generations may be limited due to systemic constraints including but not limited to enslavement, immigration, deportation, adoption, war, etc. For example: *How might systemic constraints impact the creation of your BCG? How might broaching help us navigate these limitations?*

3. Each creates their own symbols and legend to transcend traditional genogram symbols and promote a more equitable representation of themselves and family identities. We encourage supervisors to welcome the creation of symbols beyond the historic square and circle shapes symbolizing men and women and using what resonates for them (i.e., stars, hearts, ovals, triangles, emojis, etc.). For example: *What symbols do you feel represent your family and identity most accurately?*

4. The supervisor and supervisee identify at least two salient family identities intergenerationally to highlight. The RESPECTFUL Model (D'Andrea & Daniels, 2001) can facilitate the process. Each letter in the model represents important identity categories to start the discussion. After the identification of family identities, the supervisor facilitates discussion on why those identities were chosen and the meanings they hold. Be mindful that the model is not an exhaustive list of identities. For example: *Which identities from the RESPECTFUL Model resonate most with you and why? How might these salient family identities influence your personal and professional development?*

5. The supervisor and supervisee identify at least two structural or institutional factors that positively or negatively impact their family systems to open dialogue on the impact on the family intergenerationally. For example: *How do you see institutionalized racism or other structural factors influencing your family system across generations? What potential impact might these structural factors have on our work? And you, as a counselor with your clients?*

6. The supervisor then initiates a dialogue rooted in the Intersectionality framework, focusing on the social location of identities and power, privilege, and oppression seen within each genogram. For example: *Can you identify specific examples within your genogram where power, privilege, or oppression may be present? How might these instances impact you and/or your family?*

7. The dialogue continues to explore social locations between the supervisor and supervisee and how power, privilege, and oppression show up during the supervisory relationship. For example: *What are some concerns or ways that power, privilege, and oppression can show up during our work together? How do your social locations influence the way you view yourself and how you see the world?*

8. The supervisory dyad co-creates a plan to navigate conflicts that may occur in session due to socio-cultural context, power, privilege, and oppression, including how to repair potential ruptures due to cultural missteps, cultural insensitivities, and lack of cultural competence and humility. For example: *What are some ways that we can work to repair ruptures that may occur during our work together?*

9. Once the supervisees have reflected on their BCG and engaged in discussion about the socio-cultural context of their genogram, the supervisor broaches and explores biases, stereotypes, values, beliefs, and attitudes that may impact clinical practice (Day-Vines et al., 2007). The supervisor and supervisee co-construct ensures client welfare and promotes supervisee(s) professional and personal development. For example: *Let's take some time to reflect on any biases, stereotypes, attitudes, or beliefs that might impact your clinical practice. Now, we can co-construct a plan for growth and development. Don't worry; everyone has biases and/or beliefs; working through them is just part of the process. I wonder in what ways your biases may affect our supervisory relationship, and how can we navigate them together?*

10. To work from a strength-based perspective with a focus on empowerment, the supervisor and supervisee examine their genograms, discussing individual and family strengths and processing from an intergenerational perspective. They discuss how they can utilize their strengths in the supervisory relationship and, by extension, how the supervisee(s) can utilize their strengths in their clinical work. For example: *What strengths do you see in your genogram and family system that can contribute to our supervisory work? How might we amplify our strengths to enhance both our supervisory relationship and your clinical practice?*

11. The supervisor reminds the supervisee that the BCG will be an ongoing reference point throughout supervision as a working document. For example: *We will use the BCG as an ongoing reference point throughout our work together. At any point, we can make revisions or additions to our genograms, revisit discussions, keep discussions ongoing, and explore new areas.*

## Supervisory Alliance and Relationship

The intervention requires vulnerability by both the supervisor and supervisee. Attunement and attention reactions to disclosing personal information should be part of the supervisory process to include frequent check-ins about the experience and relationship. Discussing family history can elicit discomfort and, therefore, the supervisor should be vigilant for potential ruptures and or recommendations for counseling referral for the supervisee.

## Legal and Ethical Considerations

Supervisors must provide supervisees with informed consent for supervision that includes language related to broaching a range of salient identities to enhance the supervisory relationship. It is important that the supervisor recognize and acknowledge the vulnerability around self-disclosure and be aware that ethical decision-making models may need to be used if ethical issues arise during broaching.

## Reflective Questions

1. As the BCG offers a visual tool for socio-cultural identities and contexts, what new areas did you discover worthy of exploration?
2. What are gaps in your knowledge or understanding and how could it affect maintaining socio-cultural attunement with supervisees?
3. In what ways did the BCG facilitate broaching between the supervisee and supervisor?
4. How can you begin to work through biases, stereotypes, and attitudes that may arise from the BCG?
5. How does the BCG capture social location and the constructs of power, privilege, and oppression related to socio-cultural identities?

## Intervention Title: Broaching and Accountability Through the Use of Anti-Oppressive-Interpersonal Process Recall (AO-IPR)

### Author(s) and Affiliation(s)

Michael M. Gale, Ph.D., LP
Springfield College

Melanie M. Wilcox, Ph.D., ABPP, LP
University at Albany

### Supervision Format and Modality

This anti-oppressive supervision intervention was developed for individual supervision conducted in person or virtually.

### Supervisee Development

This intervention may be used at all levels of supervisee development (e.g., practicum, internship, post-graduate). Assessment of the supervisee's development begins with therapeutic skills but should also include areas of critical consciousness, self-awareness, identity development status across multiple identities (e.g., racial identity, sexual identity), and openness to feedback.

### Supervisory Goals and Learning Objectives

*Supervisees will:*

1. Utilize the Interpersonal Process Recall (IPR) (e.g., Kagan, 1980) model as a supervisory framework for identifying and discussing instances and impact of oppression within clinical practice.
2. Recognize and articulate their own and others' experiences of oppression, privilege, and power within therapeutic interactions, thus enhancing self-awareness and accountability.
3. Identify institutional, systemic, and structural issues contributing to oppression and contextualize the therapeutic relationship and client presentation.
4. Display a commitment to anti-oppressive practice and the development of critical consciousness through the reflective examination of therapy sessions and identify and rehearse anti-oppressive responses.

## Time Required

The intervention requires a minimum of 30 minutes but can be expanded based on the depth and breadth of interpersonal exploration.

## Materials

Prior to the supervision session, the supervisor should review the literature on broaching (e.g., Day-Vines et al., 2021; Jones & Branco, 2020, 2023), accountability, understanding systems and structures of oppression, and IPR. The supervisor is encouraged to provide the supervisee with materials aimed at fostering critical consciousness and an anti-oppressive orientation throughout the supervisory relationship and to highlight these materials in preparation for the intervention. Beforehand, the supervisee should obtain informed consent from clients to record sessions for training purposes. Additionally, the supervisor should obtain informed consent from the supervisee regarding the use of these recordings to facilitate supervision, including independent supervisor review and reviewing together during supervision. It is recommended that the supervisor and supervisee both review session recordings prior to the supervision session and identify segments that are salient to broaching oppression-based content. However, because all therapeutic and supervisory interactions occur within the context of overarching systems of oppression, it is not strictly necessary for prior review as relevant opportunities will arise naturally. The supervisor should come prepared with a written or mental list of guided reflection questions based on the IPR model adapted for anti-oppressive supervision.

## Intervention Instructions

1.  The supervisor begins by introducing the IPR model to the supervisee as a method of using recorded therapy sessions review to heighten awareness of thoughts, emotions, and relational dynamics occurring throughout the therapeutic process. The supervisor informs the supervisee that anti-oppressive-IPR (AO-IPR) also facilitates critical consciousness (similar to as described in Ivers et al., 2017) by broaching oppression-based considerations and facilitating accountability through identifying and rehearsing anti-oppressive responses related to heightened awareness and knowledge of systemic and structural oppression and their effects on the client and the dyad. Based on this provision of information, the supervisor seeks the supervisee's consent to participate in this reflective process within supervision, mindfully

monitoring for and addressing the supervisee's hesitance given the power differential.

2. The supervisor engages the supervisee in a discussion about personal experiences, observations, and reflections on societal, institutional, and systemic oppression, including their own participation in oppressive dynamics, whether intentional or unintentional.

3. The supervisor and supervisee utilize a relevant session recording and identify moments in the therapeutic encounter that prompt deeper reflection on the supervisee's and clients' positions relative to systems and structures of oppression and experiences of structural violence and vulnerability (Wilcox et al., 2024). The supervisor and supervisee may both pause the recording to allow for the AO-IPR process.

4. The supervisor guides the supervisee through reflective questions (such as those described in Ivers et al., 2017) to uncover underlying assumptions, biases, and power dynamics and bring focus to the supervisee's thoughts, feelings, and physiological responses that arise. The following facilitative questions can foster anti-oppressive attitudes and action:

   • In what ways did this clinical work challenge or fail to challenge oppression?
   • To what extent did the actions or disclosures of the client or supervisee reflect internalized oppression?
   • Might any of the client's or clinician's actions be interpreted as a microaggression or other form of interpersonal discrimination or bias?
   • To what extent does the client's disclosure reflect experiencing or perpetuating interpersonal discrimination or structural vulnerability? To what extent was this given focus within the session?
   • In what ways can the client's disclosure be understood through the lens of structural violence (such as in education, housing, employment, health care, criminal legal system)?
   • Based on these reflections, what additional knowledge and skills do you need to acquire, further develop, or apply to promote anti-oppression within this therapeutic work?

5. As a point of divergence from IPR as traditionally practiced (focusing on awareness and limiting the use of the teaching role), the supervisor encourages the supervisee to further consider how they might address similar situations differently in the future to more effectively challenge oppression and promote equity and then provides additional knowledge through psychoeducation and sharing of resources (e.g., how to case conceptualize from an anti-oppressive structural competencies perspective as described in Wilcox et al., 2024).

6.  The supervisor assists the supervisee in co-creating strategies for further anti-oppressive action within the individual clinical relationship, as well as in relevant areas beyond the specific clinical relationships, such as through advocacy and prevention work. For example, the supervisor could share relevant local resources that might be useful for the supervisee to share with the client or even facilitate the client's connection directly. The supervisor might also share policy advocacy opportunities and relevant training (e.g., how to contact a state legislator about a pending anti-transgender state policy to advocate against it).

7.  The supervisor continuously models broaching topics of oppression and accountability, demonstrating empathy, cultural humility, and the ability to recognize one's own biases and privileges throughout the session. The supervisee then practices these skills through role-playing scenarios, drawing from real session examples when possible.

8.  The supervisor provides constructive feedback on the supervisee's practice, focusing on areas of strength, growth, and further development. The supervisor and supervisee reflect together on the process of broaching, critical consciousness, taking accountability, and emphasizing the relevance to therapeutic relationships and the broader implications for social justice in counseling. For example, the supervisor may intentionally use immediacy to address supervisory dynamics and processes that arose within AO-IPR.

9.  The supervisor and supervisee conclude by discussing the importance of continued learning, self-reflection, and action toward becoming more effective in addressing and mitigating structural violence and vulnerability within clinical practice. They then develop an action plan that includes specific commitments to incorporating broaching and accountability into their counseling practices.

### Supervisory Alliance and Relationship

The supervisor's cultural humility and critical consciousness facilitate the development of a strong supervisory working alliance marked by safety and trust, which is vital to minimizing the risk of nondisclosure and supervisee harm (Ellis et al., 2014). This cultivated trust and safety in the supervisory dyad promotes openness and vulnerability, particularly when discussing sensitive topics such as oppression and accountability.

### Legal and Ethical Considerations

The supervisor ensures all recordings are obtained and used in compliance with ethical guidelines and legal requirements, including confidentiality and informed consent. Additionally, the supervisor attends carefully to the power imbalance inherent within the supervisory relationship. In order to avoid misuse of power leading to harmful or inadequate supervision (Ellis et al., 2014), the supervisor balances emphasizing the value of vulnerability and openness in the AO-IPR process with empowering the supervisee to voice consent or nonconsent to engage in this reflective process within supervision.

## Reflective Questions

1. How can you use the IPR process more effectively to foster critical consciousness and anti-oppressive practice in your counseling?
2. How can you ensure the counseling relationship is a space for challenging and disrupting oppression?
3. What action plans can you develop with your supervisor to integrate broaching and accountability into your ongoing counseling practice and supervisory work?

## Intervention Title: Broaching and Accountability: Practicing and Modeling Through a Real-Play

### Author(s) and Affiliation(s)

Harvey Charles Peters, Ph.D., NCC
Montclair State University

Melissa Luke, Ph.D., NCC, ACS, LMHC
Syracuse University

### Supervision Format and Modality

This anti-oppressive supervision intervention was developed for individual supervision being conducted virtually or in-person. With minor modifications, this supervision intervention can be implemented in triadic, group, or peer supervision.

### Supervisee Development

Although variations will exist depending on supervisees' exposure to and current level of training and practices concerning oppression, interpersonal violence, and subjugation, it can be used across all development levels. With that, the supervisor should implement the intervention with the supervisee's development in mind, whether that be master's practicum or internship, doctoral practicum or internship, professional development plans/remediation plans, post-graduate and pre-licensed professionals, or post-graduate and post-licensed professionals.

### Supervisory Goals and Learning Objectives

1. Explore and deepen the supervisee's understanding of the cognitive, emotional, and physiological impact of oppression, interpersonal violence, and subjugation within interpersonal relationships.
2. Reflect on the experiences of causing and receiving socio-cultural harm.
3. Practice the process of broaching and attending to socio-cultural harm in the context of the counselor-client relationship.
4. Identify future actions to promote broaching and taking accountability related to socio-cultural harm within the therapeutic relationship.

## Time Required

The intervention requires approximately 30 minutes. Based on the allotted time, supervisors can make adjustments as they see necessary. Time will be influenced by the level of reflectivity and awareness the supervisee has of associated constructs and critical consciousness. However, if this is adapted within triadic or group supervision, additional time and consideration will be necessary.

## Materials

Before the supervisor uses this intervention, the supervisor should review materials related to broaching culture and harm as well as take accountability for the intentional and unintentional impact of socio-cultural harm, oppression, interpersonal violence, and subjugation. The supervisor may provide the supervisee with resources that can aid in the attitudes and beliefs, knowledge, skills, and actions. The superior will also need space to conduct a role-play. Lastly, the supervisor should consider the working space to ensure each supervisee, whether in-person or virtual, has the space to develop their intervention in an accessible environment for various needs and abilities.

## Intervention Instructions

1.  The supervisor and supervisee will begin by discussing the cognitive, emotional, and physiological impact of oppression, interpersonal violence, and subjugation that can arise within interpersonal relationships (Malott et al., 2015). This exploration can include psychoeducation; however, the aim is to focus on one's lived experiences and meaning-making.
2.  The supervisor will begin with a mutual discussion of the cognitive, emotional, and physiological impact of oppression, interpersonal violence, and subjugation that can arise within interpersonal relationships. The supervisor will explore times they both have experienced or observed socio-cultural-related oppression, interpersonal violence, and subjugation. Questions can include: What was the experience? What was the impact? How did it feel? How did it impact others? What potential implications did it have for interpersonal relationships? The supervisor should foster a sense of bravery, openness, and perspective-taking when exploring these questions.
3.  Following the initial exploration, the supervisor will begin by modeling a series of questions. The aim is to model and build rapport for the importance and process of broaching and taking accountability for

the potential harm and upholding of oppression, whether intentional or unintentional, that can and will occur within the process of clinical practice and clinical relationships. After the supervisor models the process, the supervisee will be asked to do the same. Given the power differentials and professional nature of the relationship, the supervisor should be intentional in what they disclose and not place the supervisee in a situation where they are responsible for 'taking care' of the supervisor.

4.  The supervisor and supervisee will explore the following prompts: (a) how they caused socio-cultural harm, (b) explain the situation and impact, (c) identify how they did or did not acknowledge and apologize, and (d) explain how they took or did not take accountability (Cullors, 2022). The prompts can be used to guide the process; however, the supervisor can adapt the prompts as they see fit. Following, the dyad can explore the experience, meaning-making, and relevancy to counseling and supervision.

5.  Next, the supervisor and supervisee will take turns sharing a time they experienced socio-cultural harm. The supervisor can encourage the supervisee to consider a broad range of manifestations of socio-cultural harm. If they cannot identify a socio-cultural harm, they can select another interpersonal harm. The supervisor and supervisee will explore the following prompts: (a) How they experienced socio-cultural harm, (b) Explain the situation and impact, (c) Identify how the person did or did not acknowledge and apologize, (d) Explain how the other person did or did not take accountability, and (e) Examine the experience of receiving and not receiving an apology and someone taking accountability (Cullors, 2022). The prompts can be used to guide the process; however, the supervisor can adapt the prompts as they see fit. Following, the dyad can explore the experience, meaning-making, and relevancy to counseling and supervision.

6.  After, the supervisory dyad will discuss and explore their understanding of the importance of broaching and accountability concerning socio-cultural harm. The discussion may include and is not limited to knowledge, strengths, concerns, previous experiences, skills, and models that can be used to guide the process of broaching and taking accountability (Day-Vines et al., 2021).

7.  Subsequently, after completing both sets of discussions, the supervisor and supervisee can use one of the examples they discussed or identify a different situation for a real play (i.e., role-play based on real details). The supervisee will practice broaching and taking accountability within the context of the counselor-client relationship (Day-Vines et al., 2021). The supervisee should be prepared to: (a) broach the situation and harm, (b) acknowledge the impact, (c) take accountability, (d) attend to the client, and (e) identify actions to move forward.

8.  The supervisor will then provide the supervisee with feedback as well as explore the process, experience, and applicability moving forward. The purpose is to build upon the examples and set a foundation that builds upon various counseling broaching and cultural skills that can aid the supervisee in being able to broach and take accountability for socio-cultural harm within their therapeutic relationships. Additionally, it can establish similar dynamics within the context of the supervisory relationship.

9.  Lastly, the supervisory dyad will explore action strategies and commitments to broaching and taking accountability for socio-cultural harm within counseling and supervision (Jones & Branco, 2020; Jones et al., 2019).

## Supervisory Alliance and Relationship

Supervisors must carefully manage power dynamics, culture, vulnerability, and potential harm when exploring socio-cultural issues, requiring immediacy and attention to content and process. Regular check-ins at the end and start of sessions help assess the impact on the supervisory relationship, ensuring any issues are promptly addressed.

## Legal and Ethical Considerations

The supervisor should be aware of the implications of self-disclosure and how to partake in the demystifying of self-disclosure and the necessary professional boundaries. It is essential that the supervisor be aware of the implications of self-disclosure and work to ensure they are appropriate, culturally responsive, and not placing the supervisee in the role of taking care of the supervisor. When exploring experiences of socio-cultural harm, there is a chance that legal and ethical issues arise, which may require the use of an ethical decision-making model, consultation, peer supervision, or professional action.

## Reflective Questions

1.  What did you learn about broaching and accountability in clinical relationships?
2.  What are supports and hinderances that may impact broaching and taking accountability for socio-cultural harm?
3.  How can you attend to relational ruptures that result from socio-cultural harm?
4.  How can you practice broaching and accountability within your personal and professional lives?

CHAPTER 9

# Identifying and Addressing Barriers Through Resistance and Opposition

*Peggy L. Ceballos, Philippa Chin, Karina Crescini, Melissa J. Fickling, Natoya Haskins, Kavita Khara, Melissa Luke, and Harvey Charles Peters*

## CHAPTER 9 INTERVENTIONS

### Intervention Title: Supporting the Identification and Addressing of Barriers: Supervisors' Intentional Resistance and Opposition (SIAB-SIRO)

#### Author(s) and Affiliation(s)

Melissa Luke, Ph.D., NCC, ACS, LMHC
Syracuse University

Harvey Charles Peters, Ph.D., NCC
Montclair State University

#### Supervision Format and Modality

This supervision intervention was developed for in-person or virtual individual supervision-of-supervision, often known as "sup of sup." With modifications, it can be adapted for use in triadic or group supervision-of-supervision, as well as use in supervision of counseling.

DOI: 10.4324/9781003470656-9

## Supervisee Development

This supervision intervention is geared toward advanced supervisors who are trained in and conducting supervision-of-supervision; likely doctoral student supervisors and advanced practitioners serving as site supervisors or training directors.

## Supervisory Goals and Learning Objectives

Supervisees will:
1. Engage radical reflexivity in their examination of the micro- and macro-level content of their supervision to identify examples of barriers to anti-oppressive practices.
2. Supervisees will expand their awareness and recognition of the ways they enact and/or uphold systemic barriers impacting their supervisees and, ultimately, the clients they serve.
3. Develop strategies to resist and oppose oppressive forces within their supervisory relationships.
4. Increase their ability to transfer SIAB-SIRO into future work with their own supervisees.

## Time Required

This anti-oppressive intervention is designed for use within a 60 to 75-minute supervision-of-supervision session.

## Materials

Supervisors of supervision need to refamiliarize themselves with the concept of critical discourse, radical reflexivity, and how oppressive practices have been systemically upheld within the mental health disciplines (Jamieson et al., 2023; Locke & Budds, 2020; Smith et al., 2023). In addition, they need access to one of their supervisee's supervision sessions for review prior to supervision-of-supervision.

## Intervention Instructions

1. Prior to supervision-of-supervision, the supervisor of supervision reviews the supervisee's supervisory session and identifies no more than three to four exchanges wherein the supervisory dyad

engaged in micro- and macro-level content that may reflect barriers to anti-oppressive practices and prepares to discuss these within the upcoming supervision-of-supervision.

2.  The supervisor of supervision then introduces the supervision-of-supervision intervention to the supervisee, explaining that the focus of the intervention includes not only *what is said* within the supervisee's supervisory session but also *how words and talk are used* in the session, the *ways in which the discourse is accomplished*, specifically that upholds or challenges oppressive forces and structures.

3.  The supervisor of supervision provides the supervisee with examples of how critical discourse (Locke & Budds, 2020) and radical reflexivity (Smith & Luke, 2021, 2023) can support anti-oppressive practice and goals, helping to translate the research context into a supervisory audit of sorts.

4.  Next, the supervisor of supervision collaborates with the supervisee to identify prior supervision-of-supervision talk wherein not only what was said was impactful, but how it was said was of influence. For example, the supervisor of supervision may ask, "When you reflect on our past supervision-of-supervision sessions, when might my non-verbal or para-verbal communication accentuate or alter the meaning of what was said?" If the supervisee struggles to identify an example, the supervisor may wish to introduce one themselves (see example in Supervisory Alliance and Relationship).

5.  After discussing these, the supervisor of supervision normalizes the occurrence and suggests that they will use the supervision-of-supervision session to extend this work into the examination of the supervisee's supervision session, soliciting discussion of the supervisee's anticipatory experience of this.

6.  The supervisor reminds the supervisee that they have reviewed the recorded session previously and identified a few sections to discuss, playing the first example and inviting the supervisee to consider how the micro—and macro—discursive content may reflect systemic barriers and/or challenge and address such. For example, the supervisor may suggest, "When I listen to the exchange between you and your supervisee, I am wondering about what oppressive factors may be taken for granted and remain unchallenged by you, as well as by your supervisee," "How might hierarchies or race, ethnicity, gender, class, religion or other identities remain unaddressed in this section and leave the resultant health disparities (such as diagnosis and access to treatment) unchallenged," or "What types of challenges and barriers may have led to or upheld the unaddressed oppressive forces?"

7.  Following the processing of the supervisee's response with questions such as "What is happening right now as you realize this?" or "How is it to consider the potential impact of the identified exchange?" the supervision-of-supervision dyad collaboratively generates two or more possible strategies to redress and/or synthesize the awareness into supervisory behaviors.

8.  The supervisor-of-supervision repeats the process in steps 6 and 7 with another section of the recorded session, offering the supervisee additional feedback that may contain more immediacy and raising discrepancy to expand the supervisee's perspectives. For example, the supervisor may note, "I appreciate your insight and ability to closely examine this exchange because I think you have identified important micro—and macro—discursive aspects. At the same time, I am also hearing . . . also wondering if . . . also aware of . . . . What are your thoughts about those possibilities?" The supervisor repeats as many times as time allows and can also suggest that the supervisee review an additional recording before the next session and bring in an example of their own to discuss.

9.  The supervisor concludes the supervision-of-supervision by supporting the supervisee to consider the possibility of their own use of SIAB-SIRO with their future work supervisees. The supervisor may note, "The supervisory space can be considered a microcosm of the larger systems of which we are part, and therefore, they naturally have the same potential to reflect the systemic and oppressive factors therein, but at the same time, they offer us an opportunity to model how to identify the barriers and engage in the disruption of these. What benefits do you see in this? What challenges? And how and when could it be helpful for your supervisees' development to do so?"

## Supervisory Alliance and Relationship

As is incumbent in the supervisory experience, particularly related to reflexivity and the examination of newly discovered bias and behavior, supervisees may experience discomfort, fear, shame, threat, and avoidance. Depending on the development of the supervisee and the strength of the supervisory relationship, the supervisor of supervision may wish to engage in intentional self-disclosure, offering an example of their discursive practice in the past wherein the micro—and macro—content of their communication inadvertently countered their conscious intentions. For example, they may say, "Despite my active commitment to anti-oppressive practices, particularly in supervision, I have identified instances when my words and the supervisory talk did not reflect this. I'd like to share the example, model how I redressed it once I was aware, and then discuss how this may impact our work."

## Legal and Ethical Considerations

Given the use of recorded sessions, informed consent and the use of HIPAA-compliant technology for the recording, storage, and transfer of recordings is necessary. Although uncommon, it is possible that through the close examination of the SIAB-SIRO intervention that the supervisor could identify gatekeeping concerns. If so, the supervisor of supervision is advised to adhere to appropriate documentation, engage in the requisite ethical practices, and communicate in accordance with the policies of the supervisory context.

## Reflective Questions

1.  What can get in the way of our radical reflexivity as supervisors? Relatedly, what has assisted in your ability in the past as well as today?
2.  Describe how your expectations leading up to the use of SIAB-SIRO intervention were similar to and different from your experience of it today.
3.  What did you discover about the language and discursive content within your supervision that surprised you, and what did you learn that will help support your supervisory development?
4.  What connections may exist between systemic barriers (as well as the strategies to address them) in your recorded session and that of our supervision-of-supervision? In your supervisee's counseling?

## Intervention Title: Leveraging Reflexive Exploration to Build Anti-Oppressive Praxis: Integrating Narrative and Working Cross-Cultural Approaches

### Author(s) and Affiliation(s)

Philippa Chin, Ph.D., LPC, LMFT, NCC
Barry University

Natoya Haskins, Ph.D., LPC, NCC
University of Virginia

### Supervision Format and Modality

This supervision intervention can be implemented in triadic, group, or peer supervision.

### Supervisee Development

This intervention was developed for use within the supervision or training experience. The supervisor and supervisee will embark on a parallel process during this intervention in the development of their anti-oppressive praxis. Therefore, the supervisor must be aware of the progressive nature of the intervention, whereby the supervisor's ability to reflectively explore personal and political spheres should be more advanced than that of the students. The supervisor will need to measure the level of reflexive and anti-oppressive capabilities of the supervisee by using the Multicultural Supervision Inventory (MSI; Wong & Wong, 2020). Following the administration of the MSI, there will be an introduction and reflection on the provision or lack thereof of anti-oppressive and anti-racist training for future mental health professionals from institutions. Assessing the supervisee's ability to hold such discourse and reflect on anti-oppression will be pertinent to modifying the intervention approach from moderate (the supervisor modeling conversations and supporting self-reflexivity) to more intermediate (the supervisee integrating anti-oppression, social justice, equity, and diversity into case conceptualization and practice). This intervention was developed for introductory and intermediate levels of supervision.

### Supervisory Goals and Learning Objectives

1. Facilitate the development of counselors' anti-oppressive praxis.
2. Develop the reflexive exploration skills of personal and political spheres, describing at least one example from each that can illuminate barriers.

3. Apply the anti-oppressive approaches and reflexive skills into clinical practice.
4. Identify at least one example of your professional development as a socially just change agent equipped to analyze, resist, and transform oppression.

## Time Required

Forty-five to 60 minutes per supervision session. Each phase or step of the intervention is implemented throughout the course of several supervision sessions. The supervisor may decide to focus on one phase over several sessions, while another phase may be accomplished during one session.

## Materials

The Multicultural Supervision Inventory (MSI) is a questionnaire that assesses the multicultural supervision process across four areas: attitudes and beliefs, knowledge and understanding, skills and practice, and relationships. It may be accessed by going to http://www.drpaulwong.com/wp-content/uploads/2018/03/Multicultural-Supervision-Inventory-MSI-Wong-Wong–2000.pdf.

## Intervention Instructions

1. The supervisor and supervisee will engage in *co-constructed discourse* on personal and professional anti-oppression, social justice, equity, and diversity approaches toward clinical case conceptualization and practice. The supervisor will initially measure the level of reflexive and anti-oppressive capabilities of the supervisee by MSI. Following the assessment, the supervisor will give verbal prompts or questions to facilitate critical thought on the supervisee's personal understanding and positionality around anti-oppression. The perspectives and experiences of the supervisee are valued and discussed. Reflective questions for this step include "Can you describe your positionality around anti-oppression towards the counseling process?" and "How does oppression fit into your experiences?"
2. The supervisor and supervisee will *enter a contract* whereby they will both collaboratively consider how anti-oppressive practices show up within the supervisor/supervisee relationship, within the supervisee, and the client/counselor relationship. The supervisor and supervisee engage in active reflection of the role of anti-oppression, social

justice, equity, and diversity in the supervision relationship throughout the supervision process (Lee & Kealy, 2018). Therefore, the contract may be an evolving developmental process that may be revisited
periodically. The contract will provide some consistency in how the
anti-oppressive praxis will be incorporated into supervision. Reflective questions for this step include "How would you like to address
some of the discomfort that might be felt when discussing systemic
oppression," "How should we identify and reveal oppression within
the supervision process," and "What steps will be taken to address anti-
oppression within case conceptualization?"

3. In this step, the supervisor and supervisee *actively listen* for oppressive markers during interaction with the supervisee and the client to
   see where anti-oppressive practices may be implemented into clinical
   practice. They will actively listen for examples of exploitation, powerlessness, and other forms of systemic oppressive markers that may
   be defined as racism, sexism, classism, and ableism, or other forms
   of injustice. Then the supervisor and supervisee seek to deconstruct
   the narrative given by the client by being curious about the origins
   of the issue and the belief system involving the dominant ideology (Bernard & Goodyear, 2019). Deconstruction of the narrative
   is achieved by focusing on developing an understanding of how the
   oppressive marker is influencing the client's presenting issues. Active
   listening will create an awareness and examination of how oppression
   is experienced by the client and within the supervisory relationship.
   Reflective questions for this step include "What oppressive markers or perspectives should be considered related to the issue," "What
   oppressive markers or perspectives are important to the client's family," and "What social justice issues emerge for the supervisee and
   the supervisor?"

4. The next action involves *self-reflexivity*, which includes the use of
   the reflective processing narrative strategy, which allows individuals to observe themselves from an external perspective (Chang et al.,
   2009). The supervisor model's self-reflexivity fosters the supervisee's
   self-reflexivity. The goal of this self-reflexivity stage is to show how
   challenging it is to navigate reflexivity and how oppression causes discomfort for all to discuss during practice, which can serve as a barrier to anti-oppressive practice. Self-reflexivity helps the supervisee
   observe oneself from an external perspective. Reflective questions for
   this step include, "How are my own views on social justice, equity,
   and diversity entering this supervision space?" and "Am I considering
   how my own identity and experience have impacted the recommendations and discourse around this case?"

5. *Relational reflexivity* is the final phase. This stage implements cultural integration through the supervisor's procedural competence of relational reflexivity by having the supervisor question the supervisee about the role of oppression, equity, and diversity matters during supervision. This action involves incorporating hypothesis development and expansive conversations with the supervisee's relational reflexivity skills (e.g., how might you imagine that oppression could play a role in understanding this experience; Kahn & Monk, 2017). The supervisor should regularly question the supervisee about the role of oppressive matters during supervision. The goal of this phase is to teach the supervisee to utilize reflexivity as an anti-oppressive practice procedure in the conceptualization process. Reflective questions for this include "What are the challenges and roadblocks they experience?" and "How does their cultural identity and society's view of their identity play into the client's struggle?"

## Supervisory Alliance and Relationship

It is imperative that the supervisor have a higher level of social justice advocacy, diversity and anti-oppressive awareness, and applicability experience in comparison to their supervisee(s). The supervisor should be intentional in building a rapport at the outset of the supervisory relationship that models anti-oppression. The supervisor should be mindful of power dynamics and cultural differences that might serve as barriers to implementing this intervention; for example, supervisors from the dominant culture may need to have conversations about their own journey and their identity. Due to the potential for merely checking a box, it will be necessary to practice reflexivity of their own alongside their supervisees.

## Legal and Ethical Considerations

Supervisors are to inform supervisees of the institutional and professional ethics, policies, and procedures to which supervisors are to adhere. As such, supervisees are made aware of this intervention and the goals for their practice. Counseling supervisors are aware of and address the role of multiculturalism/diversity in the supervisory relationship. Supervisors who are not anti-oppressive or decolonizing their practice should first work on their own self-awareness, knowledge, and skills before applying this intervention, as it is imperative that the supervisor do no harm.

## Reflective Questions

1. What are some of the oppressive aspects that you/your supervisor/ your clients may experience in their daily lives?
2. How do your and my own oppressive experiences, or lack thereof, enter this supervision space?
3. How will you use these new skills to address barriers to oppression with clients?

## Intervention Title: Resisting Oppression by Exploring Identities and Using Supervision Agreements to Co-Create the Supervision Space

### Author(s) and Affiliation(s)

Kavita Khara, M.S.C.P, LCPC, NCC
Northern Illinois University

Melissa J. Fickling, PhD, LCPC, CADC, ACS
Northern Illinois University

### Supervision Format and Modality

This anti-oppressive supervisory intervention is designed for individual supervision, but it can be employed in triadic supervision if both supervisees express interest and are willing to engage in critical discussions of their identities and needs in each other's presence. The intervention is adaptable for both in-person and virtual modalities.

### Supervisee Development

The intervention can be used across all developmental levels, particularly when starting a new supervisory relationship or a new phase of an existing supervisor-supervisee relationship. This intervention necessitates a supervisor who is aligned with and socialized in an anti-oppressive framework. Depending on the supervisor's familiarity with anti-oppressive theory and practice, it is applicable at introductory, intermediate, and advanced levels. Supervisors should seek consultation or supervision from those more advanced in anti-oppressive frameworks.

### Supervisory Goals and Learning Objectives

The supervisee will:

1. Engage in mutual contribution and ownership of the working alliance and supervisee development.
2. Participate in self-directed goal setting to foster intentional growth and evolution in the supervisee's professional development.
3. Anticipate and manage the potential impact of oppression on the supervisory and counseling relationships.

## Time Required

Before initial supervision sessions, taking 30 minutes for pre-session reflection engages both the supervisor and supervisee, followed by one hour of in-session discussion on individual and mutual needs and wants for supervision, with an additional 5-minute segment per session for checking in on supervision agreements and exploring resistance opportunities.

## Materials

The supervisor provides a professional disclosure statement (PDS), a supervision agreement template, and blank journals (physical or electronic, based on preference).

## Intervention Instructions

*Readers may contact the authors directly for a sample PDS and supervision agreement template that is aligned with anti-oppressive principles.*

1.  Before the initial supervision, the supervisor should draft a PDS, analyzing their identities and positionalities regarding privilege and marginalization while establishing a clear stance on anti-oppression and showcasing how clinical supervision can serve as a form of resistance. This statement is shared with the supervisee, demonstrating the supervisor's commitment to critical self-reflection and vulnerability, providing context and experience for the supervisee's next steps. Along with the PDS, the supervisor may choose to share the supervision agreement template discussed in step five in order to provide the supervisee ample time and space to consider it prior to the first supervision session.
2.  In the initial clinical supervision session, the supervisor invites the supervisees to discuss their identities and positionalities, clarifying that immediate disclosure is not expected and expressing readiness to establish a brave space for such explorations when the supervisee feels secure. The conversation should center on how the supervisee's identities influence their clinical supervision needs and the supervisor's strategies to provide effective support. The goal is for the supervisor to leverage the supervisee's self-knowledge to identify obstacles to their development, authenticity, and power, thus fostering collaboration to challenge hindering systems in their professional growth.

3.  In the initial session, the supervisor can encourage questions and reactions to their PDS, such as "I wonder how you are feeling about our working together after reading the PDS." This ensures a focus on the supervisee's curiosities and needs rather than centering the supervisor in the exchange. By acknowledging areas for personal growth and recognizing the potential for the supervisor to learn from the supervisory relationship, power-sharing is facilitated, and relational dynamics are opened up for future discussion.

4.  If applicable, an additional document for discussion could be an evaluative measure required by training programs or employers. Encouraging a critical conversation about the uses and limitations of these documents, along with exploring ways to enhance their utility in supervision, is recommended. Transparency regarding the process, expectations, norms, and the purpose of evaluative practices can enhance supervisee autonomy and empower their expression of hopes and concerns related to this supervisory experience. For example: "Your program has provided us with this measure for evaluating your work. Are there items you are interested in focusing on this semester? Are there ways we want to assess growth that is not reflected in this document?"

5.  Historically, supervisors have drafted a "supervision contract" prior to the first supervision for the supervisor and supervisee to review together. However, supervision contracts tend to use language that is oppressive in nature. In a sample contract by Bernard and Goodyear (2019), the contract uses phrases such as expecting the supervisee to "justify" their case conceptualizations and center supervisor's expectations without consultation with the supervisee. Thus, following the discussion of identities, the supervisor and supervisee will work together to draft a supervision *agreement*, in which the following will be discussed and mutually agreed upon. We recommend starting this discussion in the first session, working in between sessions one and two, and establishing a working agreement by the end of session two.

    a.  What are the supervisee's professional goals for their current stage of development, and what does the supervisee need from the supervisor in order to meet those goals?

    b.  What type of feedback, and in which format(s), does the supervisee prefer to receive? How can the supervisor honor these needs? This may include but is not limited to written notes, verbal processing, etc.

    c.  How does the supervisee believe that clinical supervision can fill the gaps in their current experience and knowledge?

    d.  In the context of power and oppression, how does the supervisee currently experience their profession, and what do they believe needs to change? How can the supervisor and supervisee effectively utilize clinical supervision to promote this change?

    e.  How and where does the supervisee experience liberation and empowerment, and what do they need from the supervisor to feel so?

6.  The supervision agreement should be revisited and modified as the supervisee and supervisor see fit to reflect the supervisee's professional development and evolving needs. We recommend this occur more frequently in the beginning (every one or two sessions) and with less frequency over time. Revisiting and adjusting the supervision agreement ideally should not occur during summative feedback sessions.

## Supervisory Alliance and Relationship

Given the inherent power imbalance in clinical supervision, the supervisee may be more likely to identify oppression before the supervisor does (hooks, 1989). The co-creation of the supervision agreement invites both the supervisee and supervisor to redefine resistance as a site of liberation rather than a sign of inappropriate supervisee behavior. By collaboratively developing the supervision agreement, the supervisor gains a deeper awareness of the supervisee's identities and needs, fostering a holistic understanding. This process enables the supervisor to engage with the supervisee's actions through an anti-oppressive lens, acknowledging moments of disagreement as meaningful parts of the supervisee's journey toward becoming a counselor.

## Legal and Ethical Considerations

By actively resisting oppressive structures, both supervisees and supervisors can envision the supervisory space as potentially liberatory, although they must navigate statutory and regulatory requirements aimed at safeguarding the public. Embracing principles of resistance raises questions about the interplay between laws and ethics, particularly in the context of challenging legislation such as abortion bans and anti-DEI, anti-CRT, and anti-trans laws, where gender-affirming care and bodily autonomy face criminalization. Thus, blanket statements here about the merits of laws undermine anti-oppressive praxis. Critical engagement and thoughtful resistance are essential while prioritizing safety, mutuality, and autonomy.

## Reflective Questions

1. How might supremacist assumptions shape our experience together? What needs resisting in the supervisory space?

2. How have the helping professions capitulated to oppressive, colonizing power structures in conceptualizing wellness? What might we have individually and collectively internalized as a result of the profession's desire to align with power?

3. Read hooks' (1989) "Marginality as a Site of Resistance" and reflect on the following: How can we, in clinical and supervisory work, remain nourished in the margins in order to refuse (reject, resist, oppose) domination?

4. How does the supervision agreement align or not with other evaluative supervisory experiences you have had (positive/negative)?

5. As a supervisor, how does it feel to identify and let go of internalized hierarchical assumptions toward supervisees? Does it feel possible to acknowledge the wisdom of the supervisee and the limitations of your own perspective while maintaining client safety? What do you need to address in your practice in order to attend to all of these dynamics?

## Intervention Title: Recognizing and Resisting Oppression

## Author(s) and Affiliation(s)

Peggy L. Ceballos, PhD, NCC
University of Texas at San Antonio

Karina Crescini, M.A., LMHC, LPC, RPT, NCC
University of North Texas

## Supervision Format and Modality

This activity is designed to be delivered over two individual supervision sessions of 50 minutes each. However, this activity can be modified to be done virtually if the supervisor uses an online sandtray program. Similarly, the activity can be adapted for a group. Sandtray therapy is an expressive/projective modality of therapy that facilitates the processing of the user's inner world using sandtray materials (Homeyer & Sweeney, 2022). A goal of doing sandtray is to build a supervisee's self-awareness (Hartwig & Bennett., 2017), which includes examining one's core values and beliefs (Hou & Skovholt, 2019).

## Supervisee Development

This intervention is for supervisees who are in the Advanced Student Phase (Skovholt & Rønnestad, 2003). Ideally, the supervisee has already been exposed to a diversity class and is familiar with concepts such as privilege, oppression, and resistance.

Skovholt and Rønnestad's model of supervision (1992) looked at skills development and processes that are part of clinical growth across time. Throughout clinical development, supervisors must facilitate awareness of the self to enhance professional identity. Additionally, supervisors must enhance supervisees' understanding and application of cultural orientation (Ray et al., 2022). This orientation includes openness to cultural humility, cultural opportunities, and cultural comfort within counseling relationships. This level of cultural integration throughout the counseling process requires supervisees' awareness of privilege and oppression. As supervisees conceptualize the effects of oppression on clients' mental health, supervisors can facilitate supervisees' resistance to oppression.

## Supervisory Goals and Learning Objectives

Supervisees will:

1. Understand the impact of privilege and oppression on the supervisee's professional identity.
2. Understand the impact of privilege and oppression on the client's presenting problem.
3. Explore strategies to resist oppressive factors within the therapeutic process.

## Time Required

This intervention is done over two supervision sessions of 50 minutes each. It is recommended to continue to process in subsequent supervision sessions the application of anti-oppressive strategies.

## Materials

The materials for the intervention include the Power Flower Activity, adapted from Rick Arnold et al. (1991), which can be downloaded from the "Building Competence + Capacity for 2SLGBTQ" website; crayons; a sand tray; and a variety of diverse miniatures, including people, animals, nature items, landscape objects, automobiles, buildings, furniture, fantasy/mythical objects, and spiritual/religious items, among others.

## Instructions

### Supervision Session 1

#### 10 Minutes

The supervisor provides the supervisee with a copy of the power flower exercise. The supervisee chooses a color that represents privilege and a color that represents oppression. The outer petal represents the identities within each of the cultural markers that are privileged in this society. For example, under race, White is considered a privileged identity, and the supervisee will color it with the color chosen for privilege. In the inner petal, the supervisee writes their own race; if it matches the privileged identity, it is colored with the same color; if not, it is colored with the color that represents oppression. This process is repeated around the flower with the various identity markers. The result is a visual representation of one's cultural marks as related to how these identities bring privileged vs. oppressive daily experiences.

- **15 minutes**

  - The supervisor processes the power flower activity: 1—What comes up for you as you see your power flower? Any feelings? Thoughts? 2—Which of these identities are most salient to you? 3—What type of experiences come to mind with your salient identities? How do these identities affect who you are as a counselor? (This is an important question that can lead to processing how to decolonize counseling for underrepresented supervisees).

- **15 minutes**

  - After processing the supervisee's experience of their power flower, the supervisor focuses on bringing awareness about clients' experiences of oppression by asking: 1—If you could do a power flower that represents your clients, what would it look like? 2—How different/similar would their power flower be from yours? 3—How does the intersectionality of your identities and your clients' identities affect the therapeutic alliance? 4—What type of oppressive experiences are your clients exposed to? 5—How do those experiences affect their mental health? 6—How does oppression challenge your clients' self-actualizing force?

- **10 Minutes**

  - Supervisees are invited to process how was the experience of doing the power flower and how it has helped them acquire a deeper understanding of their clients. The supervisor lets the supervisee know that during the next supervision session, they will focus on the concept of resistance to counter oppressive factors.

*Session 2*

- **10 Minutes**

  - The supervisor summarizes the previous supervision session and invites the supervisee to share any reflections regarding the power flower exercise. The supervisor explains this session will focus on what it means to resist oppression and the various forms in which resistance can manifest.

- *15 Minutes*

  - The supervisor introduces the sandtray and invites the supervisee to become familiar with the sand. The supervisor can say, "You can start by touching the sand; if you feel comfortable, you can close your eyes. Take a deep breath as you touch the sand; breathe in and breathe out; do this a couple of times; breathe in and breathe out; one more time; feel your lungs expanding as you breathe in and feel the air coming out. Focus on what it feels like to have sand in your hands. What feelings come up for you? Where are these feelings manifesting in your body? How intense are the feelings? . . . When you are ready, I invite you to open your eyes (if closed) and, using the miniatures in the room, represent on one side of the tray the oppressive factors your clients are facing and the ones you face as you try to help them. Once you are finished with that side, I invite you to look at it and become aware of the feelings and thoughts that the representation of oppression brings for you. On the other side of the tray, I invite you to use miniatures to represent ways in which you and your clients can resist the oppressive forces."

- *15 Minutes*

  - Once the sand tray is built, the supervisor asks the supervisee, "Tell me about your sandtray." The supervisor proceeds to process by reflecting on important parts of the sandtray and/or making process; for example, if the supervisee is hesitant and exchanges one of the miniatures, the supervisor can reflect on this. Some processing questions could be: 1—Can you talk more about the miniatures that represent oppression? And the ones that represent resistance? 2—Which of the miniatures representing resistance are actions you can do vs. actions that you can empower your clients to do? 3—How can you integrate into the counseling process the discussion of these ways of resisting oppression? 4—How can you address resistance to bring resilience and empowerment?

- *10 Minutes*

  - The supervisor invites the supervisees to process the sandtray activity: How was the experience of doing it? The supervisees can also share how they plan to use the awareness they gained from the activity as they continue to work with clients.

## Supervisory Alliance and Relationship

Expressive art activities can evoke unconscious experiences (Homeyer & Sweeney, 2022), leading supervisees to process strong emotional reactions. Supervisors must maintain professional boundaries, clarifying that personal issues may be addressed only when relevant to the supervisee's clinical development; otherwise, the supervisor should evaluate the need for referral to personal counseling.

## Legal and Ethical Considerations

Ethically, supervisors must be knowledgeable about the techniques employed in supervision. Therefore, those wishing to incorporate expressive art activities should possess both knowledge and experience with the specific expressive arts they plan to use. Furthermore, the supervisor's consent form must include information about these activities, particularly their potential to elicit emotional reactions (Ceballos & Huan, 2020).

## Reflective Questions

1. What is the impact of oppression on the development and maintenance of mental health problems?
2. How have underserved and historically excluded communities resisted? What are the sources of resilience?
3. How can you, as a counselor, resist oppression? What is your ethical responsibility? How do you integrate resistance in your clinical work?

### Intervention Title: Diversity, Equity, Inclusion, and Anti-Oppression Supervision Case Audit

### Author(s) and Affiliation(s)

Harvey Charles Peters, Ph.D., NCC
Montclair State University

Melissa Luke, Ph.D., NCC, ACS, LMHC
Syracuse University

### Supervision Format and Modality

This anti-oppressive supervision intervention was developed for individual supervision being conducted virtually or in-person. With minor modifications, this supervision intervention can be implemented in triadic, group, or peer supervision.

### Supervisee Development

The intervention should be adapted to each supervisee's clinical and anti-oppressive development level, considering their stage—master's or doctoral practicum, internship, professional development, or post-graduate status. This approach ensures the intervention is appropriate across varying levels of training and practice in diversity, equity, inclusion, and anti-oppression.

### Supervisory Goals and Learning Objectives

1. Understand and communicate the importance of conducting a diversity, equity, inclusion, and anti-oppressive counseling case audit.
2. Develop and familiarize oneself with the key components and process of a counseling diversity, equity, inclusion, and anti-oppression case audit.
3. Apply strategies for promoting diversity, equity, inclusion, and anti-oppression in counseling practice.
4. Develop actions for implementing changes based on diversity, equity, inclusion, and anti-oppression case audit findings.

### Time Required

The intervention requires approximately 45–60 minutes. Based on the allotted time, supervisors can make adjustments as they see necessary. Time will be influenced by the level of reflectivity and awareness the supervisee has of associated constructs and critical consciousness. However, if this is adapted within triadic or group supervision, additional time and consideration will be necessary.

## Materials

Before using the intervention, the supervisor should review diversity, equity, inclusion, and anti-oppressive audits, noting their overlap with counseling case audits. The supervisor and supervisee need access to client data, including intake paperwork, case notes, and treatment plans. The supervisor should provide intervention instructions to each supervisee and ensure the working space, whether in-person or virtual, is accessible for all needs and abilities.

## Intervention Instructions

1.  The supervisor will collaborate with the supervisee to engage in a diversity, equity, inclusion, and anti-oppression (DEIAO) audit of the supervisee's caseload, practices, policies, and/or cultivated environment (Theoharis et al., 2022). Ideally, the supervisor should plan ahead and ensure the supervisee is able to collect and explore data prior to clinical supervision; however, if that is not feasible, the supervisor can work with the supervisee to explore and deconstruct the DEIAO audit in supervision. The list identified later is not an exhaustive list; rather, they are suggestions that can aid in the intentionally and individually tailored DEIAO audits.
2.  The supervisor can begin with operationalizing and contextualizing the DEIAO audit, including an overarching definition (i.e., a comprehensive assessment of a supervisee's caseload, policies, and practices related to diversity, equity, inclusion, and anti-oppression to assess for the current environment), the purpose, function, and processes (Bright & Ghouse, 2018; Griffith et al., 2022; Wells et al., 2023).
3.  The supervisor and supervisee should start by defining the scope of the DEIAO audit and setting specific assessment goals to understand the supervisee's and client's experiences with the environment and services through a DEIAO perspective.
4.  Next, the supervisor and supervisee will examine the key socio-cultural client identities captured in the supervisee's caseload (e.g., race, ethnicity, gender identity, affectional/sexual orientation, socioeconomic status, dis/ability, nationality, linguistic diversity, immigration status, religious and spiritual identity, etc.), including identities listed

on paperwork and disclosed in session. The assessment and subsequent discussion can explore what (a) social locations are present, (b) identities may be less present or overlooked, (c) factors that contribute to the current caseload (e.g., policies, social-cultural competence, broaching of identity, etc.), and (d) factors that may support or hinder diverse representation and retention of clients from diverse social locations.

5.  Following, the supervisor and supervisee can explore the current policies associated with the clinical placement or agency as well as any and all policies associated with the supervisee's clinical practice (Bright & Ghouse, 2018; Griffith et al., 2022; Wells et al., 2023). This review and discussion can focus on what policies may support and/or hinder client services, access, and experience in session. The data that can be used can include the supervisees, supervisors, and clients reported insight and experiences. For instance, exploring the accessibility of the building or virtual platform, service fee structure, attendance policy, intake and diagnostic protocols, etc. to better understand how policies can direct support and hinder client care and DEIAO efforts.

6.  Next, building upon the exploration of policies, the supervisor and supervisee can explore client cancellations, terminations, and other issues related to the retention of clients. The supervisor will encourage the supervisee to consider a wide scope of factors, such as personal, clinical, relational, organizational, cultural, and systemic. The DEIAO audit aims to gather data on socio-cultural and oppressive factors affecting client engagement and retention, especially for minoritized communities. The supervisory dyad should examine relevant local, state, and national laws, such as those impacting human rights and anti-oppression education. By analyzing client demographics and social locations, they can identify patterns in attendance based on factors like socioeconomic status, race, or parental status. The supervisor can then lead an exploration of these issues using data and literature to understand causes and develop practices to address DEIAO challenges.

7.  The supervisor and supervisee should review existing diagnoses and treatment plans to assess DEIAO relevance. They will examine how social-cultural identities and oppression appear in diagnoses, therapeutic approaches, goals, and client integration into counseling. They must evaluate whether these elements are culturally responsive and avoid reproducing inequities or oppression (e.g., diagnoses, treatment plans, therapeutic modalities, assessments).

8.  Following, the supervisory dyad should examine formal and informal processes for collecting DEIAO audit data. They will evaluate how to refine intake forms, treatment plan templates, and clinical

documentation to improve DEIAO practices. They must identify strengths, issues, and gaps, such as updating demographic sheets or including socio-cultural and anti-oppressive elements in the documentation. They should also discuss current methods for gathering client feedback on services, environment, and outcomes related to DEIAO. Collecting, analyzing, and interpreting client data is crucial for DEIAO-informed services.

9.  Lastly, the supervisory dyad can reflect on the process, discussion, and insights while actively working toward identifying actionable items for the supervisee and supervisor aimed at promoting a DEIAO culture and community focused on culturally responsive, equitable, and anti-oppressive practices and policies. The supervisory dyad can use the data, discussion, and increased insight to explore and identify how the dyad can continue to build upon strengths, address gaps and issues, and advocate within the system to uphold their commitment and responsibilities to DEIAO. The aim of the final discussion is to identify how the supervisory dyad can seek to identify, address, and disarm the oppressive practices, forces, and obstacles that impact DEIAO.

## Supervisory Alliance and Relationship

Supervisors must carefully manage the supervisory alliance when addressing diversity, equity, inclusion, and anti-oppression issues. The audit may evoke defensiveness, vulnerability, or shame, potentially causing ruptures in the relationship. Discuss potential process and relational implications before, during, and after the intervention. Address any site, agency, supervisee, or supervisor-related issues ethically and responsibly, remaining mindful of power dynamics. Supervisors should support and advocate for supervisees, especially when the data reveals diversity and equity issues, and provide additional protection and advocacy as needed.

## Legal and Ethical Considerations

Supervisors should ensure supervisees consider legal and ethical issues, particularly when handling documentation related to diversity, equity, inclusion, and anti-oppression audits. Client information must be protected per HIPAA and professional standards. Supervisors should oversee and support supervisees in managing ethical and legal issues, consulting legal counsel if necessary, and using ethical decision-making processes and documentation to support compliance. Regular review of professional standards and seeking consultation is crucial.

## Reflective Questions

1. What did you learn about yourself and your clinical placement, site, and agency from the DEIAO audit?
2. How can you continue the formal and informal process of the DEIAO audit in your professional practice?
3. What are three to five actions that you will work towards? What type of timeline do these actions require?
4. What might support and hinder your completing a DEIA audit?

CHAPTER 10

# Socioecological Advocacy and Activism Through Collective Action

*Janice A. Byrd-Badjie, Tahani Dari, Darius A. Green, Sravya Gummaluri, Melissa Luke, Sylvia Nassar, Harvey Charles Peters, Rochele Royster, and Cassandra A. Storlie*

## CHAPTER 10 INTERVENTIONS

**Intervention Title: Cultivating a Professional Identity and Practice of Advocacy and Activism**

### Author(s) and Affiliation(s)

Harvey Charles Peters, Ph.D., NCC,
Montclair State University

Melissa Luke, Ph.D., NCC, ACS, LMHC
Syracuse University

### Supervision Format and Modality

This anti-oppressive supervision intervention was developed for individual supervision being conducted virtually or in-person. With minor modifications, this supervision intervention can be implemented in triadic, group, or peer supervision.

DOI: 10.4324/9781003470656-10

## Supervisee Development

The intervention can be applied across all development levels, from master's and doctoral practicums to post-graduate professionals. The supervisor should tailor the intervention to each supervisee's development level, considering their training in socioecological systems, anti-oppression, advocacy, and activism.

## Supervisory Goals and Learning Objectives

1. Discuss and review the supervisee's understanding of and experience with advocacy and activism.
2. Facilitate the implementation of the PPCT model concerning the supervisee's advocacy and activist identity and practices.
3. Develop goals and objectives for implementing advocacy and activism with a current client or a small number of clients.

## Time Required

The intervention typically requires 45–60 minutes, with supervisors adjusting the time based on the supervisee's reflectivity and critical consciousness. Supervisors should allocate additional time and consider the group's dynamics if adapted for triadic or group supervision.

## Materials

Before using the intervention, the supervisor should review the materials to understand the content, process, and experience. Prepare handouts on advocacy, activism, socioecological theory, and anti-oppression, and have process questions readily available. Provide each supervisee with a copy of the intervention instructions. This preparation will help frame advocacy and activism within a socioecological and anti-oppressive context and accommodate various needs and abilities.

## Intervention Instructions

1. The supervisor will begin this intervention by discussing the supervisees' understanding of advocacy and activism within their professional roles and responsibilities. The supervisor can ask questions such as: (a) How do you define advocacy and activism? (b) How do you practice from an anti-oppressive lens? (c) How comfortable and competent do

you feel serving as an advocate or activist within the counselor-client relationship? (d) How do you integrate advocacy and activism within your clinical practice? (e) What opportunities for advocacy and activism exist within your clinical practice?

2. Next, the supervisor can offer a brief overview of their perspective. This step can be flexible, with some supervisors starting with modeling and psychoeducation. This can support and challenge the supervisee's understanding and allow the supervisor to demonstrate transparency and positionality. Supervisees may need guidance to move from multicultural awareness to anti-oppressive, which involves intentionally addressing and dismantling oppressive forces, structures, and policies (Peters et al., 2022).

3. After the discussion, the supervisor will guide the supervisee through an application of the Process-Person-Context-Time (PPCT) model of socioecological theory (Bronfenbrenner, 2005; Peters et al., 2022; Tudge et al., 2009; Xia et al., 2020) to aid the supervisee in the practice of anti-oppressive advocacy and activism within the current professional context. Accordingly, it is essential for the supervisor to be familiar with the PPCT model, and it may be beneficial to develop a worksheet operationalizing each component of the model.

4. Using a sheet of paper and a writing utensil or its equivalent (e.g., dry-erase board), the supervisor will guide the supervisee through the PPCT model. The aim is to support the supervisees in reflecting, conceptualizing, and documenting the socioecological factors influencing their anti-oppressive advocacy and activism within their current professional context.

5. The supervisor will explore the "process" component of the PPCT, which involves the supervisee's essential and direct interactions with key persons, objects, and symbols and the impact duration (e.g., length of therapeutic relationship) and spatial and temporal proximity (e.g., accessibility) and context (e.g., counseling space, geographic location) of these interactions (Bronfenbrenner, 2005; Peters et al., 2022). The supervisor can ask the supervisee to share and trace how the "process" influences their advocacy and activism. The supervisor can explore supervisees' cognitions, emotions, and socio-cultural considerations, starting with individual reflections and then focusing on key stakeholders such as clients and other supervisors.

6. Next, the supervisor supports the supervisee in examining the "person" component of the PPCT, which includes the characteristics the supervisee holds that can support their anti-oppressive advocacy and activism (Bronfenbrenner, 2005; Peters et al., 2022). These characteristics and factors shape how an individual processes information

and interacts with their environment. The three individual characteristics include demand characteristics (e.g., physical appearances),
resource characteristics (e.g., cognitive and emotional resources), and
force characteristics (e.g., motivation, resilience, and temperament).
The supervisee can document each of the characteristics and discuss
how they can and have informed, supported, and/or hindered the
supervisee's anti-oppressive advocacy and activism within their current professional context. The supervisor can also ask the supervisee
to speak in general or related to specific clients (e.g., have or have not
utilized advocacy and activism), which may help them in exploring
their characteristics across stakeholders.

7.  Following, the supervisor will focus on the "context" component
of the PPCT, which includes the social, cultural, and physical environments in which the supervisee operates and impacts their advocacy and activism (Bronfenbrenner, 2005; Peters et al., 2022). The
"context" includes microsystem (i.e., immediate environment and
relational compositions), mesosystem (i.e., interactions between
microsystem stakeholders, environments, and contexts), exosystem
(i.e., one or more settings that are not directly a part of but affect and
influence the supervisee's immediate setting), and macrosystem (i.e.,
primary societal and cultural values, attitudes, beliefs, and resources
that influence and surround the supervisee's immediate environment
and relational compositions). The supervisor can help the supervisee examine how personal, professional, and societal norms, values,
and relationships impact their anti-oppressive advocacy and activism
at interpersonal, community, and societal levels. The supervisee can
analyze these influences and supports or hindrances across clients and
contexts. Additionally, the supervisor can guide the effective and ethical use of ecological systems in advocacy and activism.

8.  Subsequently, the supervisor will focus on the "time" component
of the PPCT, which refers to the temporal aspects influencing the
relationship between the supervisee and their environment (Bronfenbrenner, 2005; Peters et al., 2022). The three types of time involve
microtime (i.e., time within a particular interaction or activity), meso-
time (i.e., time involving consistent interactions over a period of time),
and microtime (i.e., time related to historical events across ecological
contexts). The supervisor can explore the role and impact of time on
the supervisee's advocacy and activism, including the timing of their
identity development and training, current and historical factors, and
time within the therapeutic and supervisory relationship.

9.  After the supervisor and supervisee have worked through the PPCT and
their anti-oppressive advocacy and activism, the supervisor can process

the experience, meaning-making, and identify future goals and objectives. The supervisor can use conceptualization skills to explore goals, objectives, and implementation concerning specific clients. Such questions can include: (a) Which of your current clients may benefit from your advocacy and activism with and on behalf of the client and the oppressive issue? (b) Based on your current work with and conceptualization of the client and the discrimination or oppression they deal with, how does this oppression impact their biopsychosocial health? (c) What is the client looking for or in need of support with? (d) What supports and hinderances might you face? (e) What type of personal and professional work and development might you need to support your future advocacy and activism efforts? (f) How will you attend to your insider and/or outsider status and center the community in your advocacy and activist efforts? (g) Based on this information, what are appropriate goals and objectives you can work towards?

10. The supervisor will ideally follow up with the supervisee and use the PPCT model to continue to frame, discuss, and practice anti-oppressive advocacy and activism.

## Supervisory Alliance and Relationship

Supervisors should consider multiple factors when addressing advocacy, activism, and oppression, as these issues are deeply personal and tied to the supervisee's socio-cultural background. They must use current, culturally responsive language. Address any harmful or oppressive language, whether intentional or unintentional, and take accountability to repair ruptures in the supervisory relationship. Assess the supervisee's development level and socio-cultural identity, as their critical consciousness, privilege, and fragility influence the intervention's implementation and interpretation. Maintaining humility, openness, and adherence to anti-oppression principles is essential for building a strong supervisory alliance.

## Legal and Ethical Considerations

The supervisor should support the supervisee in examining relevant laws, policies, regulations, and the professional code of ethics regarding advocacy, activism, and civil disobedience. They must consult competencies and professional standards, using ethical decision-making models to guide the supervisee. The supervisor should also consider legal and ethical issues related to critical thought and practices in contexts challenging critical theories, affirmative healthcare, and minoritized communities.

## Reflective Questions

1. What are a few ways you can practice advocacy and activism with your current clients?
2. What might advocacy and activism for your clients look like within as well as outside the counseling room?
3. How can you actively engage in accountability practices to advance advocacy and activism for the sociocultural and systemic issues affecting the clients and communities your profession seeks to serve?

## Intervention Title: Utilizing Relational Cultural Theory (RCT) and Socioecological Theory (SET) to Develop a Holistic Conceptualization of Advocacy in Action

### Author(s) and Affiliation(s)

Cassandra A. Storlie, PhD, LPCC-S, NCC
Kent State University

Janice A. Byrd-Badjie, PhD
The Pennsylvania State University

### Supervision Format and Modality

This supervision intervention uses the tenets of Relational Cultural Theory (RCT; Jordan, 2000, 2018) and Socioecological Theory (SET; Bronfenbrenner, 2005) to support the development of awareness and actions of community-engaged counselors-in-training (CITs) during group supervision in a live, in person or virtual format. Although intended for group supervision with no less than five supervisees, this supervision intervention can be modified to individual, triadic, or peer supervision.

### Supervisee Development

This supervision intervention is intended for master's level practicum and/or internship students across mental health professions (e.g., clinical mental health counseling, social work), but specifically, those that have already taken a Multicultural Counseling, Social & Cultural Diversity, and/or Systems Theory course. However, this intervention could be modified to include doctoral practicum or internship, professional development/remediation plans, post-graduate and pre-licensed professionals, or post-graduate and post-licensed professionals. This intervention is most appropriate for Intermediate level supervisees.

### Supervisory Goals and Learning Objectives

1. Supervisees will demonstrate how to incorporate RCT and SET in their conceptualization of clients.
2. Supervisees will utilize RCT and SET as a collaborative framework in their work with historically marginalized clients/students in addressing their experiences with systemic oppression.
3. Supervisees will develop action steps related to community-engaged counseling practice to support advocacy and activism.

## Time Required

This intervention requires 60–90 minutes of group supervision. Within this timeframe, supervisors may need to adapt and adjust the amount of time they focus on various components of RCT (Jordan, 2018) and on SET (Bronfenbrenner, 2005) based on the knowledge and awareness of the supervisees. While reflective questions are asked of supervisees throughout the intervention, supervisors should be flexible in helping the supervisees understand the core components of RCT and SET before their application to clients/students.

## Materials

The materials required are a worksheet that includes components of RCT (see Figure 10.1; Jordan, 2000, 2018), another worksheet that includes components of SET (see Figure 10.2; Bronfenbrenner, 2005), and a pair of dice.

Prior to using this supervision intervention, the supervisor must have a strong foundation in their understanding of RCT (see Jordan, 2000, 2018) and SET (see Bronfenbrenner, 2005). RCT stems from feminist theory and has moved beyond to expand to all clients (Miller, 2008). RCT centers on the counseling relationship, awareness of socio-cultural

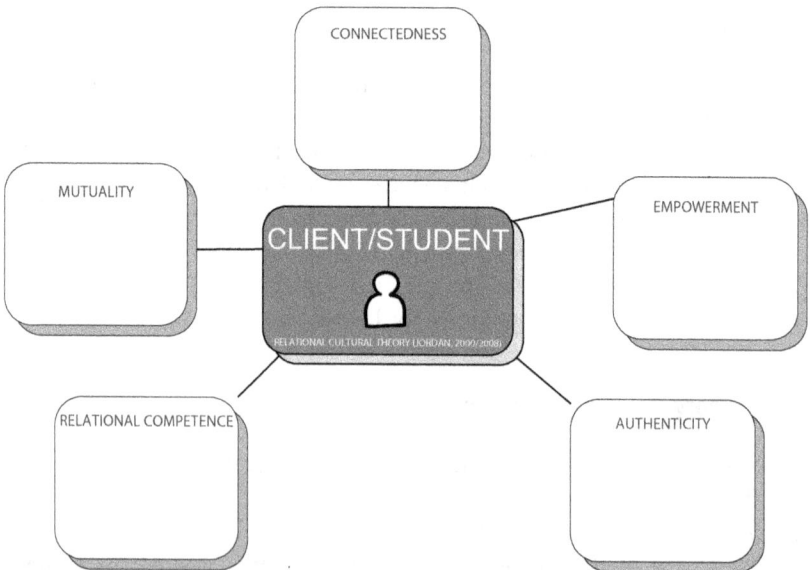

*Figure 10.1* RCT

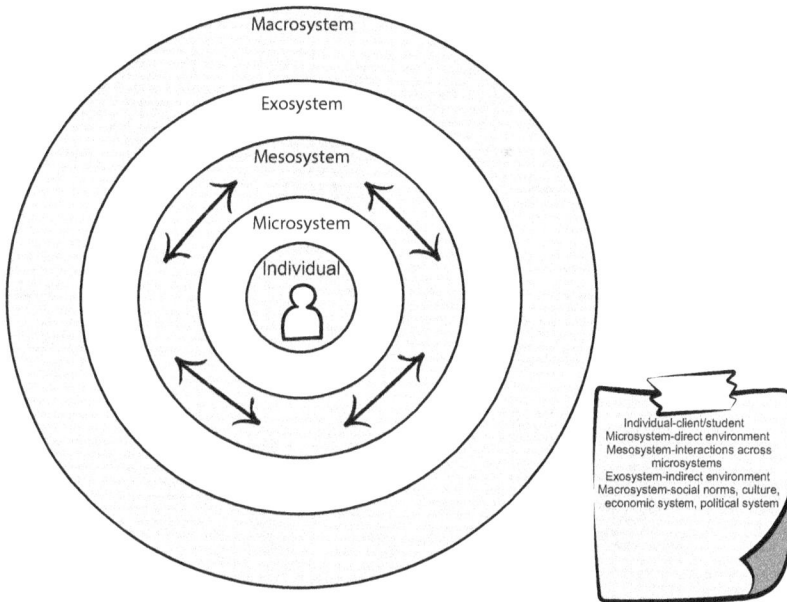

BRONFENBRENNER'S ECOLOGICAL MODEL (BRONFENBRENNER, 2005)

*Figure 10.2* SET

issues, and their influence on counseling (Jordan, 2000, 2018; Miller, 2008). Bronfenbrenner's ecological model (2005) provides contextual understanding for conceptualizing systemic factors that may influence the client's growth and development. Taken together, supervisors can provide a confluence of these theories to support discussion about advocacy with supervisees while they develop into community-engaged counselors. The supervisor will need to familiarize themselves with the worksheets, and if conducting this virtually, a Jam-board or virtual dice roller can be used.

## Intervention Instructions

1. The supervisor begins by introducing RCT and SET to supervisees, including the significant tenets of RCT (mutuality, connectedness, empowerment, authenticity, and relational competence; Jordan, 2000, 2018) and how RCT has been used in conceptualizing/working with marginalized populations. The supervisor should also review the systems associated with SET (see Bronfenbrenner, 2005) and how this theory has been used with marginalized populations.

2.  The supervisor asks supervisees to think about one client/student they have worked with for a minimum of 2–3 sessions that hold at least one or more marginalized identities. The supervisor asks the supervisees to write down the first three things that come to mind when working with this client/student. We also recommend that the supervisees reflect upon their working relationship with members of their client/student community.

3.  Next, the supervisor should pass out the two worksheets (see Figure 10.1; see Figure 10.2) and bring out the dice. The supervisor explains that each number on each dice will correspond to an RCT tenet or a SET system.

    -   Dice A—RCT
        1 = Connectedness
        2 = Mutuality
        3 = Empowerment
        4 = Relational Competence
        5 = Authenticity

    -   Dice B—SET
        1 = Individual
        2 = Microsystem
        3 = Mesosystem
        4 = Exosystem
        5 = Macrosystem
        ★It should be noted that Individual could be exchanged for Chronosystem, depending on the age of the client/student client.

4.  Each supervisee rolls each dice and addresses the corresponding RCT tenet and SET system related to their client/student. For example, if a supervisee rolls a 5, 2—they would then discuss (and/or write) how authenticity on a microsystem level impacts their client/student, particularly regarding their marginalized identity. If a 6 is rolled, the dice should be rolled again. The dice rolling should occur with each supervisee until most tenets and systems are addressed. Throughout this process, the supervisor poses reflective questions to the group, such as: How does this SET system look different for clients who do not share this marginalized identity? How might those from a privileged identity perceive this RCT tenet?

5.  Next, the supervisor asks the group supervisees to reflect on the first three things that came to mind when initially thinking of their client/student. The supervisor allows time for each supervisee to holistically

discuss their client/student and how RCT and SET can provide additional context and complexity to their presenting problems. Supervisors may suggest opportunities for advocacy and activism during this time (e.g., writing letters to state officials via legislative advocacy or participating in an organized community event). Supervisors can assist in helping supervisees draw the connection between RCT, SET, and a holistic case conceptualization.

6. Recognizing that supervisees range in their development of critical consciousness, the supervisor can then invite supervisees to reflect on this experience and add anything that would help in conceptualizing and/or advocating for (and with) their client/student. Once the supervisee engages in reflection, other supervisees may also provide constructive feedback.

7. At the conclusion of the intervention, the supervisor can direct a conversation on community-engaged counseling practices. For example, the supervisor can state: "Now that you have begun to more readily understand the systemic factors that affect clients/students, what is one community-engaged action step you can use in your counseling practice to support advocacy and activism against the oppressive factors your client/student may be going through?"

★ For more advanced supervisees, supervisors can introduce intersectionality (Crenshaw, 1991) and how the dice is a metaphor for understanding oppression (how the dice lands "by chance," who decides who is rolling the die, etc.).

## Supervisory Alliance and Relationship Considerations

Supervisors must consider various factors when guiding supervisees to engage in critical reflexivity, advocacy, and examining the influence of oppression on all aspects of their client/student's development (i.e., academic, personal/social, career). Supervisors can consider their supervisees' professional identity development, cultural identity development, and level of critical consciousness. Supervisors should remember supervisees in internships are still novices in their ability to integrate theory (e.g., counseling and culture) and should provide feedback that encourages and challenges them. Additionally, supervisees should be encouraged to reflect on where they are in their cultural identity development and how this awareness impacts their relationships with clients/students and in the supervisory relationship. Notably, Washington and colleagues (2023) summarized critical takeaways from various articles on supervision and shared the opportunities for supervisors to discuss the significance of racial issues in counseling and supervision, highlight how oppression can influence client/student's presenting issues, illuminate cultural sensitivity and awareness in treatment recommendations and the essentiality of examining cultural biases and racial identity.

Finally, supervisors and supervisees can exhibit behavioral defenses to presumed threats to their own privileged identities when engaging in supervision interventions, inviting one to critically examine cultural differences. Watt's (2015) Privileged Identity Exploration Model can provide the language to assist supervisees and supervisors in naming the defenses that arise when discussing power, privilege, and oppression. Harmful and oppressive language and practices used by anyone within the supervisory relationship must be named and discussed and accountability should be core to the relationship.

## Legal and Ethical Considerations

Supervisors have ethical responsibilities within the supervisory relationship that are central to ensuring its success. Namely, the supervisor serves as a model for ethical counseling practice by examining legal and ethical issues related to the client and within the supervisory relationship. Additionally, supervisees are assessed on their confidentiality and privacy practices (e.g., record keeping, clinical notes), professionalism, and cultural competence. The call for supervisees and supervisors to integrate community-engaged counseling practices warrants advanced-level conversations about the ethical and legal issues that may arise in this work. Supervisees are encouraged to regularly reference their professional codes of ethics (e.g., American Counseling Association Code of Ethics, 2014), ethical decision-making models, or any other discipline-specific ethics–related documents relevant to the specific counseling practice. Considering that many unique ethical dilemmas may arise, supervisors should be well versed on state—and national-level laws related to advocacy and using critical theories in practice.

## Reflective Questions

1.  Where do you see opportunities for continued community-engaged counseling practices in your work with clients/students?
2.  How might you infuse RCT and SET in examining treatment recommendations for clients/students?
3.  In what ways can you work with your students/clients on activism against oppressive practices?

**Intervention Title: Integrating Arts-Based Supervision for Intersectional Cultural Insight and Socioecological Advocacy**

## Author(s) and Affiliation(s)

Rochele Royster, Ph.D., ATR-BC
Syracuse University

## Supervision Format and Modality

This arts-based supervision intervention was developed for in-person, group supervision (six to ten supervisees) and incorporates a reflective approach and emphasizes collaborative, anti-oppressive practices and self-awareness.

## Supervisee Development

This supervisory intervention can be used across all levels of supervisee development, but it is particularly helpful for Skill Development, Self-Reflection, Cultural Competence, and Supervision Process (reflexive and feedback). This intervention is best employed with supervisees with intermediate and advanced levels of skills.

## Supervisory Goals and Learning Objectives

Supervisees will:

1.  Enhance their reflective practice and critical thinking skills by presenting a case study with a focus on socioecological advocacy (individual, relationship, community, and societal factors) and anti-oppressive principles.
2.  Demonstrate active listening, cultural humility, and meaning-making through the art process in a discursive setting.
3.  Engage in a structured process of art-making, sharing, self-reflection, and dialogue within the context of supervision. Encourage supervisees to critically examine their reactions, assumptions, and interpersonal dynamics, fostering a deeper understanding of their professional roles as therapists.

## Time Required

This intervention requires one hour weekly for 6–10 weeks.

## Materials

This intervention requires art supplies for the supervisees to express themselves artistically, including colored pencils, paint, oil pastels, and pen and ink.

## Intervention Instructions

Background: This arts-based, anti-oppressive approach, rooted in cultural humility and inclusivity, fosters an intersectional cultural lens that validates diverse perspectives and dismantles hierarchal power dynamics. The resulting artwork becomes a catalyst for examining and dispelling ethnocentric and related dominance-centric assumptions, facilitating a deeper understanding of one's culture within the broader reality. Moreover, the group dynamic nurtures a profound sense of community and belonging, fostering reciprocal support among members dedicated to addressing each other's needs. This collective experience engenders a feeling of belonging and community, vital for the therapist's personal and professional growth, mirroring essential aspects of human development. In alignment with anti-oppressive supervision principles (particularly that of Principle 9), this intervention is a holistic approach that recognizes the intricate interplay between individual, environmental, and cultural factors, emphasizing their interdependence and influence on mental health, social determinants of mental health, and wellness.

Intervention Actions:

1. The supervisor familiarizes themselves with Bronfenbrenner's ecological perspective, merging community-wide public health strategies with individual-level considerations. Supervisors can describe the symbiotic nature of health on an individual and collective level, paralleling Anti-Oppressive Principle 9 and the concept of liberation, where mutual freedom is interconnected and interdependent and considers the interplay between individual, environmental, and cultural factors.

2. To implement the (ME) portion of the intervention at the Individual Level, the supervisor supports one supervisee at a time to:

    a. Select a Case: Choose a client case that involves systemic oppression, cultural diversity, or socioecological factors impacting the client's well-being. Use art-based responses to express aspects of the story. This could include creating a visual representation, such as a drawing or painting, that captures the complexities of the client's experience and the supervisee's embodied feelings and sensations. Encourage supervisees to focus on images that accompany their felt experiences.

For example, the supervisor can say, "What is happening in your image? How are you experiencing the feeling in your body?"

b.  Background Information: Provide a brief overview of the client's background, including relevant cultural, social, and environmental factors. Using Bronfenbrenner's ecological systems model, highlight any instances of systemic injustice or oppression the client may be facing. Discuss social determinants and root causes impacting the client's mental health.

c.  Use of Art-Based Response: Participants in the group supervision circle create art responses to the case study that was shared, expressing aspects of the case through an art-based response. This could include creating a visual representation in the form of drawing or other artistic medium that captures the complexities of the narrative that was shared.

d.  Anti-Oppressive Analysis: In the presentation, group members share their art and aspects of the narrative that resonated with them. Group members may ask questions, find connections, or make comments that intend to guide the supervisee to critically analyze how systemic oppression or societal factors contribute to the client's challenges. Explore the power dynamics at play and identify opportunities for advocacy.

e.  Self-Reflection: Prompt the supervisees to reflect on their own cultural humility and biases. How might their own background and social locations influence their understanding of the client's experiences, and how can they remain attuned to these factors?

f.  Actions: Discuss potential advocacy or activism actions that could be taken within the therapeutic relationship or in collaboration with external systems to address systemic issues impacting the client.

g.  Supervisory Feedback: Provide constructive feedback on the case presentation, highlighting the effectiveness of the art-based response, the depth of anti-oppressive analysis, and the supervisee's cultural humility. Discuss any areas for further exploration or development.

3.  To implement the (WE) portion of the intervention at the Community Wide level, the supervisor facilitates:

a.  Integration into Practice: Encourage consideration of how the insights gained from this reflective case presentation can be integrated into their ongoing clinical and/or community practice, fostering a commitment to socioecological advocacy and anti-oppressive approaches.

b.  Encourage participants to become co-participants in community art installation, photo-voice exhibit, or public art display as [art therapy] to focus on community voice to amplify civic engagement, advocacy, and empowerment.

c.  Engage the community through an art action that is important to the community (community art workshops, skill shares, movement, and art sessions, etc.) with a shared intention or focus for the action (gun violence awareness, literacy, Black maternity health, repair, community care, lead exposure, etc.; Royster, 2021).

## Supervisory Alliance and Relationship

As the foundation of effective supervision lies in a collaborative and open supervisory alliance, fostering trust, empathy, respect, cultural humility, and flexibility, it is particularly significant for supervisees of color and other marginalized communities to acknowledge the importance of cross-cultural supervision and embracing an intersectional cultural lens to honor diverse perspectives and experiences.

## Legal and Ethical Considerations

Supervision of and using arts-based approaches, whether in clinical or community contexts, requires compliance with licensing laws and regulations. Supervisors must possess the necessary credentials and stay abreast of legal requirements for overseeing emerging therapists. In addition, arts-based activism involves navigating power and privilege, particularly when engaging with marginalized communities or advocating for social change. Community care and voice should be the catalyst for any community art action, and this requires a process of self-awareness, cultural humility, and maintaining grounding principles of community psychology.

## Reflective Questions

Use to guide the supervisees in deepening their understanding of the intervention's impact on both individual and systemic levels, fostering continuous growth and development in their therapeutic practice.

1.  Individual Level:
    How did the art-based response enhance your understanding of the client's narrative and the intersectional factors influencing their mental health and social determinants of mental health?
    Reflect on your own cultural biases and how they might have influenced your interpretation of the case. How did you remain aware

of these factors when thinking of an intervention or goal setting for your client?

2. Case Presentation:

   Share an aspect of the case that stood out to you during the presentation. How did the art responses from group members contribute to your understanding?

   Explore power dynamics within the client's narrative. How did societal factors contribute to their challenges, and where do opportunities for socioecological advocacy lie?

3. Self-Reflection:

   Reflect on your own journey in cultural humility throughout this intervention. How did your background influence your understanding of the client's experiences, and how did you navigate these influences? Consider any personal biases that may have emerged during the art-making process. How can you remain attuned to these biases in future sessions?

4. Actions:

   Discuss potential advocacy or activism actions within the therapeutic relationship or external systems. How can you address systemic issues impacting the client with them and community members as participants and stakeholders in the process?

   Explore the role of art in advocating for socioecological change. How can artistic expression contribute to challenging oppressive structures?

5. Supervisory Feedback:

   What feedback resonated with you during the group discussion? How can this feedback inform your ongoing development as a therapist?

   Discuss any areas of growth identified by the supervisor and group members. How can you integrate this feedback into your practice?

6. Integration into Practice:

   Consider how insights gained from this reflective case presentation can be integrated into your ongoing clinical and community practice.

   Identify specific strategies for fostering socioecological advocacy and anti-oppressive approaches in your work.

**Intervention Title: Supervision for Mental Health Practitioner Activist Self-Efficacy and Praxis**

### Author(s) and Affiliation(s)

Sravya Gummaluri, MA, LAC (NJ), NCC
The George Washington University, Washington, DC

Darius A. Green, Ph.D., LPCC, NCC
University of Colorado, Colorado Springs

### Supervision Format and Modality

This anti-oppressive clinical supervision intervention was developed for in-person or virtual individual supervision; however, it can be adapted for use in other supervision formats, such as peer, group, and triadic supervision.

### Supervisee Development

This intervention can be adapted for use by supervisees across all developmental levels; however, the particular focus of this intervention is on doctoral practicum and internship students and post-graduate and pre- and post-licensed professionals. This intervention is intended for supervisees at an intermediate developmental level.

### Supervisory Goals and Learning Objectives

This clinical supervision intervention aims to empower practitioners-in-training to develop self-efficacy in praxis to engage in direct action and activism in response to oppressive policy and legislation directed towards marginalized communities.

The supervisee will:

1. Discuss their understanding of anti-oppression, activism, and legislation harming marginalized communities as it relates to their personal and professional lives.
2. Articulate an understanding of the core tenets of a critical abolitionist framework.
3. Develop an action plan to engage in policy/legislative activism for a cause they have identified.

4.  Engage in at least one aspect of the constructed action plan and discuss progress on this plan in supervision.

## Time Required

This intervention requires the academic year for doctoral students and one year for post-graduate and pre- and post-licensed professionals, with the goal being an ongoing engagement in policy and legislative activism. The timeline to complete this intervention is determined by the supervisee's needs and level of critical consciousness surrounding the topics of anti-oppression, activism, legislation, and policy, current engagement in activism, and timelines indicated in their action plan.

## Materials

The supervisor compiles anti-oppressive interdisciplinary literature on abolition, legislation, policy, and activism relating to mental health, therapy, and various avenues for activism. Additionally, material to develop critical consciousness is information on relevant state laws and the possible consequences of engaging in activism. The supervisor can use this information to discuss how engaging in activism can impact a clinician's licensure. Before presenting these materials to the supervisee, the supervisor familiarizes themselves with the literature and completes the Critical Abolitionist Legislative Action Plan (see below). Some examples of foundational literature include:

*   *The 10 Principles of Anti-Oppression* (Peters & Luke, 2022)
*   Articles on Abolition in Mental Health Practice

    *   *Abolitionist Praxis for Substance Use Clients who Experience Anti-Drug Policing* (Green & Sperandino, 2024)
    *   *Towards an abolitionist practice of psychology: Reimagining psychology's relationship with the criminal justice system* (Klukoff et al., 2021)

*   Seminal Books on Decolonization and Activism for Critical Action and Praxis

    *   *Decolonizing Therapy* (Mullan, 2023)
    *   *Freedom is a Constant Struggle* (Davis, 2016)

## Intervention Instructions

1.  This intervention first explores the supervisor's and supervisee's positionalities on oppressive legislation and policy harming marginalized

*Table 10.1* Critical Abolitionism for Legislative Action Plan

| Prompt | Sub Question(s)/Reflections | Notes | Proposed Actions |
|---|---|---|---|
| What are your salient identities, moral, and guiding values? Where do they stem from? | | | |
| What concerns are present in your clients and the communities you serve related to oppressive legislation and policy? What do you want to change? Why? | • How do these identified concerns connect to counseling, wellness in marginalized individuals, activism, and social justice? | | |
| What is your overall goal in addressing the legislative/policy-related issue above? | | | |
| List objectives to meet your activism goal. | • Consider making these objectives SMART.<br>• Consider addressing multiple levels and domains of advocacy (e.g., individual, community, systemic levels, community-based advocacy). | | |
| Using the core tenets of a critical abolitionist framework, identify and categorize potential actions toward addressing your objectives. | • Identify the abolition tenet guiding each action step. | | |
| Which resources would be helpful in accomplishing these objectives? | • Consider identifying community resources such as agencies or grassroots organizations working on the issue you have identified. | | |
| How can supervision support your objectives for collective action for the issue you have identified? | | | |
| How might you assess the degree to which objectives are met (be specific)? | | | |

communities. Following, the supervisor and supervisee explore their definitions of activism, their level of engagement in social justice activism, as well as hopes to engage in future activism. Activism is operationalized as the engagement in direct collective sociopolitical actions by helping professionals in the pursuit of social justice in response to oppressive sociopolitical stressors through collaboration with marginalized and dominant communities (Lee et al., 2018; Jew & Tran, 2022). The goal of this step is engagement in critical reflexivity to enhance critical consciousness as outlined by *Principle 1*. The supervisor and supervisee reflect on the following prompts: (a) What salient identities do you identify with? (b) How has your surrounding sociocultural political context shaped your experience and existence within these identities? (c) What are your perceived implications of recent oppressive legislation and policy? (d) How do you define advocacy and activism? and (e) What are your experiences in engaging in activism?

2.  The supervisor presents anti-oppressive learning material to the supervisee to build critical consciousness surrounding historical and current socio-political context, oppression, and harmful rhetoric, and will select three pieces most helpful in their activism goals. Additionally, *Decolonizing Therapy* will be foundational literature to read. Biweekly check-ins on supervisee progress can be used with the following questions: (a) What critical aspects of the current reading can be applied in your work with and activism for marginalized clients? (b) What difficulties did you experience in applying the reading? and (c) What action can you take towards implementing the reading towards resisting identified oppressive legislation?

3.  Core tenets of a critical abolitionist framework are summarized in contemporary literature (see Green & Sperandio, 2024) and include: Dismantling and divesting from carcerality, abolitionist dreaming, creating safety, interpersonal and systemic accountability, fostering community, and transformative and healing justice. Supervisors should collaboratively engage in critical dialogue with the supervisee around these core tenets to ensure understanding.

4.  Supervisees will be provided with a copy of the Critical Abolitionism for Legislative Action Plan developed by the authors for supervisees to develop self-efficacy in activism (see Table 10.1).

5.  The supervisee engages in the action plan and checks in with the supervisor throughout the year. The action plan should be adapted and revised throughout supervision to fit the supervisee's development.

## Supervisory Alliance and Relationship

Social and cultural identity, and their affiliated privilege and oppression, are central to the supervisory alliance when it comes to using supervision to support engagement in legislative activism. In-depth discussions around culture and identity enhance self-efficacy in multicultural-related tasks (Phillips et al., 2017). Thus, supervisors play a pivotal role in enhancing supervisees' critical consciousness as it relates to their intersecting identities and the cultural identities of those targeted via oppressive legislation through proactively, collaboratively, and iteratively discussing engagement in their Critical Abolitionism for Legislative Action Plan.

## Legal and Ethical Considerations

While a critical abolitionist praxis is essential in combating oppressive legislation, it does not come without its legal and ethical challenges. Mental health professions are steeped within broader carceral systems that can create ethical and legal dilemmas for practitioners. For example, carceral systems possess the ability to criminalize activism as a form of pushing back against challenges to those systems (i.e., arresting individuals who engage in public demonstrations). Thus, it is essential for supervisors to centralize the tenet of safety as it applies to threats of physical, psychological, and legal harm by brainstorming and strategizing ways to mitigate harm while engaging in legislative activism.

## Reflective Questions

1. How can you integrate liberatory frameworks such as critical abolitionism into your activism and theoretical approach with clients?
2. How can you empower clients to resist oppressive legislation?
3. What challenges do you anticipate encountering in your activism, and how do you plan to navigate these?
4. Which strategies might you use to build and sustain support in your activism?
5. How might you develop and maintain a community of care for yourself while engaging in activism?

## Intervention Title: Cultivating a Professional Identity and Practice of Advocacy

### Author(s) and Affiliation(s)

Tahani Dari, PhD
University of Detroit Mercy

Sylvia Nassar, PhD
North Carolina State University

### Supervision Format and Modality

This anti-oppressive supervision intervention is designed to be applied to peer group supervision.

### Supervisee Development

One core aspect of supervision involves helping counselors develop their skills as active and effective advocates for their clients (Peters et al., 2022). The MSJCCs (Ratts et al., 2016) suggest that clinical supervision should include mentorship on the institutional, community, and policy elements of counseling practice, given the importance of understanding cultural and systems to best serve diverse clients.

While this intervention is developed for master's level supervisees, it can also be applied to doctoral-level group supervision. Across each group, supervisee development, particularly relative to multiculturalism and social justice, should be considered throughout the semester-long intervention.

### Supervisory Goals and Learning Objectives

The supervisee will:

1. Explore the ways the ways in which their privileged and marginalized statuses are internalized by supervisees and, in their interpersonal relationships, contextualized in privilege and marginalization.
2. Identify the ways in which their respective institutions and communities facilitate equity and perpetuate marginalization.
3. Learn about and be able to explain the historical underpinnings of past and present laws and public policies on community well-being.

## Time Required

The intervention takes place throughout a full semester, requiring 90 minutes for each supervision session. Based on the allotted time, supervisors can make adjustments as necessary. The level of reflectivity and awareness that supervisees possess regarding associated constructs and their level of critical consciousness will influence the more specific amount of time required.

## Instructions

Supervisors should recognize the importance of inviting clients and communities to have their voices heard as a part of every program, policy, planning effort, and evaluation to advance equity and access to mental health services.

The intrapersonal level activity should occur at the very beginning of the semester, followed by the interpersonal level activity. At the conclusion of those activities (i.e., within the first month of the semester), the community and public policy level activities are assigned for supervisees to work on independently or in groups. The culmination of the latter activities, i.e., the community and public policy case study presentations, should occur during the last month of the semester.

1. *Intrapersonal Level (Activity A)*

- Supervisors invite supervisees to reflect on critical incidents where they encountered manifestations of oppression or witnessed systemic barriers affecting clients' access to resources or services. Supervisors should support both privileged and marginalized supervisees in reflecting on what it is like to live in a variety of oppressive situations and marginalized identities within society. This can help supervisees to unlearn their own privilege and approach their clients with greater empathy.

    - Supervisor Process Questions:

        - What aspects of your identity do you consider to be socially acceptable?
        - What aspects of your identity are you less likely to share with others?
        - Which aspects of your identity feel internally congruent to you?
        - Which aspects of your identity do you take for granted?
        - What might advocacy for your clients look like at the intrapersonal level?

- This self-reflective process will elicit information from supervisees that supervisors should incorporate into future steps in the process. The process will also facilitate critical thinking skills relative to advocacy and activism among both supervisees and supervisors and, in turn, allow for respective application to clients' presenting issues.

## 2. *Interpersonal Level (Activity B)*

One core aspect of supervision involves helping counselors develop their skills as active and effective advocates for their clients.

To practice interpersonal skills, supervisors can request that supervisees facilitate group discussions. During group meetings, supervisees can conceptualize and practice advocacy with and on behalf of clients by brainstorming strategies that could help them address how to support their clients' personal growth:

Supervisor Process Questions:

- How can clients determine which people serve as support systems for them?
- How can counselors support clients in fostering stronger supportive relationships with others in similar social positions?
- What language and/or communication skills can we teach our clients to help them communicate more meaningfully with peers about their privilege or marginalization?
- What kinds of evidence-based interventions are culturally appropriate and sensitive to the backgrounds, experiences, and worldviews of both privileged and marginalized clients?
- What might advocacy for your clients look like at the interpersonal level?

In addition to having them facilitate group discussions, the supervisor can lead supervisees in teamwork and peer support work. Working in teams (ideally of three), each team will select a marginalized population and explore systemic barriers that each has faced, as well as relevant challenges and opportunities for the population in its engagement with the counseling profession.

Outcomes will include:

- Finding a minimum of six (6) scholarly references regarding their chosen population.
- Creating a presentation about this group's history and needs.
- Identifying implications for counselors working with this population.

### 3. Community Level (Activity C)

Another key aspect of multicultural and social justice competent counselors is to effect change within institutional and other community structures. Thus, supervisors should encourage supervisees to consider their role as agents of change within their larger socioecological context and explore opportunities for collaborative action with community stakeholders.

To further supervisees' knowledge and expand their classroom learning into practice, in the same teams as in Activity B, students will schedule a visit with a community agency that works with their chosen population to explore how this population's mental health counseling needs are met, and ways in which the agency advocates for with and on its behalf. Supervisees will then integrate what they learned into a presentation that incorporates the MSJCC Principles (or related professionally specific multicultural and social justice standards/competencies) and other relevant codes of ethics. This presentation should build on what they learned in the previous EBP presentation by illustrating how the actual practice compares to their research. Supervisees should reflect on both experiences (library research versus field research). Each presentation should last approximately 20 minutes and must include a list of references, contacts, and resources.

Supervisor Process Question:

- What might advocacy for your clients look like at the community level?

### 4. Public Policy Level (Activity D)

Federal, state, and local policies can seriously affect clients' lives. Counselors can encounter public policies that inhibit fair and equitable treatment of community members, and they can advocate for client development for or on behalf of their clients.

Supervisors can help supervisees learn about conducting needs assessments to inform decision-making and enhance access to mental health services (by removing barriers for clients).

Trainees can learn about asset mapping, or identifying strengths in the community, to support community members in identifying the effects of existing policies on their lives and well-being and also allow them to identify areas for improvement. For example, supervisees can be assigned to research and present case studies of real communities that have utilized asset mapping to address policy impacts. Another way to introduce supervisees to asset mapping is by inviting guest speakers to share insights on how they used asset mapping to improve community well-being.

Supervisor Process Questions:

- Identify one attitudinal barrier and one environmental barrier to a specific population is facing.
- What resources exist in the community to help reduce this barrier? How did you identify or locate these resources?
- Which institutions and individuals would you consider partnering with to make improvements on this issue? In formulating your response, consider the local resources in your community.
- What challenges do you anticipate facing during the process? What steps might help you overcome these challenges? What are the benefits?
- What might advocacy for your clients look like at the public policy level?

## Supervisory Alliance and Relationship

The MSJCC embodies aspirational competencies (Ratts et al., 2016). When applying the MSJCC to supervision, it's crucial for the supervisor to approach with cultural humility (Del Re et al., Submitted). This includes emphasizing that everyone in the supervisory relationship is growing and developing within it. The supervisor, acknowledging their inherent privilege and power, takes primary responsibility for addressing emergent issues (Day-Vines, 2000). However, the supervisee's input is critical, and the supervisor should create an environment where this input is not only welcomed and valued but essential for multicultural and social justice competence development for both parties.

## Legal and Ethical Considerations

While the public policy-focused activity will explore and facilitate knowledge about laws and policies that serve to marginalize and oppress supervisees and their respective clients, additional laws may be particularly relevant to the advocacy initiatives identified by supervisees through several of the proposed activities. It is important that supervisees understand how any and all of these laws may either diverge from or converge with the professional ethics codes, recognize the need to apply relevant decision-making models, and consult when necessary.

## Reflective Questions

1. Reflecting on your identities and experiences, how do you think your background influences your perception of systemic barriers?
2. Consider a recent interaction with a client. Were there any implicit biases or assumptions that you may have brought into the session?
3. What specific strategies can you implement in your daily counseling practice to address systemic barriers impacting your clients?

# Redistributing Social, Cultural, and Political Capital Through Access and Opportunity

*Rehman Abdulrehman, Rawan Atari-Khan, Janice A. Byrd-Badjie, Deepika Raju Nantha Kumar, Melissa Luke, Harvey Charles Peters, Alex L. Pieterse, Ahmad Rashad Washington, and Monnica T. Williams*

## CHAPTER 11 INTERVENTIONS

### Intervention Title: Examining Social, Cultural, and Political Capital Within Group Supervision

### Author(s) and Affiliation(s)

Harvey Charles Peters, Ph.D., NCC,
Montclair State University

Melissa Luke, Ph.D., NCC, ACS, LMHC
Syracuse University

### Supervision Format and Modality

This anti-oppressive supervision intervention was developed for group supervision being conducted virtually or in-person. With minor modifications, this supervision intervention can be implemented in triadic supervision.

DOI: 10.4324/9781003470656-11

## Supervisee Development

This intervention is suitable for all development levels, including master's and doctoral practicums, internships, and post-graduate stages. The supervisor should adapt it to each supervisee's level of exposure to anti-oppression and their social, cultural, and political capital.

## Supervisory Goals and Learning Objectives

1. Identify and discuss the presence of social, cultural, and political capital within group supervision.
2. Examine the impact of social, cultural, and political capital across group levels (intrapersonal, interpersonal, group-as-whole, supra-group).
3. Explore actionable items to ensure social, cultural, and political capital within group supervision centers equity and anti-oppression.

## Time Required

The intervention requires approximately 60–90 minutes, depending on the proposed adaptions to the group supervision intervention. Based on the allotted time, supervisors can make adjustments as they see necessary. Time will be influenced by the number of group members, the level of discussion, and any adaptions to the intervention. If this is adapted within triadic supervision, less time may be required. The intervention is written by between 6–12 group members.

## Materials

Before using this intervention, the supervisor should review the materials and familiarize themselves with the content, process, and experience related to the intervention. This includes familiarization with social, cultural, and political capital. Furthermore, if a supervisor uses one of the provided adaptions, they may need to familiarize themselves with Virginia Satir's sculpting intervention (Costa, 1991; Satir et al., 1991). The supervisor should consider the working space to ensure each supervisee, whether they attend in person or virtually, has the space to develop their intervention in an accessible environment for various needs and abilities. Lastly, supervisors may consider having access to the proposed facilitation questions and any additional processing questions they deem essential for their unique group supervision.

## Intervention Instructions

1. The supervisor will begin supervision by discussing each group member's personal and professional definition or understanding of social capital, cultural capital, and political capital. *Social capital* can be briefly defined as resources, relationships, and networks that individuals and groups have within a social structure, including social connections, norms, and values (Alexander et al., 2016). *Cultural capital* can be briefly defined as an individual's knowledge, skills, education, and cultural assets, which can play a vital role in one's social status, opportunities, and ability to navigate particular social and cultural contexts (Alexander et al., 2016). *Political capital* can be briefly defined as the influence, power, and resources individuals or groups possess within systems, including political networks, relationships with influential individuals, organizational affiliations, and knowledge of political processes (Alexander et al., 2016).

2. Following a discussion, group members can share their experiences of social capital, cultural capital, and political capital within the context of group supervision. The supervisor should allocate time for exploring each aspect of social, cultural, and political capital, with both the supervisor and supervisees participating in the discussion.

3. Next, the supervisor will facilitate a discussion about these topics. The supervisor should separate each topic to ensure each question focuses on social, cultural, and political capital individually instead of concurrently. Discussion questions can include: (a) Who appears to have the most and least social, cultural, and political capital, and on what basis? (b) How have we observed social, cultural, and political capital effectively and ineffectively used in group supervision? (c) How has identity, culture, and power played into social, cultural, and political capital in group supervision, your professional training, and your professional communities and praxis? (d) In what ways can we work to redistribute social, cultural, and political capital equitably within group supervision? (e) How can the supervisor better utilize and attend to social, cultural, and political capital within group supervision? and (f) How can we work towards enacting practices that foster relationships and an environment aimed at naming and repairing the negative impact through the redistribution of social, cultural, and political capital within group supervision?

4. Following this, the supervisor should ensure they attend to the discussion and feedback and identify how they will be accountable as the supervisor in integrating this feedback and insight moving forward. The supervisor can take time to intentionally reflect and identify action strategies for themselves as well as the group; however, it is essential the supervisor follow through on any and all actions named.

### Adaption: Satir Sculpting

1. One potential adaption can come from Virginia Satir's family theory and practice (Costa, 1991; Satir et al., 1991). The aim of this adapted intervention is to create multiple sculptures representing group members' current relational dynamics and experience of social, cultural, and political capital within the group.

2. To begin, the group selects an individual to guide the process, instructing fellow group members to arrange themselves according to their internal perceptions of their relationships, emotions, and roles within group supervision, explicitly focusing on social, cultural, and political capital. The selected individual will physically sculpt and arrange the group members to create a series of sculptures that serve as a unified piece.

3. It is through the physical representation of the individual and collective sculpture; group members can gain insight into their group system and dynamics. Each sculpture can provide a tangible and visual representation of the group's structure, emotional connections, and dynamics.

4. In practice, the group will: (a) select an individual to facilitate and sculpt the group, (b) identify the focus based on capital (i.e., social, cultural, and political), (c) assign each group member a role or symbolic representation, (d) create a physical culture by positioning all group members according to their role and or symbolic representation, and (e) observe and take note of the sculpture. After each of the series of sculptures, it is essential to: (a) explore the group members' thoughts and emotions regarding the sculpture and positions, (b) communicate and process shared understanding of group members' experiences, (c) facilitate repositioning and experimentation by allowing others to move positions and shape to alter dynamics and create solutions, and (d) reflect upon and foster closure for the interventions.

5. Depending on time and goals, the group could select three members to create sculptures representing social, cultural, and political capital. After completing each sculpture, the facilitator would process the sculptors' and members' insights. The supervisor would then explore how different sculptures reflect varied experiences of the group's social, cultural, and political capital.

6. Next, the supervisor can invite the group to engage in a group sculpture to capture the desired equitable and anti-oppressive use of social, cultural, and political capital within group supervision. The group would work together to co-sculpt the dynamics and environment they hope to cultivate.

7. Finally, the group should explore their experiences and identify strategies to cultivate equitable and anti-oppressive use of social, cultural, and political capital. The group can revisit these dynamics periodically throughout group supervision to ensure continued focus and improvement.

## Supervisory Alliance and Relationship

There are multiple considerations for supervisors. Given this intervention focuses on group supervision, group dynamics and experiences related to social, cultural, and political power are essential for understanding the group's stage of group development (i.e., forming, storming, norming, performing, and adjourning). The current stage of group development and relationships at various group levels (i.e., intrapersonal, interpersonal, group-as-whole, supra-group) are important considerations for the group supervisor (Atieno Okech & Rubel, 2007).

## Legal and Ethical Considerations

The supervisor should help the supervisee address group dynamics, power, and strengths through the lens of social, cultural, and political capital. Interventions might uncover experiences of harm, such as microaggressions or isms (e.g., racism, ableism), which require attention due to potential legal and ethical issues. The supervisor should review relevant professional standards and literature and seek consultation or peer supervision for guidance on these matters.

## Reflective Questions

1. What have been the most impactful experiences with social, cultural, and political capital?
2. How have you seen social, cultural, and political capital used effectively, ethically, and equitably?
3. How have you seen social, cultural, and political capital misused?
4. What does an equitable, ethical, and anti-oppressive use of social, cultural, and political capital look like in practice?
5. What role does intersectionality play in social, cultural, and political capital?

### Intervention Title: Engaging Frantz Fanon and Exploring His Relevance to Counselor Education

### Author(s) and Affiliation(s)

Ahmad Rashad Washington, Ph.D.
The University of Louisville

### Supervision Format and Modality

Although this approach to anti-oppressive supervision is designed for in-person group supervision, it can be for individual or triadic supervision.

### Supervisee Development

Given the depth and intensity of the topics explored in this advanced-level intervention, doctoral practicum or internship students are the ideal population. Ideally, these doctoral students would have taken an introductory/intermediate multiculturalism course prior to this supervision experience.

### Supervisory Goals and Learning Objectives

1. Students will offer a comprehensive definition of racism, one that understands racism fundamentally as a power dynamic between Whites and racially subordinated groups.
2. Students will offer a comprehensive definition of antiBlackness, one that understands antiBlackness, fundamentally, as an irreconcilable antagonism between non-Black people and Black people.
3. Students will effectively contrast racism and antiBlackness.
4. Students will provide at least two tangible examples of how racism and antiBlackness, as power dynamics, are enacted socially (e.g., interpersonal interactions), culturally (e.g., entertainment and advertisement), and politically (e.g., political discourses and political policies.

### Time Required

Group supervisors should allot a minimum of two group supervision sessions, each lasting at least 60 minutes. To maximize effectiveness, supervisor to student ratio should not exceed 12:1. Supervisor and students should use discretion to determine whether the goals have or have not been achieved and whether additional sessions are required to unpack assigned content.

## Materials

Prior to beginning, the supervisor should familiarize themselves with the reading materials (three book chapters and one peer-reviewed manuscript) that guide the intervention. The first chapter is entitled *The Negro and Language* from Frantz's Fanon (1952) important text *Black Skin, White Masks.* The second chapter, again written by Frantz Fanon (1961), is called *Concerning Violence* and is taken from *The Wretched of the Earth.* The supervisor should also become acquainted with the chapter *The Self in America,* from Cushman's (1995) book *Constructing the Self, Constructing America.* Yosso's (2005) article *Whose Culture Has Capital? A Critical Race Theory Discussion of Community Cultural Wealth* represents the last pedagogical resource that will support students during this supervision intervention. To assist the supervisor, excerpts from these readings are provided in what follows; however, the supervisor should not focus exclusively or narrowly on these excerpts at the expense of other meaningful and resonating quotes dispersed throughout these texts:

> The colonized is elevated above his jungle status in proportion to his adoption of the mother country's cultural standards. He becomes whiter as he renounces his blackness, his jungle.
>
> (Fanon, 1952, p. 18)

> In capitalist societies the educational system, whether lay or clerical, the structure of moral reflexes handed down from father to son, the exemplary honest of workers who are given a medal after fifty years of good and loyal service, and the affection which springs from harmonious relations and good behavior—all of these aesthetic expressions of respect for the established order serve to create around the exploited person an atmosphere of submission and of inhibition which lightens the task of policing considerably.
>
> (Fanon, 1961, p. 38)

> As if to show the totalitarian character of colonial exploitation the settler paints the native as a sort of quintessence of evil. Native society is not simply described as a society lacking in values. It is not enough for the colonist to affirm that those values have disappeared from, or still better never existed in, the colonial world. The native is declared insensible to ethics; he represents not only the absence of values, but also the negation of values. He is, let us dare to admit, the enemy of values, and in some sense he is the absolute evil. He is the corrosive element, destroying all

that comes near him; he is the deforming element, disfiguring all that has to do with beauty or morality; he is the depository of maleficent powers.

(Fanon, 1961, p. 41)

The moral uncertainty about the proper way to be human move the white population to desperate measures in an attempt to define the self of their era. The nineteenth-century American white identity strategy was based on the psychological processes used to define "the other." It was difficult for the young, increasingly diverse nation to develop a consensus as to what the self was. It was easier to develop a sense of what the self was not—the supposedly lazy, stupid Negro or the supposed heathen, savage Indian. The white self was defined as being unlike the Negro slave and unlike the untamed; it was *not* lazy, stupid, savage, and uncivilized. Of course, in order to use African Americans and Native Americans to help define the white self, these racial groups had to be actively redefined in specific ways. Whites accomplished this particular definition through the vehicles of popular theatre and political discourse.

(Cushman, 1995, pp. 40–41)

In addressing the debate over knowledge within the context of social inequality, Pierre Bourdieu (Bourdieu & Passeron, 1977) argued that the knowledges of the upper and middle classes are considered capital valuable to a hierarchical society. If one is not born into a family whose knowledge is already deemed valuable, one could then access the knowledges of the middle and upper class and the potential for social mobility through formal schooling. Bourdieu's theoretical insight about how a hierarchical society reproduces itself has often been interpreted as a way to explain why the academic and social outcomes of People of Color are significantly lower than the outcome of Whites. The assumption follows that People of Color "lack" the social and cultural capital required for social mobility. As a result, schools often work from this assumption in structuring ways to help "disadvantaged" students whose race and class background has left them lacking necessary knowledge, social skills, abilities and cultural capital.

(Yosso, 2005, p. 70)

## Intervention Instructions

1. The supervisor begins by inviting the students to discuss how they define racism. Students should be encouraged to elaborate on what informs their definition of racism and how that definition has evolved. After students have had the opportunity to define racism, the supervisor prompts students to define antiBlackness. Once antiBlackness has been adequately operationalized, the supervisor asks the group to compare and contrast racism and antiBlackness. The supervisor should be attentive to how students define racism and antiBlackness and make a note

of how often and to what extent students define racism and antiBlackness as individual, random acts of bias and discrimination derived from bigoted thinking. For example, helping students understand that racism is an ideology rooted in the belief that essential differences between the races exist while antiBlackness is a structural dynamic that tethers Blackness to "slaveness" and its constitutive elements (e.g., gratuitous violence, natal alienation, general dishonor) (Patterson, 2018).

2.  Next, the supervisor uses the previously mentioned excerpts, or other excerpts from the texts, to stimulate conversation with the students about how the authors defined racism and antiBlackness. Students are encouraged to: (a) work through Fanon and Cushman's theorizations about racism and antiBlackness, as relations of domination, (b) consider how these theorizations differ from dominant conceptions in society, (c) ponder how Fanon and Cushman's theorizations can be integrated into their operational definitions, and d) envision how a more comprehensive understanding of racism and antiBlackness would help them respond clinically to discussions of racism and antiBlackness.

3.  Finally, the supervisor utilizes Yasso's conceptualization of the cultural community wealth of racially marginalized and socio-politically subordinated groups to examine the myriad ways these groups deploy cultural community wealth to resist social, cultural, and political hegemony and promote intracommunal health and wellness, asking questions like: (a) Given the hegemony of White American culture in every conceivable American institution, how do narrow, interpersonal definitions of racism and antiBlackness obscure the institutional and structural nature of race-based oppression in this country? (b) how has constructing "the cultural other" been an indispensable part of how this country has come to define itself and legitimate its own social, cultural, and political agendas? (c) how are the battles over education curriculum in this country, in states like Florida, confrontations between conflicting and irreconcilable paradigms (e.g., accounts of history that are deemed fair and accurate to the extent they represent America as exceptional and valorize White, Anglo-Saxon, protestant viewpoints versus accounts of history that reflect the lived experiences of Black, Indigenous, queer perspectives)?

## Supervisory Alliance and Relationship

Given the nature of these conversations, the supervisor should deliberately cultivate an environment conducive to honest and intellectually rigorous discussion. The supervisor should model a disposition of curiosity and openness and share how their own ideas about racism and antiBlackness continue to evolve. The supervisor should proactively acknowledge that for many people, these conversations evoke discomfort, shame, and embarrassment and that those emotions are developmentally appropriate considering how we have been socialized in this country. However, the supervisor should not neglect to highlight counseling's Eurocentric roots (Cushman, 1995; Katz, 1985), its inherently political nature, and how our refusal and/or unwillingness to engage these ideas with nuance and sophistication reproduce the status quo.

## Legal and Ethical Considerations

Clinical supervisors have an ethical obligation to take the professional mandate of operating as agents of social justice and social change seriously. Supervisors are expected to embody and demonstrate an orientation towards social justice and social change in their teaching, research, and professional and community service. Clinical supervisors are uniquely positioned to: (a) expose counseling students to content that deepens their understanding of anti-oppressive theoretical frameworks and (b) design supervision dynamics that encourage counseling students to actively integrate these frameworks into their burgeoning practice.

## Reflective Questions

1. Reflecting on Fanon's and Cushman's writings, how do you see cultural narratives about race and identity influencing both counselors and clients within a therapeutic setting?
2. How might cultural narratives affect your understanding of a client's lived experiences, especially when those experiences are shaped by systemic oppression?
3. In considering the definitions of racism and antiBlackness as presented by Fanon and Patterson, how do you understand the ways that antiBlackness operates beyond individual acts of discrimination?
4. Based on Yasso's concept of community cultural wealth, what strengths and resources can you identify within marginalized communities that counteract systemic oppression?
5. How can you leverage this understanding of community cultural wealth to foster resilience and empowerment in your clients during counseling sessions?

## Activity Title: Integrating Structural Competencies to Redistribute Capital in the Supervisory Relationship

### Author(s) and Affiliation(s)

Rawan Atari-Khan, PhD, Licensed Psychologist
Marquette University

Alex L. Pieterse, PhD, Licensed Psychologist
Boston College

### Supervision Format and Modality

This anti-oppressive supervision intervention was developed for individual or triadic supervision to be conducted in-person or virtually.

### Supervisee Development

This supervision intervention can be used across all developmental levels. When implementing this intervention, the supervisor should pay particular attention to the supervisee's prior knowledge about social, cultural, and political capital as informed by structural oppression. Supervisees with less knowledge about these forms of capital may need more support from the supervisor, particularly when integrating structural competencies into their case conceptualizations. This intervention serves as an introductory or intermediate-level activity, aiming to provide supervisees with a foundational understanding of the influence of structural inequities on access to social, cultural, and political capital and its potential effects on mental health.

### Supervisory Goals and Learning Objectives

Supervisees will:

1. Reflect on how structures of oppression and privilege impact access to social, cultural, and political capital.
2. Discuss the impact of access (or lack thereof) to social, cultural, and political capital on the dynamics within the supervisory relationship.
3. Understand how structures of oppression influence mental health and psychological functioning.

4.  Integrate structural competencies and intergenerational context into case conceptualizations for clients/patients.

## Time Required

Approximately 45–60 minutes upon initial implementation, varying based on discussion length and the supervisee's prior knowledge. Because one goal of the intervention is to teach supervisees how to implement structural competencies into their case conceptualizations, the intervention can serve as a guiding framework for ongoing supervision to be revisited as needed.

## Materials

Supervisors should familiarize themselves with the Supervision Structural Inequity Inventory (SSII) and Structural Competencies Model (Wilcox et al., 2024), engage in their own identity reflection, and be familiar with models of social justice in supervision, which require the supervisor to engage in ongoing self-evaluation (Dollarhide et al., 2021). Accessibility requirements for the SII should be considered, which may include providing hard copies or electronic documents. Supervisors should prepare information to introduce the intervention and may develop additional discussion questions beyond those provided to facilitate engagement.

## Intervention Instructions

1.  The supervisor introduces the purpose of this exercise as it relates to redistributing social, cultural, and political capital within the supervisory relationship.
2.  The supervisor and supervisee(s) independently complete the SSII (see Appendix A).
3.  After the completion of the SSII, the supervisor initiates a discussion regarding experiences in completing the inventory. The supervisor leads in describing their own experiences, aiming to exemplify appropriate self-disclosure. Discussion questions might include:
    a.  What were your impressions upon completing the inventory?
    b.  Were there any items that brought up an unexpected reaction?
    c.  Did you encounter any items that you did not fully understand and that require further discussion?
4.  Following this discussion, the supervisor and supervisee(s) can explore how structural inequities relate to their experiences with social, cultural, and political capital. To begin, the supervisor shares the following

definitions to guide the discussion: *Social capital*—resources, relationships, and networks that individuals and groups have within a social structure, including social connections, norms, and values; *Cultural capital*—individuals' knowledge, skills, education, and cultural assets, which can play a vital role in one's social status, opportunities, and ability to navigate particular social and cultural contexts; *Political capital*—influence, power, and resources individuals or groups possess within systems, including political networks, relationships with influential individuals, organizational affiliations, and knowledge of political processes (Alexander et al., 2016; Swartz, 2012). Discussion questions might include:

   a.   Where does each of our social, political, and cultural capital come from?
   b.   Is any of this capital related to how each of us is protected by structural and systemic forces described in the SSII? Are there other forces to consider?

5.   Following this discussion, the supervisor consolidates the information shared and comments on any disparities in capital apparent within the supervisory relationship. Next, the supervisor touches base with the supervisee(s) to assess whether there is consensus or divergent viewpoints regarding their observations and encourages them to share their insights.

6.   After an exploration of power imbalances in the supervisory relationship, the supervisor and supervisee(s) explore the following together:

   a.   How might this imbalance be harmful to our supervisory relationship?
   b.   How might we redistribute capital between us to make it more equitable?
   c.   How might this power imbalance affect our work with clients?

7.   As an extension to this intervention, the supervisor and supervisee(s) may utilize the SSSI-Client Version (see Appendix B) to leverage their understanding of access to social, political, and cultural capital when formulating case conceptualizations. This can facilitate discussions on how to approach clinical work by conceptualizing client distress and functioning within the Structural Competencies Framework (Wilcox et al., 2024). Please refer to Figure 1, the Case Conceptualization diagram in Wilcox et al. 2024. When applying the SSSI to an understanding of the client's presentation supervisor and supervisee(s) should reflect on the following questions:

   a.   How has my social, cultural, and political capital influenced my understanding of the client's distress?
   b.   How might my social, cultural, and political capital inform my ability to empathically enter the client's lived experience?

### Supervisory Alliance and Relationship

Before implementation, supervisors should cultivate an effective supervisory alliance by creating an atmosphere of trust and acceptance. This step is crucial because the intervention requires supervisee(s) to disclose their socio-cultural identities, which may amplify concerns related to the power imbalance in supervision. In doing so, the supervisor can model identity disclosure, including how structures of privilege and oppression have impacted their personal and professional development. This intervention can also serve as a tool to enhance trust and safety already cultivated within the supervisory relationship.

### Legal and Ethical Considerations

Supervisors should support supervisee autonomy in sharing their socio-political realities and recognize this may lead to the supervisee disclosing experiences of recent harm. Therefore, the supervisor should be ready to provide necessary support, seek peer consultation, and refer to legal and ethical professional standards when necessary.

### Reflective Questions

1. How has your understanding of the role and purpose of counseling been influenced by using the SSII?
2. What aspects of social, cultural, and political capital have been the most difficult for you to examine, and how do you understand that difficulty?
3. How has the use of the SSII facilitated your experience of the supervision relationship?

## APPENDIX

### Appendix A Supervision Structural Inequity Inventory

While reflecting on your personal and professional experiences, please evaluate the salience of each statement with a response ranging from 0 (not at all) to 100 (very much):

1. My identities and positionality allow me to be protected and favored by structures and systems in the U.S. that privilege White/Caucasian people.
2. My identities and positionality allow me to be protected and favored by structures and systems in the U.S. that privilege heterosexuals.

3. My identities and positionality allow me to be protected and favored by structures and systems in the U.S. that privilege cis-gender men/males.
4. My identities and positionality allow me to be protected and favored by structures and systems in the U.S. that privilege Christians.
5. I have felt threatened and/or harmed by federal, state, and local legislation passed.
6. I have been harmed by racial segregation and redlining policies.
7. I have easy access to fresh and healthy food.
8. I can afford fresh and healthy food.
9. I have access to sidewalks and parks where I feel physically safe.
10. I am worried about being the target of violence in my neighborhood.
11. I can afford to live in a safe neighborhood.
12. I am worried about being the target of violence in any other space I frequently occupy.
13. I have access to reliable and affordable healthcare.
14. I have reading, writing, and speaking proficiency in English.
15. I had many options for which university or college I would attend for my bachelor's degree.

## Appendix B Supervision Structural Inequity Inventory— Client Version

While reflecting on your client's lived experience please evaluate the salience of each statement with a response ranging from 0 (not at all) to 100 (very much):

1. The clients' identities and positionality allow them to be protected and favored by structures and systems in the U.S. that privilege White/ Caucasian people.
2. The clients' identities and positionality allow them to be protected and favored by structures and systems in the U.S. that privilege heterosexuals.
3. The clients' identities and positionality allow them to be protected and favored by structures and systems in the U.S. that privilege cis-gender men/males.
4. The clients' identities and positionality allow them to be protected and favored by structures and systems in the U.S. that privilege Christians.
5. The client has felt threatened and/or harmed by federal, state, and local legislation.
6. The client has been harmed by racial segregation and redlining policies.

7. The client has easy access to fresh and healthy food.
8. The client can afford fresh and healthy food.
9. The client has access to sidewalks and parks where they feel physically safe.
10. The client is worried about being the target of violence in their neighborhood.
11. The client can afford to live in a safe neighborhood.
12. The client is worried about being the target of violence in any other space they frequently occupy.
13. The client has access to reliable and affordable healthcare.
14. The client has reading, writing, and speaking proficiency in English.
15. The clients' ability allows them to be protected and favored by structures and systems in the U.S. that privilege able-bodied people.
16. The clients' citizenship status allows them to be protected and favored by structures and systems in the U.S. that privilege people with citizenship.
17. The clients' body size allows them to be protected and favored by structures and systems in the U.S. that privilege people with slim bodies.
18. The clients' skin tone allows them to be protected and favored by structures and systems in the U.S. privilege light skin/fair complexion.
19. My client belongs to a group that has experienced generational oppression and discrimination in U.S. society.

## Intervention Title: Celebrate Everything: A Conversation About Equity in Federal Holidays

### Author(s) and Affiliation(s)

Rehman Abdulrehman, Ph.D.
University of Manitoba

Monnica T. Williams, Ph.D., ABPP
University of Ottawa

### Supervision Format and Modality

This anti-oppressive supervision intervention was developed for group supervision conducted virtually or in person. It is important for each person in the group to share their own thoughts and insights in order to foster group cohesion and reciprocal vulnerability. The voices of racialized and marginalized participants should be prioritized, but racialized and marginalized people should not be compelled to speak for all members of their cultural group.

### Supervisee Development

This supervision can be used across all developmental levels.

### Supervisory Goals and Learning Objectives

1. Engage supervisees in a critical discussion about federal holidays, examining which holidays are recognized and their implications for sustaining a White-centered social infrastructure.

2. Facilitate conversations that highlight how holidays centered around White and colonial narratives create inequities in cultural representation, ultimately limiting access to resources for marginalized communities.
3. Guide supervisees in critically evaluating the unexamined acceptance of federal holidays and their role in reinforcing privilege among racial, cultural, and religious groups.

4.  Develop actionable strategies with supervisees for redistributing social, cultural, and political capital by redefining the holidays celebrated within their practice and advocating for a more inclusive social infrastructure.

5.  Empower supervisees to propose and implement changes that reflect a diverse society in the celebrations and practices within their professional environments.

## Time Required

This intervention requires approximately 60 minutes, depending on the number of group members, level of discussion, and any adaptions to the intervention.

## Materials

Before using this intervention, the supervisor should review the currently recognized federal and regional holidays and the history of each holiday. They should also familiarize themselves with the content, process, and experience related to the intervention. They should create a handout or slide featuring the Celebrate Everything proposed holiday calendar (see box later on).

## Intervention Instructions

Most recognized holidays have roots in religious observances and events that emphasize Eurocentric, Christian, and privileged heritage, including those often deemed secular, such as Christmas and Easter. This exercise invites trainees to reflect on these holidays, considering who benefits and who is marginalized. Federal holidays provide paid time off for employees, while municipalities spend tax money on decorations and create a social structure that favors those who adopt these holidays. Consequently, this exercise highlights historical and current inequities in the distribution of capital, resources, access, and opportunities for those who do not celebrate these holidays. This exercise is based on the work of Abdulrehman (2024) and his project called Celebrate Everything, which advances a plan to ensure that most groups are represented in our social observances.

1.  The supervisor will deliver the following questions. Supervisees will get into groups of 2/3 and spend 5–10 minutes answering each of the following questions:

- Take a look at your yearly calendar. How many federal holidays are there? What are they celebrating and why?
- In what ways are these holidays biased based on race, gender, ethnicity, religion, and/or other social locations?
- Consider the various ethnic and cultural groups in your community. You can go online and look up the demographics of your city or state/province to better understand the diversity of your community. Which holidays are most important to each of these groups? Why are these important to know as an anti-oppressive clinician?
- Which of the cultural holidays you identified can be added to our calendar, and how would we accommodate this within your clinical practice?

2. Reassemble as a larger group and go around the room, allowing someone from each group to respond to how they answered the questions posed.
3. Next, present the information from the Celebrate Everything project. Following the presentation, facilitate a group discussion on how well supervisees identified key holidays to include on the calendar. Emphasize the importance of incorporating holidays for marginalized communities, even if they are not part of the supervisees' own community. Acknowledging these holidays fosters representation for marginalized groups and educates those unfamiliar with their perspectives and experiences. This serves as both an exercise in representation and a commitment to anti-oppression and anti-racism.
4. Next, using Abdulrehman (2024) project called "Celebrate Everything," the supervisor will review, contextualize and discuss the following information.

- The supervisor can state, "A key to ensuring cultural representation across all segments of society is to ree-valuate how we utilize public financial and social resources (capital) to foster a truly multicultural society (Abdulrehman, 2024). It is essential that citizens from all communities feel represented under a shared cultural umbrella. Celebrated holidays contribute to shared social capital, enabling marginalized individuals to draw on the strength of their larger communities (Bartlett et al., 2022). Recognizing at least one major holiday or observance from each socio-cultural community promotes inclusivity, and it can help educate those outside these communities, thereby reducing ignorance and addressing the roots of bias, racism, and oppression."

- Following, the supervisor can state, "Celebration fosters connection and allows us to address ignorance and hate, in a more functional and positive way the anxiety and stress that typically come with this kind of discussion. The goal is also to celebrate these holidays the way that the marginalized communities celebrate them, turning what is typically perceived as foreign into local, exotic into normal, and what is other/them into us, thereby increasing relatability between different groups. To be clear, this is different from global festivals where "international cultures" can be stereotyped. Rather, this is an initiative to shift thinking and practice to local intersectional identities, to move beyond tokenism, and to empower positive socio-cultural identities in everyone."

- Last, the supervisor can share, "Our current calendar of holidays primarily centers on dominant social locations, such as Christian, Eurocentric, and heterosexist holidays. The goal now is to ensure equity and representation by doing the same with other socio-cultural groups. The best way to do this is to ensure that major religious or cultural holidays are acknowledged publicly by the government, businesses, schools, the media, and private organizations. Since religious holidays (not unlike Christmas and Easter) are celebrated both religiously and culturally (secularly) by people in cultural communities, it is important that religious and cultural holidays are included in the calendar and professional ethos."

5. Next, the supervisor will place the following information from the Celebrate Everything project on a slide or handout for the group to review together. The supervision group can begin with holidays based on race, ethnicity, and religion and then can follow up with other socio-cultural holidays.

# CELEBRATE EVERYTHING HOLIDAYS TO INCLUDE

What follows are holidays to add to our current calendar. Though already on our calendars, Christmas is mentioned here to show that many communities of color fall under this umbrella, yet there are still ways to make it more inclusive.

## *Religious Holidays*

## *Christianity*

Communities who are not White but come from countries with a Christian heritage or culture (e.g., Latino, African, European, and Filipino communities) will be included in the current celebration of holidays such as Christmas and Easter. Consider the different ways these are celebrated by cultural communities and bring those into our current practice to allow everyone celebrating these holidays to feel more included (e.g., popcorn ceremony for the Ethiopian community). But because these holidays already exist, cultural communities from Christian-based countries will already have representation. Our focus will be to include holidays listed in what follows, as they are not currently represented, including different cultural aspects to already celebrated holidays is easier to do, and we do some of this already. These holidays are where we need to initially place our focus on increasing equity and inclusion.

## *Judaism*

- Rosh Hashanah
- Yom Kippur (observed not celebrated)

## *Islam*

- Ramadan and Eid al Fitr (month-long observance, day celebrated at the end)
- Eid al Adha

## *Hinduism*

- Diwali (also celebrated by Sikhs, Jains, and Buddhists)

### Buddhism

- Vesak (birth of Buddha). Many Buddhists also belong to other cultural communities and celebrate other holidays on this list.

### Sikhism

- Baisakhi (Vasakhi)

### Baha'i

- Nowruz (Iranian or Persian New Year; also celebrated culturally by Persian, Kurdish, & Afghan communities). But Baha'is also celebrate many Muslim and Christian holidays as well.

### Cultural Holidays

It is important to ensure the representation of cultural holidays from communities that may not belong to any religious community or have intersecting identities that are very important to them. Some that fall in that category include:

### East Asian Community

- Lunar New Year (a less inclusive term was Chinese New Year)

### Indigenous Community

- National Indigenous People's day. This will be the most important day to celebrate, as it celebrates the First Peoples of Canada and the U.S., and can be a step toward reconciliation.

### Black Community

- Kwanzaa. Celebrated by some in the Black community, this is an annual celebration of African American culture, culminating in a feast on the 6th day—called Karamu. Created by activist Maulana Karenga to have a holiday reflective of African American culture, it is celebrated by some Canadians as well.

6. Next, supervisees can look into various holidays and the subsequent practices. In doing so, supervisees can look into the history, who is included or excluded, and outline how we can collectively honor and celebrate within our personal and professional spaces and communities.

7. Last, the entire supervision group can discuss how they will work towards continuing to identify diverse socio-cultural holidays and foster a commitment to diversity, equity, and inclusion as a means to re-center historically silenced and excluded holidays and communities within their clinical contexts (e.g., counseling, supervision, class, etc.). Moreover, the discussion should also include how they can integrate such anti-oppressive practices into their clinical sites and client advocacy.

## Supervisory Alliance and Relationship Considerations

There are multiple considerations for supervisors. Given this intervention is a group exercise, group dynamics and experiences related to social, cultural, and political power are essential for understanding how learners may respond to the prompts and to one another.

## Legal and Ethical Considerations

Consultation with communities is always encouraged, as it allows clarification of how these observances can be acknowledged respectfully and fully (Abdulrehman, 2024).

## Reflective Questions

1. How might new holidays change how we understand and appreciate the many different cultural groups around us?

2. How does failure to recognize a holiday that is important to a specific cultural group advance inequity in capital and resources within clinical and supervisory spaces?

3. What feelings and biases do you notice at the prospect of changing our calendar as advanced by Celebrate Everything?

4. How can you use your privilege to advance change in your own personal and professional community? (See Williams et al., 2023a for a discussion on civil courage.)

### Intervention Title: What's Your Capital?: Utilizing Community Cultural Wealth as a Strengths-Based Framework to Guide Supervisors and Counselors-in-Training

### Author(s) and Affiliation(s)

Janice A. Byrd-Badjie, Ph.D.
The Pennsylvania State University

Deepika Raju Nantha Kumar, M.Ed, NCC
The Pennsylvania State University

### Supervision Format and Modality

This intervention utilizes the Community Cultural Wealth (Yosso, 2005) framework to guide a strengths-focused conversation about cultural capital between supervisors and supervisees. This intervention is written to be facilitated live, in-person, and during individual supervision. However, the intervention can be modified and applied to group, triadic, or peer supervision. Additionally, the intervention can be adapted to virtual and case report modalities.

### Supervisee Development

This supervision intervention is intended for masters-level practicum and/or internship students; however, we suggest supervisors consider the supervisee's developmental awareness of social systems, power, privilege, and oppression before facilitating. Specifically, we recommend supervisees who have taken a Multicultural Counseling, Social & Cultural Diversity, and/or Systems Theory course. This intervention can be adapted for individuals who are in doctoral practicum or internship, have professional development/remediation plans, are post-graduate and pre-licensed professionals, or are post-graduate and post-licensed professionals. This intervention is intended for individuals at the introductory stage of becoming a counselor (e.g., masters-level practicum and/or internship students) or those refining their counseling skills (e.g., post-graduate/pre-licensed).

### Supervisory Goals and Learning Objectives

1. Supervisees will increase their understanding of how one's identity impacts all facets of their life, including barriers and opportunities.

2. Supervisees will demonstrate the use of Community Cultural Wealth (Yosso, 2005) as a framework to guide conversations about supervisees and client/student strengths.
3. Supervisees will develop at least three action steps for self and client/student—empowerment, critical consciousness, and advocacy.

## Time Required

This intervention requires 60 minutes for activity completion (i.e., 30 minutes for Worksheet 1 and 30 minutes for Worksheet 2) and discussion. Supervisors are encouraged to adjust the time during the one-hour meeting based on the supervisee's self-awareness and knowledge of the framework. Supervisors should be prepared to describe the framework to the supervisees, provide examples, and answer questions.

## Materials

- The intervention will require access to Worksheet 1 (see Figure 11.1), which explores one's cultural identities, and Worksheet 2 (see Figure 11.2, adapted from Yosso's (2005) Community Cultural Wealth. It will also necessitate access to Yosso's (2005) article.

  - Yosso, T. (2005). Whose culture has capital? A critical race theory discussion of community cultural wealth, *Race Ethnicity and Education*, *8*(1), 69–91. https://doi.org10.1080/1361332052000341006

- Before engaging in this intervention, supervisors are encouraged to complete the worksheets independently to familiarize themselves with the intervention, model the necessity of reflection to their supervisees, and build rapport by sharing their responses with their supervisees. If time and resources are available, supervisors can discuss their responses to these prompts with a professional peer to increase self-awareness and challenge any biases or blind spots that surface during the reflective process that may impact the supervisory relationship. Additionally, supervisors should review the Community Cultural Wealth (Yosso, 2005) framework and assign it as a reading for the supervisee before facilitating the intervention. Supervisors and supervisees are encouraged to read more about how this framework has been used with marginalized populations (Anandavalli, 2021; Clemons, 2024).

## Intervention Instructions

1. Supervisors should introduce the concepts supervisees will engage with on each worksheet. Firstly, the supervisor will describe cultural

identities and provide examples (e.g., show their completed worksheet) to guide the process. Secondly, supervisors can review Yosso's (2005) Community Cultural Wealth framework and engage in questions the supervisee may have. Supervisors are encouraged to ask questions about the framework and can ask supervisees about their perceptions to gauge understanding. For example, what are some of your thoughts about how community cultural wealth is described? In what ways does community cultural wealth show up for you and/or the clients you work with? How does community cultural wealth help you understand your cultural strengths?

2.  The supervisor will give supervisees time to complete Worksheet 1 (see Figure 11.1), which explores their cultural identities.

3.  Once Worksheet 1 is completed, the supervisor and supervisee will share each other's completed worksheets and engage in conversation using the reflective prompts. They are encouraged to discuss the way their identities impact the supervisory relationship and their relationships with clients. For instance, how do power, privilege, and oppression show up in your daily life? Looking at our responses to these questions, how may power and privilege affect our relationship and communication?

4.  Next, the supervisor will provide the supervisee time to complete Worksheet 2 (see Figure 11.2), which explores Community Cultural Wealth (Yosso, 2005).

5.  Once Worksheet 2 is completed, the supervisor and supervisee will share each other's completed worksheets and engage in conversation using the reflective prompts. They are encouraged to discuss what Community Cultural Wealth (Yosso, 2005) they hold and how previous discussions about their identities influence barriers created by systems of oppression and/or opportunities informed by privilege related to this capital.

6.  After the intervention, supervisors can engage supervisees in conversation about the intervention and explore how it can be used with current or future clients/students. For example, how might this intervention be helpful to the young Black girl you're counseling who is taking personal responsibility for negative characterizations she hears about herself/other Black girls in the school? How might this exercise help your linguistically diverse clients recognize the wealth of being multilingual while also validating the negative emotions that arise from daily microaggressions? Supervisors are encouraged to remind supervisees of the resources (Anandavalli, 2021; Clemons, 2024), outlining

how the Community Cultural Wealth (Yosso, 2005) framework can be used in clinical and school counseling settings.

## Supervisory Alliance and Relationship

Supervisors are encouraged to consider many factors when guiding supervisees through this intervention, which warrants being critically reflexive and considering one's privilege and social-political location. Firstly, supervisors should consider where the supervisee is in their professional and cultural identity development. Supervisors are reminded that masters-level supervisees are often newly out of their bachelor's programs. Much of their perceptions of learning are still rooted in a banking education model, a one-way flow of information from teacher to student. Asking students to think critically, challenge systems they have navigated all their lives, and create new perspectives can bring about privileged identity defenses or cognitive dissonance. Secondly, the supervisor should consider the supervisee's ability to engage in critical discourse about power, privilege, and oppression. Supervisors are encouraged to reference scholarship about concerns that supervisees of color encounter in cross-cultural supervisory relationships (Washington et al., 2023) and the issues that supervisors of color face (Singh & Chun, 2010). Finally, the supervisor should consider the supervisee's receptiveness to receiving and implementing feedback. Conversations about community expectations related to feedback and communication styles should be addressed early in the supervisory relationship.

## Legal and Ethical Considerations

Supervisors and supervisees have ethical responsibilities within the supervisory relationship that are crucial to fostering environments that support supervisee growth and ensure client/student safety. As noted previously, supervisors are constantly modeling dispositions that reflect positive ethical practices for their supervisees. Because this intervention centers on personal disclosures, supervisors are encouraged to remind supervisees of what confidentiality looks like in the supervisory relationship and how that looks similar or different from what it looks like in the counseling relationship. Secondly, supervisors are encouraged to discuss concepts like transference and countertransference with the supervisee, which can manifest in both counseling and supervisory relationships. Thirdly, supervisors are encouraged to revisit their profession's code of ethics, ethical decision-making models, and any discipline-specific resources related to their professional identity.

### Reflective Questions

1. In what ways do your clients' communities demonstrate unique forms of cultural wealth, such as familial support, linguistic skills, or resistance strategies, that contribute to their resilience and well-being?
2. In what ways can you help clients recognize and utilize their community assets to navigate systemic barriers?
3. How can we build a culture of valuing and developing cultural wealth within the supervisory space?

## APPENDIX

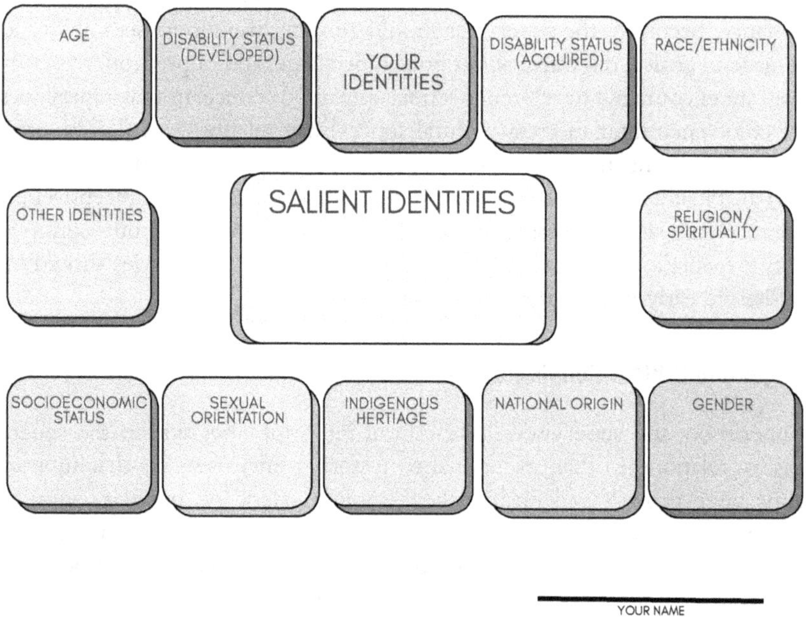

*Figure 11.1* Worksheet 1

1. What are some strengths that you derive from these identities? How do these strengths support your social-emotional well-being?
2. What aspects of your identity provide sources of influence?
3. What aspects of your identity are marginalized and influence the barriers and oppression you face?

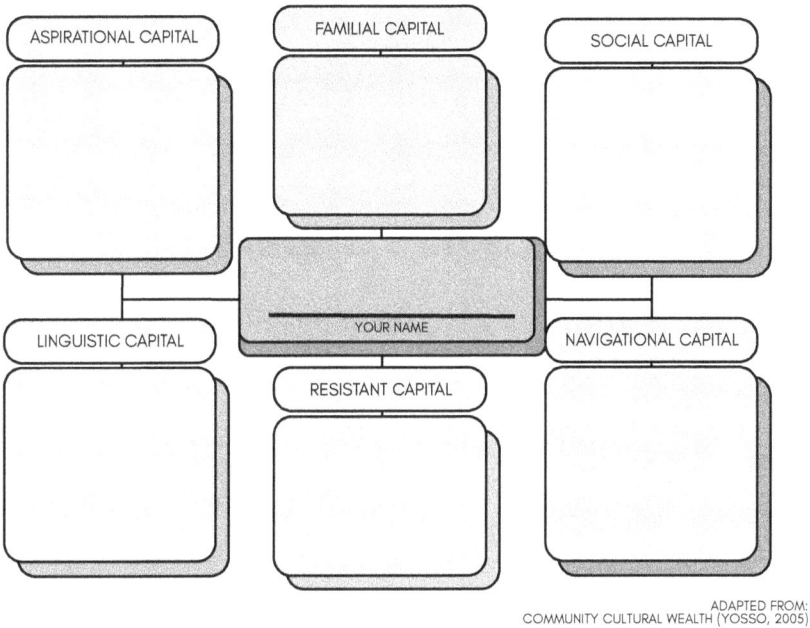

ADAPTED FROM:
COMMUNITY CULTURAL WEALTH (YOSSO, 2005)

*Figure 11.2* Worksheet 2

1.  What strengths come from the identified community cultural capital?
2.  How do the strengths identified help you navigate barriers, marginalization, and oppression?

### Key Definitions:

*   Aspirational capital: capability to hold onto hope for oneself and others despite the barriers posed by systems of oppression.
*   Familial capital: heritage and cultural wealth that is inherited through traditions, stories, and kinship.
*   Social capital: networks and community within various spaces.
*   Linguistic capital: narration of stories, experiences, and skills using a variety of ways of communicating and different languages of communication.
*   Resistant capital: unique ways to resist and disrupt the systems of oppression.
*   Navigational capital: gaining skills and guidance on navigating systems of oppression with an understanding that the systems were not created to serve individuals with systemically marginalized identities.

# CHAPTER 12

# Anti-Oppressive Supervision

## A Personal and Professional Call to Action

*Harvey Charles Peters and Melissa Luke*

## CLOSING AND IMPLICATIONS

Our book, *Interventions for Anti-Oppressive Clinical Supervision: Navigating Critical Praxis,* began as an ambitious effort to bridge the considerable gap between contemporary theory and the praxis of anti-oppressive supervision (Lee, 2023; Peters et al., 2022). Despite continued attention to multicultural supervision (Kemer et al., 2022; Watkins et al., 2019) and social justice-related supervision (Asakura & Maurer, 2018; Dollarhide et al., 2021; Ellison et al., 2024; Hair, 2015), as well as an increased focus on anti-racist (Abdulrehman, 2024; Johnson et al., 2022) and culturally humble (Ertl et al., 2023; Jones & Branco, 2020; Watkins, 2023; Wilcox et al., 2023) approaches in clinical supervision, there remained a lack of resources, training, and opportunities to connect these to anti-oppressive methods (Ali & Lee, 2019; Bradley et al., 2023). Likewise, there were few accessible contemporary scholarly resources that support the praxis of anti-oppressive clinical supervision more broadly across mental health professions (Legha, 2023a, 2023b; Okech et al., 2023a; Peters et al., 2022). With the publication of this book, however, the deficiency has been reduced. Educators, supervisors, clinicians, students, and supervisees alike now have a comprehensive resource to edify and guide their anti-oppressive supervisory praxis.

In Chapter 1, we (editors) reviewed and synthesized the anti-oppressive-related supervision scholarship across counseling, psychology, social work, marriage and family therapy, and other allied fields and infused this into the development of the Anti-Oppressive Supervision Model (AOSM). The AOSM is grounded in the 10 research-derived principles of anti-oppression (Peters & Luke, 2022) and extends the Discrimination Model

DOI: 10.4324/9781003470656-12

(Bernard, 1979, 1997), the most widely used and researched model of clinical supervision to date. Across each of the 10 anti-oppressive principles that serve as the entry point into the AOSM, we offer a plethora of detailed examples as to how supervisory needs may present across intervention, conceptualization, and personalization foci, and how each can be addressed using the teacher, counselor, and consultant role postures. Similar to other extensions of the Discrimination Model (Luke & Bernard, 2006), this is followed by exemplars of AOSM points or entry, focus, and role combinations that the supervisor may use to accomplish their clinical supervisory goals and objectives. We believe that readers will find the book and AOSM helpful when adapting and adopting this material into their current understanding and praxis of anti-oppressive supervision. We also have confidence that to do so, anti-oppressive supervisors will honor their ethical and clinical commitments to the continuation of their own personal and professional skill development in the service of their supervisees and the clients with whom they work (ACA, 2014; APA, 2017). Our hope is that the range of provided examples can highlight common intra—and inter-personal experiences associated with this work and offer both preventative and responsive approaches to address in supervision should they arise.

This is followed by Chapters 2–11, wherein selected expert contributing supervisors shared their innovative and forward-looking anti-oppressive supervisory interventions. Individually, the chapters focus on a different anti-oppressive principle (Peters & Luke, 2022), with each chapter containing five inimitable anti-oppressive supervisory interventions that collectively span what Bernard and Goodyear (2019) identify as the relationships within and the delivery areas of supervision, namely individual, triadic, and group contexts; in-person, virtual, or hybrid modalities; drawing from a range of theoretical frameworks; and intended for specific supervisory development levels. Understanding the necessity of a clear context for and a description of the requisite materials and steps of implementation (Bean et al., 2014; Prasath & Copeland, 2021), all contributing authors were asked to provide this so readers will be able to immediately apply the anti-oppressive supervisory interventions into their supervisory praxis. As many of the interventions offer ideas for further extension or adaptation, we hope that supervisors draw on this anti-oppressive grounding by purposefully adjusting and infusing the material to the unique and evolving needs of their supervisees, their own supervisory styles and frameworks, and their emergent anti-oppressive supervision practices. Building on the limited peer-reviewed creative supervisory interventions (Bradley et al., 2023), the supervision praxis literature can benefit from additional examples of anti-oppressive supervisory interventions for supervisors and educators to incorporate into their respective supervisory settings. As such, we encourage readers to codify and begin to evaluate the impact of their own anti-oppressive supervisory interventions (and seek mechanisms and venues for distribution). Despite the diversity of identities and social locations of contributing supervisory authors, we recognize the proportionally under-representation of practitioner-supervisors, as well as supervisors practicing outside of the United States, and particularly encourage representation and inclusion of these perspectives in the anti-oppressive supervisory intervention literature.

Relatedly, we encourage readers, supervisors, and supervision scholars to consider how the AOSM and subsequent anti-oppressive supervisory interventions can be synthesized into ongoing supervision training and professional development. As all mental health disciplines have discipline-specific training standards for supervision (APA, 2014; Borders, 2014; Henriksen et al., 2019; Ogbeide & Bayles, 2023), increasingly addressing anti-oppressive principles (reference), we suggest that educators and program specialists consider conducting an anti-oppressive content audit of their current training and related materials (Bright & Ghouse, 2018; Griffith et al., 2022; Theoharis et al., 2022; Wells et al., 2023) to identify areas in need of update, expansion, and/or revision and then identify areas of Chapter 1 that can be included to fill the gaps, as well as seeking additional resources. In addition, many professional organizations, community agencies and institutions, as well as primary investigators for federal mental health training grants, are called to provide professional development for the clinical supervisors with whom they work (Elliott, 2016; Leventhal et al., 2004). As such, we encourage these professional development providers to incorporate the AOSM and subsequent anti-oppressive supervision interventions into the workshops, brown bags, and seminars that they provide.

For those supervision trainers who seek interactive and experiential training, the AOSM, as presented, can be adapted for case vignettes for the experiential anti-oppressive training of attendees. Naturally, presenters should intentionally attend to both process and content related to the 10 anti-oppressive principles and be careful to allot the necessary time and space for relationship-building within the training. For example, the authors conducted an online two-day, six-hour anti-oppressive supervisory training for site supervisors in the community, and once the initial content was determined, they reflected on the andrologies most appropriate with anti-oppressive principles and supervisory learning goals. In doing so, we recognized that the interpersonal aspects and necessary reflection and processing required additional time, necessitating abbreviating some of the content. Participant evaluations were positive, revealing significant recognition of and appreciation for the processes modeled, as well as the substance of the materials and resources shared.

Although many of the anti-oppressive supervision interventions are extensions of empirically evaluated and/or research-supported supervisory practices, to our knowledge, few if any of the interventions have been directly researched themselves. While we always encourage supervisor practitioners to gather their own process and outcome evaluations, we hope to inspire a link between anti-oppressive supervisory praxis and research, where practicing supervisors consider research methods such as single case designs, multiple case study (Dillman Taylor & Blount, 2021; Merriam, 1998; Yin, 2017), and collaborative transformative action research (Steen et al., 2023) as means to not only measure their direct supervisory work but also as viable mechanisms to provide data for research that is disseminated more broadly. Moreover, supervision and anti-oppressive scholars can employ other more familiar quantitative (e.g., descriptive, correlational, experimental) and qualitative (e.g., phenomenology, narrative, discourse analysis, consensual qualitative research) methodologies to investigate and explore what comprises anti-oppressive supervision, how anti-oppressive supervision interventions compare to other historic supervisory approaches, as well as the development processes subsumed within becoming both an anti-oppressive supervisor and anti-oppressive mental health practitioner. We encourage researchers to specifically employ critical and anti-oppressive research methodologies, such as critical analytic synthesis (Peters & Luke, 2022), Indigenous methodology (Kovach, 2021; Snow et al., 2016), Intersectional methodology (Esposito & Evans-Winters, 2021), decolonial methodology (Rhee, 2020), and post-structuralist methodology (St. Pierre, 2021, 2023), in this work.

Ideally, *Interventions for Anti-Oppressive Clinical Supervision: Navigating Critical Praxis* is the beginning of a resilient link between anti-oppressive supervision theory and praxis, with an understanding that both are continually re/surfacing and advancing. Just as we recognize that this work builds upon the foundation laid by the supervision and anti-oppressive giants that came before, we anticipate that this work will inspire future anti-oppressive supervision scholarship and praxis that is essential for the development of the mental health fields, our literatures, and most importantly supervisors, supervisees, and practitioners, as well as the clients with whom we work. We stand in solidarity with all those who bravely advocate for and engage in anti-oppressive supervision, changing people and systems in the process.

We end our book with a "call to action" concerning the future of anti-oppressive clinical supervision across interdisciplinary mental health and allied professions. We call upon readers across professional roles and contexts to join us in shaping the future of anti-oppressive clinical supervision. It is our position that the future of clinical supervision rests upon a significant paradigm shift centering anti-oppressive praxis and activism at its core, bridging theory and practice to address deeply rooted historical systemic inequities faced by mental health professionals and those we seek and claim to serve. To effectively advance anti-oppressive supervision, each of the mental health professions must move beyond traditional training modalities, techniques, interventions, and frameworks to actively implement models like the AOSM. Moreover, educators, supervisors, and leaders across professional contexts can use our book and the extant scholarship to conduct critical and systematic reviews of training materials, processes, practices, protocols, and policies to identify gaps and oppressive issues where anti-oppressive principles can be integrated, thereby aligning training with the evolving theorization and praxis of anti-oppressive clinical supervision. Such work necessitates continuous adaptation, reflexivity, and evaluation to ensure these principles and subsequent material become integral to supervision praxis across each of the mental health professions.

For example, we see the need for educators and schools as well as agencies and organizations to critically examine unpaid internships and fellowships and their ethical and equitable implications (see Hood et al., 2024; Wilcox et al., 2021; Zilvinskis et al., 2020). Unpaid training opportunities often perpetuate financial and systemic barriers, disproportionately impacting the holistic personal and professional being of marginalized students and supervisees from historically oppressed sociocultural backgrounds (Hood et al., 2024; Wilcox et al., 2021; Zilvinskis et al., 2020), especially those who are most affected by the multiplicity within the matrix of domination (Crenshaw, 1989; Collins, 2022). By sustaining structures and systems that privilege those who can afford to work or require supervision to take out significant loans without compensation, the current internship and fellowship systems reinforce capitalistic and oppressive inequities rather than dismantle them. To align with an anti-oppressive philosophy, we call educators, supervisors, and professional leaders to advocate for paid, accessible training pathways that recognize the labor and contributions of trainees and supervisees, ensuring a more just and sustainable professional landscape (Hood et al., 2024; Wilcox et al., 2021; Zilvinskis et al., 2020). Although only one example, we believe it showcases the need to deconstruct and reconstruct the longstanding training and supervision structures and systems in place across each of the professions to holistically and ecologically align with anti-oppression.

Lastly, we ask readers across professional roles and contexts to look toward the future of anti-oppressive clinical supervision. In doing so, we

emphasize the crucial role of research in developing, refining, expanding, and validating anti-oppressive supervisory practices, training, and
theorization, including those outlined in our book. As noted previously,
urge scholars to employ critical, intersectional, community-centered, and
anti-oppressive methodologies using qualitative, quantitative, and mixed-
method paradigms to explore the impact and effectiveness of these interventions, building an evidence base that supports anti-oppression and
systemic change (Bhattacharya, 2017; Esposito & Evans-Winters, 2021;
Hays & Singh, 2023; Kovach, 2021; Rhee, 2020; Rodney et al., 2024;
Snow et al., 2016; St. Pierre, 2021, 2023; Winkle-Wagner et al., 2019).
More specifically, we call for research that does not merely reproduce existing frameworks but pushes boundaries by developing new interventions
and frameworks, adapting evolving paradigms, and evaluating outcomes
in real-world contexts. This includes examining how anti-oppressive
interventions and frameworks influence the sense of agency, critical consciousness, and anti-oppressive professional identity development of trainees, supervisees, and supervisors. It is vital that supervision scholars also
explore essential constructs identified in clinical supervision and expand
upon them within the context of anti-oppression and related paradigms
such as anti-racism and decolonization. This includes but is not limited
to examining the experiences of marginalized supervisees and supervisors
within anti-oppressive supervision (e.g., Degenstein et al., 2023), navigating parallel processes within anti-oppressive supervision (e.g., Stein &
Cullen, 2024), developing anti-oppressive supervision instruments (e.g.,
Li et al., 2024), exploring anti-oppressive metacognition in the context
of supervision (e.g., Zalzala & Gagen, 2023), and assessing the impact and
harm of performative and inadequate anti-oppressive supervision (e.g.,
Hutman et al., 2023). Additionally, it is crucial for scholars to investigate
the longitudinal effects of these frameworks on professional growth, supervisory relationships, and client outcomes. To achieve this, collaborative
efforts must intentionally and critically include diverse partners, including
but not limited to students, supervisees, agencies, clinicians, educators,
and policymakers, in order to bridge the gap between siloed academic
and practitioner communities. Our call to action is clear. By embracing
a research-informed, critical, and inquisitive approach to clinical supervision, we can collectively transform clinical supervision and our profession into spaces of equity, justice, liberation, and healing. Centering
anti-oppression in both research and practice is not just an aspiration, it is
the pathway to creating a tangible reality that fosters a more just, compas-
sionate, anti-oppressive, liberatory, and truly equitable mental health field
for all.

# References

Abdulrehman, R. Y. (2024). *Developing anti-racist cultural competence.* Hogrefe/American Psychological Association.

Abramson, L. Y., Seligman, M. E. P., & Teasdale, J. D. (1978). Learned helplessness in humans: Critique and reformulation. *Journal of Abnormal Psychology, 87*(1), 49–74.

Accurso, E. C., Taylor, R. M., & Garland, A. F. (2011). Evidence-based practices addressed in community-based children's mental health clinical supervision. *Training and Education in Professional Psychology, 5*(2), 88. https://doi.org/10.1037/a0023537

Adkins-Jackson, P. B., Jackson Preston, P. A., & Hairston, T. (2023). 'The only way out': How self-care is conceptualized by Black women. *Ethnicity & Health, 28*(1), 29–45. https://doi.org/10.1080/13557858.2022.2027878

Ahmed, R., Bruce, S., & Jurcik, T. (2018). Towards a socioecological framework to support mental health caregivers: Implications for social work practice and education. *Social Work in Mental Health, 16*(1), 105–122. https://doi.org/10.1080/15332985.2017.1336744

Alexander, J. C., Thompson, K., & Edles, L. D. (2016). *Contemporary introduction to sociology: Culture and society in transition.* Routledge.

Ali, S., & Lee, C. C. (2019). Using creativity to explore intersectionality in counseling. *Journal of Creativity in Mental Health, 14*(4), 510–518. https://doi.org/10.1080/15401383.2019.1632767

American Counseling Association. (2014). *ACA code of ethics.* https://www.counseling.org/resources/aca-code-of-ethics.pdf

American Psychological Association (APA). (2006). *Guidelines and principles for accreditation of programs in professional psychology (G&P).* http://www.apa.org/ed/accreditation/about/policies/guiding-principles.pdf

American Psychological Association (APA). (2014). *Guidelines for clinical supervision in health service psychology*. http://apa.org/about/policy/guidelines-supervision.pdf

American Psychological Association (APA). (2017). *Multicultural guidelines: An ecological approach to context, identity, and intersectionality*. http://www.apa.org/about/policy/multicultural-guidelines.pdf

Anandavalli, S. (2021). Strengths-based counseling with international students of color: A community cultural wealth approach. *Journal of Asia Pacific Counseling, 11*(1), 111–124. https://doi.org/10.18401/2021.11.1.7

Anekstein, A. M., Hoskins, W. J., Astramovich, R. L., Garner, D., & Terry, J. (2014). "Sandtray supervision": Integrating supervision models and sandtray therapy. *Journal of Creativity in Mental Health, 9*(1), 122–134. https://doi.org/10.1080/15401383.2014.876885

Arnold, R., Burke, B., James, C., Martin, D., & Thomas, B. (1991). *Educating for a change*. Doris Marshall Institute for Education and Action and Between the Lines Press.

Arredondo, P., Toporek, R., Brown, S. P., Jones, J., Locke, D. C., Sanchez, J., & Stadler, H. (1996). Operationalization of the multicultural counseling competencies. *Journal of Multicultural Counseling and Development, 24*(1), 42–78. https://doi.org/10.1002/j.2161-1912.1996.tb00288.x

Asakura, K., & Maurer, K. (2018). Attending to social justice in clinical social work: Supervision as a pedagogical space. *Clinical Social Work Journal, 46*(4), 289–297. https://doi.org/10.1007/s10615-018-0667-4

Ashley, W., & Lipscomb, A. E. (2018). Culturally affirming clinical supervision in graduate field education: Enhancing transformative dialogue in the supervisory dyad. https://doi.org/10.5430/irhe.v3n3p22

Atieno Okech, J. E., & Rubel, D. (2007). Diversity competent group work supervision: An application of the supervision of group work model (SGW). *The Journal for Specialists in Group Work, 32*(3), 245–266. https://doi.org/10.1080/01933920701431651

Baltrinic, E. R., & Luke, M. (2022). Empathy: A fundamental and multidimensional teaching disposition in counselor education. *Teaching & Supervision in Counseling, 4*(2), article 1. https://trace.tennessee.edu/tsc/vol4/iss2/1

Bandura, A. (1977). Self-efficacy: Toward a unifying theory of behavioral change. *Psychological Review, 84*(2), 191–215. https://doi.org/10.1037/0033-295X.84.2.191

Bandura, A. (1989). Human agency in social cognitive theory. *American Psychologist, 44*, 1175–1184. https://doi.org/10.1037/0003-066X.44.9.117

Banks-VanAllen, C. E., Midgley, B. D., & Brown, S. R. (2023). Single cases and the laws of subjectivity. *Theory & Psychology, 33*(6), 792–813. https://doi.org/10.1177/09593543231185354

Bartlett, A., Faber, S., Williams, M., & Saxberg, K. (2022). Getting to the root of the problem: Supporting clients with lived-experiences of systemic discrimination. *Chronic Stress, 6,* 1–10. https://doi.org/10.1177/24705470221139205

Bayne, H. B., & Branco, S. F. (2018). A phenomenological inquiry into counselor of color broaching experiences. *Journal of Counseling & Development, 96*(1), 75–85. https://doi.org/10.1002/jcad.12179

Bean, R. A., Davis, S. D., & Davey, M. P. (Eds.). (2014). *Clinical supervision activities for increasing competence and self-awareness.* Wiley.

Bernard, J. M. (1979). Supervisor training: A discrimination model. *Counselor Education and Supervision, 19,* 60–68.

Bernard, J. M. (1997). The discrimination model. In C. E. Watkins, Jr. (Ed.), *Handbook of psychotherapy supervision* (pp. 310–327). Wiley.

Bernard, J. M., & Goodyear, R. K. (2019). *Fundamentals of clinical supervision* (6th ed.). Pearson Education.

Bernard, J. M., & Luke, M. (2015). A content analysis of 10-years of the clinical supervision literature in counselor education. *Counselor Education & Supervision, 54*(4), 242–257. https://doi.org/10.1002/ceas.12024

Berry, J. W. (1997). Immigration, acculturation, and adaptation. *Applied Psychology, 46*(1), 5–34. https://doi.org/10.1111/j.1464-0597.1997.tb01087.x

Bhattacharya, K. (2017). *Fundamentals of qualitative research: A practical guide.* Routledge.

Bjorøy, A., Madigan, S., & Nylund, D. (2016). The practice of therapeutic letter writing in narrative therapy. In *The handbook of counselling psychology* (pp. 332–348). SAGE. https://doi.org/10.4135/9781529714968.n21

Borders, L. D. (2014). Best practices in clinical supervision: Another step in delineating effective supervision practice. *American Journal of Psychotherapy, 68*(2), 151–162. https://doi.org/10.1176/appi.psychotherapy.2014.68.2.151. PMID: 25122982

Borders, L. D., & Brown, L. L. (2022). *The new handbook of counseling supervision.* Routledge.

Borders, L. D., Dianna, J. A., & McKibben, W. B. (2023). Clinical supervisor training: A ten-year scoping review across counseling, psychology, and social work. *The Clinical Supervisor, 42*(1), 164–212. https://doi.org/10.1080/07325223.2023.2188624

Borders, L. D., Lowman, M. M., Eicher, P. A., & Phifer, J. K. (2022). Trauma-informed supervision of trainees: Practices of supervisors trained in both trauma and clinical supervision. *Traumatology.* https://doi.org/10.1037/trm0000382

Bourdieu, P., & Passeron, J. (1977). *Reproduction in education, society, and culture.* SAGE Publications.

Bradley, L., Mendoza, K., Hollingsworth, L., Johnson, P., Duffey, T., & Daniels, J. (2023). Creative supervision: Ten techniques to enhance supervision. *Journal of Creativity in Mental Health*, 1–13. Advance Online Publication. https://doi.org/10.1080/15401383.2023.2176391

Bradley, N., Stargell, N., Craigen, L., Whisenhunt, J., Campbell, E., & Kress, V. (2019). Creative approaches for promoting vulnerability in supervision: A relational–cultural approach. *Journal of Creativity in Mental Health*, *14*(3), 391–404. https://doi.org/10.1080/15401383.2018.1562395

Bright, K., & Ghouse, N. J. (2018). Taking AIM: Integrating organization development into the creation of a diversity, equity, and inclusion audit. In S. Baughman, S. Hiller, K. Monroe, & A. Pappalardo (Eds.), *Proceedings of the 2018 library assessment conference: Building effective, sustainable, practical assessment* (pp. 589–599). Association of Research Libraries. https://www.libraryassessment.org/wp-content/uploads/2019/09/64-Bright-Ghouse-TakingAIM.pdf

Bronfenbrenner, U. (2005). *Making human beings human: Bioecological perspectives on human development*. SAGE Publications.

Bronfenbrenner, U., & Morris, P. A. (1998). The ecology of developmental processes. In R. M. Lerner (Ed.), *Handbook of child psychology* (5th ed., Vol. 1, pp. 993–1028). Wiley.

Brutzman, B., Bustos, T. E., Hart, M. J., & Neal, J. W. (2022). A new wave of context: Introduction to the special issue on socioecological approaches to psychology [editorial]. *Translational Issues in Psychological Science*, *8*(2), 177–184. https://doi.org/10.1037/tps0000337

Burkard, A. W., Johnson, A. J., Madson, M. B., Pruitt, N. T., Contreras-Tadych, D. A., Kozlowski, J. M., Hess, S. A., & Knox, S. (2006). Supervisor cultural responsiveness and unresponsiveness in cross-cultural supervision. *Journal of Counseling Psychology*, *53*(3), 288–301. https://doi.org/10.1037/0022-0167.53.3.288

Burnes, T. R., & Manese, J. E. (2019). Introduction. In *Cases in multicultural clinical supervision: Models, lenses, and applications* (pp. xxvii–1). Cognella Academic Publishing.

Bussey, S. R. (2024a). Skills to enhance the efficacy of anti-racist supervision. *Journal of Social Work : JSW*, *24*(3), 397–414. https://doi.org/10.1177/14680173231225124

Bussey, S. R. (2024b). The toll of supervising from an anti-racist framework: Reflections from a qualitative study. *The Clinical Supervisor*, *43*(1), 109–135. https://doi.org/10.1080/07325223.2023.2270970

Calderwood, K. A., & Rizzo, L. N. (2023). Co-creating a transformative learning environment through the student-supervisor relationship: Results of a social work field placement duo-ethnography. *Journal of Transformative Education*, *21*(1), 138–156. https://doi.org/10.1177/15413446221079590

Calhoun, A. J., Martin, A., Adigun, A., Alleyne, S. D., Aneni, K., Thompson-Felix, T., Asnes, A., de Carvalho-Filho, M. A., Benoit, L., & Genao, I. (2023). Anti-black racism in clinical supervision: Asynchronous simulated encounters facilitate reflective practice. *MedEdPublish*, *13*(4). https://doi.org/10.12688/mep.19487.2

Capobianco, S. L. (2020). Examining international education research and practice through a queer theory lens. *Frontiers: The Interdisciplinary Journal of Study Abroad*, *32*(1), 12–32. https://doi.org/10.36366/frontiers.v32i1.432

Carnes-Holt, K., Meany-Walen, K., & Felton, A. (2014). Utilizing sandtray within the discrimination model of counselor supervision. *Journal of Creativity in Mental Health*, *9*(4), 497–510. https://doi.org/10.1080/15401383.2014.909298

Cass, V. C. (1979). Homosexual identity formation: A theoretical model. *Journal of Homosexuality*, *4*(3), 219–235. https://doi.org/10.1300/J082v04n03_01

Castonguay, L., & Hill, C. E. (2023). Introduction to becoming better psychotherapists. In L. G. Castonguay & C. E. Hill (Eds.), *Becoming better psychotherapists: Advancing training and supervision* (pp. 3–10). American Psychological Association. https://doi.org/10.1037/0000364-001

Ceballos, P. L., & Huan, L. (2020). Child centered play therapy and strategies for supervision. In L. Fazio-Griffith & R. Marino (Eds.), *Techniques and interventions for play therapy and clinical supervision* (pp. 120–132). IGI Global.

Champe, J., & Rubel, D. (2012). Application of focal conflict theory to psychoeducational groups: Implications for process, content, and leadership. *The Journal for Specialists in Group Work*, *37*, 71–90. https://doi.org/10.1080/01933922.2011.632811

Chan, C. D., Cor, D. N., & Band, M. P. (2018). Privilege and oppression in counselor education: An intersectionality framework. *Journal of Multicultural Counseling and Development*, *46*(1), 58–73. https://doi.org/10.1002/jmcd.12092

Chang, C. Y., Hays, D. G., & Milliken, T. F. (2009). Addressing social justice issues in supervision: A call for client and professional advocacy. *The Clinical Supervisor*, *28*(1), 20–35. https://doi.org/10.1080/07325220902855144

Clark, M., Moe, J., Chan, C. D., Best, M. D., & Mallow, L. M. (2022). Social justice outcomes and professional counseling: An 11-year content analysis. *Journal of Counseling and Development*, *100*(3), 284–295. https://doi.org/10.1002/jcad.12427

Clark-Gordon, C., Bowman, N., Goodboy, A., & Wright, A. (2019). Anonymity and online self-disclosure: A meta-analysis. *Communication Reports*. http://doi.org/10.1080/08934215.2019.1607516

Clemons, K. L. (2024). It takes a village: A conceptual model for black American community partnerships. *Professional School Counseling, 28*(1). https://doi.org/10.1177/2156759X231225222

Coleiro, A. C., Creaner, M., & Timulak, L. (2023). The good, the bad, and the less than ideal in clinical supervision: A qualitative meta-analysis of supervisee experiences, *Counselling Psychology Quarterly, 36*(2), 189–210. https://doi.org/10.1080/09515070.2021.2023098

Collins, P. H. (2015). Intersectionality's definitional dilemmas. *Annual Review of Sociology, 41,* 1–20. https://doi.org/10.1146/annurev-soc-073014-112142

Collins, P. H. (2022). *Black feminist thought: Knowledge, consciousness, and the politics of empowerment.* Routledge.

Collins, P. H., & Bilge, S. (2020). *Intersectionality.* John Wiley & Sons.

Combs, G., & Freedman, J. (2012). Narrative, poststructuralism, and social justice: Current practices in narrative therapy. *The Counseling Psychologist, 40*(7), 1033–1060. https://doi.org/10.1177/0011000012460662

Commission on Accreditation for Marriage and Family Therapy Education (COAMFTE). (2014). *Accreditation standards: Graduate & post-graduate marriage and family therapy training programs.* Author.

Commission on Rehabilitation Counselor Certification. (2023). *Code of professional ethics for certified rehabilitation counselors.* Author. https://crc-certification.com/wp-content/uploads/2023/04/2023-Code-of-Ethics.pdf

Constantine, M. G., & Sue, D. W. (2007). Perceptions of racial microaggressions among black supervisees in cross-racial dyads. *Journal of Counseling Psychology, 54*(2), 142–153. https://doi.org/10.1037/0022-0167.54.2.142

Cormier, S. R., Manson, J. L., & Overley, L. C. (2023). Relational-cultural play therapy supervision: Integrating RCT into the supervision of play therapists. *International Journal of Play Therapy, 32*(3), 135–145. https://doi.org/10.1037/pla0000194

Costa, L. (1991). Family sculpting in the training of marriage and family counselors. *Counselor Education and Supervision, 31*(2), 121–131. https://doi.org/10.1002/j.1556-6978.1991.tb00150.x

Council for Accreditation of Counseling and Related Educational Programs (CACREP). (2023). *2024 CACREP standards.* Author.

Council on Social Work Education. (2022). *Educational policy and accreditation standards for baccalaureate and master's social work programs.* https://www.cswe.org/accreditation/standards/2022-epas/

Crenshaw, K. (1989). Demarginalizing the intersection of race and sex: A black feminist critique of antidiscrimination doctrine, feminist theory, and antiracist politics. *University of Chicago Legal Forum, 14,* 538–554. https://chicagounbound.uchicago.edu/uclf/vol1989/iss1/8

Crenshaw, K. (1991). Mapping the margins: Identity politics, intersectionality, and violence against women. *Stanford Law Review, 43*(6), 1241–1299.

Crenshaw, K. (2013). Demarginalizing the intersection of race and sex: A black feminist critique of antidiscrimination doctrine, feminist theory and antiracist politics. In *Feminist legal theories* (pp. 23–51). Routledge.

Cullors, P. (2022). *An abolitionist's handbook: 12 steps to changing yourself and the world.* St. Martin's Press.

Cushman, P. (1995). *Constructing the self, constructing America: A cultural history of psychotherapy.* Addison-Wesley Pub.

D'Andrea, M., & Daniels, J. (2001). RESPECTFUL counseling: An integrative multidimensional model for counselors. In D. B. Pope-Davis & H. L. K. Coleman (Eds.), *The intersection of race, class, and gender in multicultural counseling* (pp. 417–466). SAGE.

Davis, A. Y. (2016). *Freedom is a constant struggle : Ferguson, Palestine, and the foundations of a movement* (F. Barat, Ed.). Haymarket Books.

Day-Vines, N. L. (2000). Ethics, power, and privilege: Salient issues in the development of multicultural competencies for teachers serving African American children with disabilities. *Teacher Education and Special Education, 23*(1), 3–18. https://doi.org/10.1177/088840640002300104

Day-Vines, N. L., Cluxton-Keller, F., Agorsor, C., & Gubara, S. (2021). Strategies for broaching the subjects of race, ethnicity, and culture. *Journal of Counseling & Development, 99*(3), 348–357. https://doi.org/10.1002/jcad.12380

Day-Vines, N. L., Cluxton-Keller, F., Agorsor, C., Gubara, S., & Otabil, N. A. A. (2020). The multidimensional model of broaching behavior. *Journal of Counseling & Development, 98*(1), 107–118. https://doi.org/10.1002/jcad.12304

Day-Vines, N. L., Wood, S. M., Grothaus, T., Craigen, L., Holman, A., Dotson-Blake, K., & Douglass, M. J. (2007). Broaching the subjects of race, ethnicity, and culture during the counseling process. *Journal of Counseling and Development, 85*(4), 401–409. https://doi.org/10.1080/07325223.2020.183032710.1002/j.1556-6678.2007.tb00608

DeBlaere, C., Singh, A. A., Wilcox, M. M., Cokley, K. O., Delgado-Romero, E. A., Scalise, D. A., & Shawahin, L. (2019). Social justice in counseling psychology: Then, now, and looking forward. *The Counseling Psychologist, 47*(6), 938–962. https://doi.org/10.1177/0011000019893283

Degenstein, M., Tangen, J., & Danielson, J. (2023). Supervision experiences of trans/gender expansive counselors-in-training: An interpretative phenomenological analysis. *Counselor Education and Supervision, 62*(4), 410–422. https://doi.org/10.1002/ceas.12284

DeKruyf, L., & Pehrsson, D. E. (2011). School counseling site supervisor training: An exploratory study. *Counselor Education and Supervision*, *50*(5), 314–327. https://doi.org/10.1002/j.1556-6978.2011.tb01918.x

del Mar Fariña, M., & O'Neill, P. (2022). The structural clinical model: Disrupting oppression in clinical social work through an integrative practice approach. *Clinical Social Work Journal*, 1–12. https://doi.org/10.1007/s10615-022-00841-3

Del Re, J., Dari, T., Neyland-Brown, L., Suarez, A. & Walker, T. (Submitted). *Understanding post-graduate supervisees' experiences and perceptions of multicultural competence and cultural humility: A consensual qualitative study.*

DiAngelo, R. (2018). *White fragility: Why it's so hard for white people to talk about racism*. Beacon Press.

Dillman Taylor, D., & Blount, A. J. (2021). Case study research. In S. V. Flynn (Ed.), *Research design in the behavioral sciences: An applied approach* (pp. 275–298). Springer.

Dollarhide, C. T., Hale, S. C., & Stone-Sabali, S. (2021). A new model for social justice supervision. *Journal of Counseling & Development*, *99*(1), 104–113. https://doi.org/10.1002/jcad.12358

Doran, G. T. (1981). There's a S.M.A.R.T. way to write management's goals and objectives. *Management Review*, *70*, 35–36.

Ekstein, R., & Wallerstein, R. S. (1958). *The teaching and learning of psychotherapy*. International Universities Press.

Elliott, T. R. (2016). External funding and competing visions for academic counseling psychology. *The Counseling Psychologist*, *44*(4), 525–535. https://doi.org/10.1177/0011000016634867

Ellis, M. V., Berger, L., Hanus, A. E., Ayala, E. E., Swords, B. A., & Siembor, M. (2014). Inadequate and harmful clinical supervision: Testing a revised framework and assessing occurrence. *The Counseling Psychologist*, *42*(4), 434–472. https://doi.org/10.1177/0011000013508656

Ellison, S. E., Tierney, P., & Taylor, M. (2024). A target model for social justice supervision. *Teaching and Supervision in Counseling*, *6*(3), 1–12. https://doi.org/10.7290/tsc06czbz

Ertl, M. M., Ellis, M. V., & Peterson, L. P. (2023). Supervisor cultural humility and supervisee nondisclosure: The supervisory working alliance matters. *The Counseling Psychologist*, *51*(4), 590–620. https://doi.org/10.1177/00110000231159316

Esposito, J., & Evans-Winters, V. (2021). *Introduction to intersectional qualitative research*. SAGE.

Falender, C. A., & Shafranske, E. P. (2021). *Clinical supervision: A competency-based approach* (2nd ed.). American Psychological Association.

Falender, C. A., Shafranske, E. P., & Falicov, C. J. (Eds.). (2014). *Multiculturalism and diversity in clinical supervision: A competency-based approach.* American Psychological Association. https://doi.org/10.1037/14370-000

Fanon, F. (1952). *Black skin, white masks.* Grove Press.

Fanon, F. (1961). *The wretched of the earth.* Grove Press.

Fickling, M. J., Tangen, J. L., Graden, M. W., & Grays, D. (2019). Multicultural and social justice competence in clinical supervision. *Counselor Education and Supervision, 58*(4), 309–316. https://doi.org/10.1002/ceas.12159

Finn, J. L. (2020). *Just practice: A social justice approach to social work.* Oxford University Press.

Frank, D. A., & Cannon, E. P. (2010). Queer theory as pedagogy in counselor education: A framework for diversity training. *Journal of LGBT Issues in Counseling, 4*(1), 18–31. https://doi.org/10.1080/15538600903552731

French, B. H., Lewis, J. A., Mosley, D. V., Adames, H. Y., Chavez-Dueñas, N. Y., Chen, G. A., & Neville, H. A. (2020). Toward a psychological framework of radical healing in communities of color. *The Counseling Psychologist, 48*(1), 14–46. https://doi.org/10.1177/0011000019843506

Friedlander, M. L., & Heatherington, L. (Eds.). (2023). Good supervision, better therapy: Trainees' accounts of how supervisors helped them manage difficult therapy situations. In L. G. Castonguay & C. E. Hill (Eds.), *Becoming better psychotherapists: Advancing training and supervision* (pp. 239–265). American Psychological Association. https://doi.org/10.1037/0000364-012

Gallant, J. P., & Thyer, B. A. (1989). The "bug-in-the-ear" in clinical supervision. *The Clinical Supervisor, 7*(2–3), 43–58. https://doi.org/10.1300/J001v07n02_04

Gamby, K., Burns, D., & Forristal, K. (2021). Wellness decolonized: The history of wellness and recommendations for the counseling field. *Journal of Mental Health Counseling, 43*(3), 228–245. https://doi.org/10.17744/mehc.43.3.05

Ganske, K. H., Gnilka, P. B., Ashby, J. S., & Rice, K. G. (2015). The relationship between counseling trainee perfectionism and the working alliance with supervisor and client. *Journal of Counseling & Development, 93*(1), 14–24. https://doi.org.umiss.idm.oclc.org/10.1002/j.1556–6676.2015.00177.x

Gantt-Howrey, A., Becnel, A., Shi, Y., & Lau, J. (2023). Use of the MSJCC: A content analysis of ACA journals. *Counselor Education and Supervision, 62*(1), 40–51. https://doi.org/10.1002/ceas.12259

Gerstenblith, J. A., Kline, K. V., Hill, C. E., & Kivlighan, D. M., Jr. (2022). The triadic effect: Associations among the supervisory working alliance, therapeutic working alliance, and therapy session evaluation. *Journal of Counseling Psychology*, *69*(2), 199–210. https://doi.org/10.1037/cou0000567

Gibson, K., Pollard, T. M., & Moffatt, S. (2021). Social prescribing and classed inequality: A journey of upward health mobility? *Social Science & Medicine*, *280*, 114037. https://doi.org/10.1016/j.socscimed.2021.114037

Gladding, S. T. (2016). *The creative arts in counseling* (5th ed.). American Counseling Association.

Goodman, R. D., & Gorski, P. C. (Eds.). (2015). *Decolonizing "multicultural" counseling through social justice*. Springer.

Goodrich, K. M., & Luke, M. (2011). The LGBTQ responsive model for supervision of group work. *The Journal for Specialists in Group Work*, *36*(1), 22–40. https://doi.org/10.1080/01933922.2010.537739

Goodrich, K. M., & Luke, M. (2016). *Group counseling with LGBTQI persons* (pp. 71–73). American Counseling Association.

Goodrich, K. M., Luke, M., & Smith, A. J. (2016). Queer humanism: Toward an epistemology of socially just, culturally responsive change. *The Journal of Humanistic Psychology*, *56*(6), 612–623. https://doi.org/10.1177/0022167816652534

Goodyear, R. K. (2014). Supervision as pedagogy: Attending to its essential instructional and learning processes. *The Clinical Supervisor, 33*, 82–99. https://doi.org/10.1080/07325223.2014.918914

Graham, M. A., & Pehrsson, D. (2009). Bibliosupervision: A creative supervision technique. *Journal of Creativity in Mental Health*, *4*(4), 366–374. https://doi.org/10.1080/15401380903372661

Graham, M. A., Scholl, M. B., Smith-Adcock, S., & Wittmann, E. (2014). Three creative approaches to counseling supervision. *Journal of Creativity in Mental Health*, *9*(3), 415–426. https://doi.org/10.1080/15401383.2014.899482

Grant, K. L., Mason, E. C. M., Springer, S., & Shaikh, A. (2023). Application of principles of anti-oppression to the teaching of group counseling. *The Journal for Specialists in Group Work*, *48*(2), 109–127. https://doi.org/10.1080/01933922.2023.2197162

Graybill, E., Baker, C. N., Cloth, A. H., Fisher, S., & Nastasi, B. K. (2018). An analysis of social justice research in school psychology. *International Journal of School & Educational Psychology*, *6*(2), 77–89. https://doi.org/10.1080/21683603.2017.1302850

Green, D. A., & Sperandio, K. R. (2024). Abolitionist praxis for substance use clients who experience anti-drug policing. *Professional Counselor*, *14*(1), 48–63. https://doi.org/10.15241/dag.14.1.48

Griffith, E. E., Holmstrom, K. M., & Malone, C. (2022). Diversity, equity, and inclusion in the auditing profession: Individual auditor experiences and contributions. *Equity and Inclusion in the Auditing Profession: Individual Auditor Experiences and Contributions.* http://dx.doi.org/10.2139/ssrn.4097145

Gutierrez, D. (2018). The role of intersectionality in marriage and family therapy multicultural supervision. *The American Journal of Family Therapy, 46*(1), 14–26. https://doi.org/10.1080/01926187.2018.1437573

Häberlein, L., & Hövel, P. (2023). Importance and necessity of stakeholder engagement. In E. González-Esteban, R. A. Feenstra, & L. M. Camarinha-Matos (Eds.), *The ETHNA system project* (LNCS 13875, pp. 38–53). Springer. https://10.1007/978-3-031-33177-0_3

Hair, H. J. (2015). Supervision conversations about social justice and social work practice. *Journal of Social Work, 15*(4), 349–370. https://doi.org/10.1177/1468017314539082

Hammer, T., Chan, C., Kavanaugh, K., & Hadwiger, A. (2021). Merging tenets of relational-cultural theory, feminism, and wonder woman for counseling practice. *Journal of Creativity in Mental Health, 16*(3), 274–284. https://doi.org/10.1080/15401383.2020.1768993

Hansen, J. T. (2014). *Philosophical issues in counseling and psychotherapy.* Rowan & Littlefield.

Hardy, K. V., & Bobes, T. (2016). *Culturally sensitive supervision and training: Diverse perspectives and practical applications.* Routledge. https://doi.org/10.4324/9781315648064

Hardy, K. V., & Laszloffy, T. A. (1995). The cultural genogram: Key to training culturally competent family therapists. *Journal of Marital and Family Therapy, 21*(3), 227–237. https://doi.org/10.1111/j.1752-0606.1995.tb00158.x

Hartwig, E. K., & Bennett, M. M. (2017). Four approaches to using sandtray in play therapy supervision. *International Journal of Play Therapy, 26*(4), 230–238. https://doi.org/10.1037/pla0000050

Hays, D. G., & Singh, A. A. (2023). *Qualitative inquiry in clinical and educational settings* (2nd ed.). Cognella.

Hays, P. A. (2001). *Addressing cultural complexities in practice: A framework for clinicians and counselors* (pp. vii, 3–16, 239). American Psychological Association. https://doi.org/10.1037/10411-000

Hays, P. A. (2022). *Addressing cultural complexities in counseling and clinical practice: An intersectional approach.* American Psychological Association.

Heffron, M. C., Reynolds, D., & Talbot, B. (2016). Reflecting together: Reflective functioning as a focus for deepening group supervision. *Infant Mental Health Journal, 37*(6), 628–639.

Heitz, H. K., & Rappaport, B. (2023). Feminist therapy: Supervision as a pathway towards equitable, affirming care for nonbinary clients. *Women & Therapy, 46*(1). https://doi.org/10.1080/02703149.2023.2190230

Heller, L., & Lapierre, A. (2012). *Healing developmental trauma: How early trauma affects self-regulation, self-image, and the capacity for relationship*. North Atlantic Books.

Henriksen, R. C., Henderson, S. E., Liang, Y. W., Watts, R. E., & Marks, D. F. (2019). Counselor supervision: A comparison across states and jurisdictions. *Journal of Counseling & Development, 97*(2), 160–170. https://doi.org/10.1002/jcad.12247

Hernández, P., & McDowell, T. (2010). Intersectionality, power, and relational safety in context: Key concepts in clinical supervision. *Training and Education in Professional Psychology, 4*(1), 29–35. https://doi.org/10.1037/a0017064

Heron, J. (2001). *Helping the client: A creative practical guide* (5th ed.). SAGE.

Hill, C. E., & Norcross, J. C. (2023). Skills and methods that work in psychotherapy: Observations and conclusions from the special issue. *Psychotherapy*. Advance Online Publication. https://doi.org/10.1037/pst0000487

Hilts, D., Peters, H. C., Liu, Y., & Luke, M. (2022). The model for supervision of school counseling leadership. *Journal of Counselor Leadership and Advocacy*. https://doi.org/10.1080/2326716X.2022.2032871

Hoffman, J. & Hoffman, J. (2004). *Learning racial identity development using human sculpture*. Sculpting Race Handout.

Holloway, E. L. (1995). *Clinical supervision A systems approach*. SAGE Publications.

Holloway, E. L. (2016). *Supervision essentials for a systems approach to supervision*. American Psychological Association.

Homeyer, L. E., & Sweeney, D. S. (2022). *Sandtray therapy: A practical manual*. Routledge/Researching for LGBTQ2S+ Health. https://www.buildingcompetence.ca/workshop/power_flower/

Homeyer, L. E., & Sweeney, D. S. (2023). *Sandtray therapy: A practical manual* (4th ed.). Routledge. https://doi.org/10.4324/9781003221418

Hood, C. O., Schick, M. R., Cusack, S. E., Fahey, M. C., Giff, S. T., Guty, E. T., Hellman, N., Henry, L. M., Hinkson, K., Long, E. E., McCoy, K., O'Connor, K., Padron Wilborn, A., Reuben, A., Sackey, E. T., Tilstra-Ferrell, E. L., Walters, K. J., & Witcraft, S. M. (2024). Short-changing the future: The systemic gap between psychology internship stipends and living wages. *Training and Education in Professional Psychology, 18*(1), 49–58. https://doi.org/10.1037/tep0000449

Hook, J. N., Davis, D. E., Owen, J., & DeBlaere, C. (2017). *Cultural humility: Engaging diverse identities in therapy*. American Psychological Association.

Hook, J. N., Davis, D. E., Owen, J., Worthington, E. L., & Utsey, S. O. (2013). Cultural humility: Measuring openness to culturally diverse clients. *Journal of Counseling Psychology*, *60*(3), 353–366. https://doi.org/10.1037/a0032595

Hook, J. N., Watkins, C. E., Jr., Davis, D. E., Owen, J., Van Tongeren, D. R., & Ramos, M. J. (2016). Cultural humility in psychotherapy supervision. *American Journal of Psychotherapy*, *70*(2), 149–166. https://doi.org/10.1176/appi.psychotherapy.2016.70.2.149

hooks, b. (1989). Marginality as site of resistance. In R. Ferguson, M. Gever, T. T. Minh-ha, & C. West (Eds.), *Out there: Marginalization and contemporary cultures* (pp. 341–343). MIT Press.

Hou, J.-M., & Skovholt, T. M. (2019). Characteristics of highly resilient therapists. *Journal of Counseling Psychology*, *67*(3). https://doi.org/10.1037/cou0000401

Howard, S., Alston, S., Brown, M., & Bost, A. (2023). Literature review on regulatory frameworks for addressing discrimination in clinical supervision. *Research on Social Work Practice*, *33*(1), 84–96. https://doi.org/10.1177/10497315221121827

Hutchens, N., Block, J., & Young, M. (2013). Counselor educators' gatekeeping responsibilities and students' first amendment rights. *Counselor Education & Supervision*, *52*(2), 82–95. https://doi.org/10.1002/j.1556-6978.2013.00030

Hutman, H., Ellis, M. V., Moore, J. A., Roberson, K. L., McNamara, M. L., Peterson, L. P., Taylor, E. J., & Zhou, S. (2023). Supervisees' perspectives of inadequate, harmful, and exceptional clinical supervision: Are we listening? *The Counseling Psychologist*, *51*(5), 719–755. https://doi.org/10.1177/00110000231172504

Inman, A. G., Hutman, H., Pendse, A., Devdas, L., Luu, L., & Ellis, M. V. (2014). Current trends concerning supervisors, supervisees, and clients in clinical supervision. In C. E. Watkins & D. L. Milne (Eds.), *The Wiley international handbook of clinical supervision* (pp. 61–102). Wiley-Blackwell. https://doi.org/10.1002/9781118846360.ch4

Ivers, N. N., Rogers, J. L., Borders, L. D., & Turner, A. (2017). Using interpersonal process recall in clinical supervision to enhance supervisees' multicultural awareness. *The Clinical Supervisor*, *36*(2), 282–303. https://doi.org/10.1080/07325223.2017.1320253

Ivey, A. E., Ivey, M. B., & Zalaquett, C. P. (2023). *Intentional interviewing and counseling: Facilitating client development in a multicultural society* (10th ed.). Cengage.

Jacobson, D., & Mustafa, N. (2019). Social identity map: A reflexivity tool for practicing explicit positionality in critical qualitative research. *International Journal of Qualitative Methods*, *18*. https://doi.org/10.1177/16094069198700

Jamieson, M. K., Govaart, G. H., & Pownall, M. (2023). Reflexivity in quantitative research: A rationale and beginner's guide. *Social and*

*Personality Psychology Compass, 17*(4), e12735. https://doi.org/10.1111/spc3.12735

Jencius, M., & Baltrinic, E. R. (2016). Training counselors to provide online supervision. In T. Rousmaniere & E. Renfro-Michel (Eds.), *Using technology to enhance clinical supervision* (pp. 251–268). Wiley.

Jew, G., & Tran, A. G. T. T. (2022). Understanding activist intentions: An extension of the theory of planned behavior. *Current Psychology, 41*(7), 4885–4897. https://doi.org/10.1007/s12144-020-00986-9

Johnson, D. R., & Emunah, R. (Eds.). (2009). *Current approaches in drama therapy*. Charles C Thomas.

Johnson, K. F., Sparkman, N. M., Meca, A., & Tarver, S. Z. (Eds.). (2022). *Developing anti-racist practices in the helping professions: Inclusive theory, pedagogy, and application* (1st ed.). Palgrave Macmillan.

Jones, C. T., & Branco, S. F. (2020). The interconnectedness between cultural humility and broaching in clinical supervision: Working from the multicultural orientation framework. *The Clinical Supervisor, 39*(2), 198–209. https://doi.org/10.1080/07325223.2020.1830327

Jones, C. T., & Branco, S. F. (2023). Cultural humility and broaching enhancements: A commentary on "getting off the racist sidelines: An antiracist approach to mental health supervision and training" (Legha, 2023). *The Clinical Supervisor, 42*(2), 248–262. https://doi.org/10.1080/07325223.2023.2252415

Jones, C. T., Welfare, L. E., Melchior, S., & Cash, R. (2019). Broaching as a strategy for intercultural understanding in clinical supervision. *The Clinical Supervisor, 38*(1), 1–16. https://doi.org/10.1080/07325223.201 8.1560384

Jordan, J. V. (2000). The role of mutual empathy in relational/cultural therapy. *Journal of Clinical Psychology, 56*, 1005–1016. https://doi.org/10.1002/1097-4679(200008)56:8%3C1005::aid-jclp2%3E3.0.co;2-l

Jordan, J. V. (2018). *Relational-cultural theory*. American Psychological Association.

Kadushin, A. (1985). *Supervision in social work*. Columbia University Press.

Kadushin, A., & Harkness, D. (2014). *Supervision in social work* (5th ed.). Columbia University Press.

Kagan, N. I. (1976). *Interpersonal process recall: A method of influencing human interaction*. Michigan State University.

Kagan, N. I. (1980). Influencing human interaction: Eighteen years with IPR. In A. K. Hess (Ed.), *Psychotherapy supervision: Theory, research, and practice* (pp. 262–283). Wiley.

Kagan, N. I., & Kagan, H. (1990). IPR-A validated model for the 1990s and beyond. *The Counseling Psychologist, 18*(3), 436–440. https://doi.org/10.1177/0011000090183004

Kahn, S. Z., & Monk, G. (2017). Narrative supervision as a social justice practice. *Journal of Systemic Therapies, 36*(1), 7–25. http://dx.doi.org.proxy.wm.edu/10.1521/jsyt.2017.36.1.7

Katz, J. H. (1985). The sociopolitical nature of counseling. *The Counseling Psychologist, 13*(4), 615–624. https://doi.org/10.1177/0011000085134005

Katz, J. H. (1990). *Some aspects of white culture in the United States.* https://www.cascadia.edu/discover/about/diversity/documents/Some%20Aspects%20and%20Assumptions%20of%20White%20Culture%20in%20the%20United%20States.pdf

Katz, J. H. (2003). *White awareness: Handbook for antiracism training.* University of Oklahoma Press.

Kemer, G. (2020). A comparison of beginning and expert supervisors' supervision cognitions. *Counselor Education and Supervision, 59*(1), 74–92. https://doi.org/10.1002/ceas.12167

Kemer, G. (2024). Cohesive model of supervision: An empirically based approach. *Counselor Education and Supervision.* https://doi.org/10.1002/ceas.12320

Kemer, G., Li, C., Attia, M., Chan, C. D., Chung, M., Li, D., Neuer Colburn, A., Peters, H. C., Ramaswamy, A., & Sunal, Z. (2022). Multicultural supervision in counseling: A content analysis of peer-reviewed literature. *Counselor Education and Supervision, 61*(1), 2–14. https://doi.org/10.1002/ceas.12220

Kendall, F. (2006). *Understanding white privilege: Creating pathways to authentic relationships across race.* Routledge.

Kennard, D. (2020). *Somatic and attachment focused EMDR (SAFE).* Personal Transformation Institute.

Keum, B. T., & Wang, L. (2020). Supervision and psychotherapy process and outcome: A meta-analytic review. *Translational Issues in Psychological Science.* Advance Online Publication. http://dx.doi.org/10.1037/tps0000272

Killian, T., Peters, H. C., & Floren, M. (2023). Development and validation of the multicultural and social justice counseling competencies-inventory. *Measurement and Evaluation in Counseling and Development, 56*(4), 329–346. https://doi.org/10.1080/07481756.2022.2160357

King, K. M. (2021). I want to, but how? Defining counselor broaching in core tenets and debated components. *Journal of Multicultural Counseling & Development, 49*(2), 87–100. http://doi.org/10.1002/jmcd.12208

King, K. M., & Borders, L. D. (2019). An experimental investigation of white counselors broaching race and racism. *Journal of Counseling and Development, 97*(4), 341–351. https://doi.org/10.1002/jcad.12283

King, K. M., Borders, L. D., & Jones, C. T. (2020). Multicultural orientation in clinical supervision: Examining impact through dyadic data. *The*

*Clinical Supervisor*, 1–24. https://doi.org/10.1080/07325223.2020.176 3223

King, K. M., & Jones, K. (2019). An autoethnography of broaching in supervision: Joining supervisee and supervisor perspectives on addressing identity, power, and difference. *The Clinical Supervisor, 38*(1), 17–37. https://doi.org/10.1080/07325223.2018.1525597

Klukoff, H., Kanani, H., Gaglione, C., & Alexander, A. (2021). Toward an abolitionist practice of psychology: Reimagining psychology's relationship with the criminal justice system. *The Journal of Humanistic Psychology, 61*(4), 451–469. https://doi.org/10.1177/00221678211015755

Knudson-Martin, C., McDowell, T., & Bermudez, J. M. (2019). From knowing to doing: Guidelines for socioculturally attuned family therapy. *Journal of Marital and Family Therapy, 45*(1), 47–60. https://doi.org/10.1111/jmft.12299

Kovach, M. (2021). *Indigenous methodologies: Characteristics, conversations, and contexts*. University of Toronto Press.

Kuo, H. J., Landon, T. J., Co Kuo, H. J., Landon, T. J., Connor, A., & Chen, R. K. (2016). Managing anxiety in clinical supervision. *The Journal of Rehabilitation, 82*(3), 18–27.

Lawson, G., Hein, S. F., & Stuart, C. L. (2010). Supervisors' experiences of the contributions of the second supervisee in triadic supervision: A qualitative investigation. *The Journal for Specialists in Group Work, 35*(1), 69–91. https://doi.org/10.1080/01933920903225844

Lee, A., & Luke, M. (2018). Addressing intra—and inter-personal ambiguity in first group supervision. In J. Jordon, B. L. Perkins, C. Cox, & R. Lee (Eds.), *Handbook of experiential teaching in counselor education: A resource guide for counselor educators* (pp. 304–309). CreateSpace Independent Publishing.

Lee, E. (2023). Unsettling discourses of cross-cultural social work practice: Moving from theoretical debates to interrogating and transforming praxis. *The British Journal of Social Work*. https://doi.org/10.1093/bjsw/bcad163

Lee, E., & Kealy, D. (2018). Developing a working model of cross-cultural supervision: A competence-and alliance-based framework. *Clinical Social Work Journal, 46*, 310–320. http://dx.doi.org.proxy.wm.edu/10.1007/s10615-018-0683-4

Lee, M. A., Jorgensen Smith, T., & Henry, R. G. (2018). Power politics: Advocacy to activism in social justice counseling. *Journal for Social Action in Counseling and Psychology, 5*(3), 70–94. https://doi.org/10.33043/JSACP.5.3.70-94

Lee, M. C. Y., & Thackeray, L. (2023). Relational processes and power dynamics in psychoanalytic group supervision: A discourse analysis. *The*

*Clinical Supervisor, 42*(1), 123–144. https://doi.org/10.1080/07325223
.2022.2164537

Legha, R. K. (2023a). Antiracist mental health supervision and training
2.0 edition: Cementing a foundation of safety for self-disclosure. *The
Clinical Supervisor, 42*(2), 299–328. https://doi.org/10.1080/07325223
.2023.2279521

Legha, R. K. (2023b). Getting off the racist sidelines: An antiracist
approach to mental health supervision and training. *The Clinical Supervisor, 42*(2), 213–236. https://doi.org/10.1080/07325223.2023.2204302

Leventhal, G., Baker, J., Archer, R. P., Cubic, B. A., & Hudson, B. O. (2004).
Federal funds to train clinical psychologists for work with underserved
populations: The bureau of health professions graduate psychology education grants program. *Journal of Clinical Psychology in Medical Settings, 11*(2),
109–117. https://doi.org/10.1023/B:JOCS.0000025722.32323.49

Li, C., Kemer, G., Sunal, Z., & Chen, C.-C. (2024). A scoping review
of the development and validation procedures of 59 supervision measures published between 1984 and 2023. *The Clinical Supervisor, 43*(2),
164–220. https://doi.org/10.1080/07325223.2024.238904

Li, D., & Ai, Y. (2020). Ethics acculturation of international counseling
students. *Journal of International Students, 10*(4), 1103–1109. https://doi.
org/10.32674/jis.v10i4.1442

Li, D., & Liu, Y. (2020). International counseling doctoral students' teaching preparation: A phenomenological study. *Counselor Education and
Supervision, 59*(3), 200–215. https://doi.org/10.1002/ceas.12184

Li, D., Liu, Y., & Lee, I. (2018). Supervising Asian international counseling students: Using the integrative developmental model. *Journal of
International Students, 8*(2), 1129–1151. https://doi.org/10.32674/jis.
v8i2.137

Liberati, R., & Agbisit, M. (2017). Using art-based strategies in group-based
counselor supervision. *Journal of Creativity in Mental Health, 12*(1), 15–30.
https://doi.org.umiss.idm.oclc.org/10.1080/15401383.2016.1189369

Littrell, J. M., Lee-Borden, N., & Lorenz, J. (1979). A developmental
framework for counseling supervision. *Counselor Education and Supervision, 19*(2), 129–136. https://doi.org/10.1002/j.1556-6978.1976.
tb02021.x

Liu, Y., & Li, D. (2023). Anti-oppressive research in group work. *The Journal for Specialists in Group Work, 48*(2), 128–145. https://doi.org/10.108
0/01933922.2023.2170507

Locke, A., & Budds, K. (2020). Applying critical discursive psychology
to health psychology research: A practical guide. *Health Psychology and
Behavioral Medicine, 8*(1), 234–247. https://doi.org/10.1080/21642850
.2020.1792307

Luke, M. (2008a). Props in a box. In L. L. Foss, J. Green, K. Wolfe-Stiltner, & J. L. DeLucia-Waack (Eds.), *School counselors share their favorite group activities: A guide to choosing, planning, conducting and processing* (pp. 111–113). Association for Specialists in Group Work.

Luke, M. (2008b). Supervision: Models, principles, and process issues. In A. Drewes & J. Mullen (Eds.), *Supervision can be playful: Techniques for child and play therapist supervisors* (pp. 7–25). Rowman and Littlefield.

Luke, M. (2016). Finding shay. In B. Jones, T. Duffey, & S. Haberstroh (Eds.), *Child and adolescent counseling case studies: Fostering developmental, relational, systemic & multicultural contexts* (pp. 81–86). Springer Publishing.

Luke, M. (2019). Supervision in the counselor education context. In J. Okech & D. Rubel (Eds.), *Counselor education in the 21st century* (pp. 35–52). American Counseling Association.

Luke, M., & Bernard, J. M. (2006). The school counseling supervision model: An extension of the discrimination model. *Counselor Education and Supervision*, *45*(4), 282–295. https://doi.org/10.1002/j.1556-6978.2006.tb00004.x

Luke, M., Ellis, M. V., & Bernard, J. M. (2011). School counselor supervisors' perceptions of the discrimination model. *Counselor Education and Supervision*, *5*(5), 328–343. https://doi.org/10.1002/j.1556-6978.2011.tb01919.x

Luke, M., & Goodrich, K. M. (Eds.). (2015a). *Group work experts share their favorite group supervision activities* (Vol. 1). Association of Specialists in Group Work.

Luke, M., & Goodrich, K. M. (Eds.). (2015b). *Group work experts share their favorite group supervision activities* (Vol. 2). Association of Specialists in Group Work.

Luke, M., & Peters, H. C. (2020). Supervision as the signature pedagogy for counseling leadership. *Teaching and Supervision in Counseling*, *2*(2), article 4. https://doi.org/10.7290/tsc020204

Luke, M., Peters, H. C., & Goodrich, K. M. (2023). Reflections on the application of the principles of anti-oppression in group work. *The Journal for Specialists in Group Work*, *48*(2), 185–192. https://doi.org/10.1080/01933922.2023.2204054

Mack, B. M. (2021). Resiliency-focused supervision model: Addressing stress, burnout, and self-care among social workers. *Advances in Social Work*, *20*(3), 596–614. https://doi.org/10.18060/23897

Maier, S. F., & Seligman, M. E. (1976). Learned helplessness: Theory and evidence. *Journal of Experimental Psychology: General*, *105*(1), 3–46. https://doi.org/10.1037/0096-3445.105.1.3

Malott, K. M., Paone, T. R., Schaefle, S., & Gao, J. (2015). Is it racist? Addressing racial microaggressions in counselor training. *Journal of*

*Creativity in Mental Health, 10*(3), 386–398. https://doi.org/10.1080/1 5401383.2014.988312

Mastoras, S. M., & Andrews, J. J. W. (2011). The supervisee experience of group supervision: Implications for research and practice. *Training and Education in Professional Psychology, 5*(2), 102–111. https://doi.org/10.1037/a0023567

McCombs, B. L. (2014). Using a 360 degree assessment model to support learning to learn. In R. D. Crick, C. Stringher, & K. Ren (Eds.), *Learning to learn for all: Theory, practice and international research: A multidisciplinary and lifelong perspective* (pp. 241–270). Routledge.

McNeill, B. W., & Stoltenberg, C. D. (2016). *Supervision essentials for the integrative developmental model.* American Psychological Association.

McNeill, B. W., Stoltenberg, C. D., & Romans, J. S. (1992). The integrated developmental model of supervision: Scale development and validation procedures. *Professional Psychology: Research and Practice, 23*(6), 504–508. https://doi.org/10.1037/0735-7028.23.6.504

Menakem, R. (2017). *My grandmother's hands: Racialized trauma and the pathways to mending our hearts and bodies.* Central Recovery Press.

Merlin, C., & Brendel, J. M. (2017). A supervision training program for school counseling site supervisors. *The Clinical Supervisor, 36*(2), 304–323. https://doi.org/10.1080/07325223.2017.1328629

Merriam, S. B. (1998). Qualitative research and case study application in education. Jossey-Bass.

Middleton, T. J., Toole, K. M., Culpepper, D., Hughes, D. Parsons-Christian, E., & Dollarhide, C. T. (2023). Decolonizing & decentering oppressive structures: Practical strategies for social justice in school and clinical counseling. *Journal of Counselor Leadership and Advocacy.* https://doi.org/10.1080/2326716X.2023.2237023

Miller, J. B. (2008). Telling the truth about power. *Women & Therapy, 31,* 145–161. https://doi.org/10.1080/02703140802146282

Mitchell, M. D., & Butler, S. K. (2021). Acknowledging intersectional identity in supervision: The multicultural integrated supervision model. *Journal of Multicultural Counseling and Development, 49*(2), 101–115. https://doi.org/10.1002/jmcd.12209

Moe, J., Perera, D., & Rodgers, D. (2023). Promoting wellness at the intersections of gender, race and ethnicity, and sexual-affectional orientation identities. *Journal of Mental Health Counseling, 45*(3), 231–246. https://doi.org/10.17744/mehc.45.3.04

Morgaine, K., & Capous-Desyllas, M. (2020). *Anti-oppressive social work practice: Putting theory into action* (2nd ed.). Cognella Academic Publishing.

Mosley, D. V., McNeil-Young, V., Bridges, B., Adam, S., Colson, A., Crowley, M., & Lee, L. (2021). Toward radical healing: A qualitative metasynthesis exploring oppression and liberation among black queer people. *Psychology of Sexual Orientation and Gender Diversity, 8*(3), 292–313. https://doi.org/10.1037/sgd0000522

Mosley, D. V., Neville, H. A., Chavez-Dueñas, N. Y., Adames, H. Y., Lewis, J. A., & French, B. H. (2020). Radical hope in revolting times: Proposing a culturally relevant psychological framework. *Social and Personality Psychology Compass, 14*(1). https://doi.org/10.1111/spc3.12512

Mullan, J. (2023). *Decolonizing therapy: Oppression, historical trauma, and politicizing your practice.* W. W. Norton.

Mullen, B., Champagne, T., Krishnamurty, S., Dickson, D., & Gao, R. X. (2008). Exploring the safety and therapeutic effects of deep pressure stimulation using a weighted blanket. *Occupational Therapy in Mental Health, 24*(1), 65–89. https://doi.org/10.1300/j004v24n01_05

Mullen, J. A., Luke, M., & Drewes, A. (2007). Supervision can be playful too: Play therapy techniques that enhance supervision. *International Journal of Play Therapy, 16*(1), 69–85. https://doi.org/10.1037/1555-6824.16.1.69

Musson Rose, D., & Baffour, T. (2023). Tools to accelerate anti-racist supervision practices in social work practicum-based education settings. *Social Work Education*, 1–7. https://doi.org/10.1080/02615479.2023.2273254

Myers, J. E., & Sweeney, T. J. (2004). The indivisible self: An evidence—based model of wellness. *Journal of Individual Psychology, 60*(3), 234–245. https://core.ac.uk/download/pdf/149232976.pdf

Myers, J. E., & Sweeney, T. J. (2008). Wellness counseling: The evidence-base for practice. *Journal of Counseling & Development, 86*(4), 482–493. https://doi.org/10.1002/j.1556-6678.2008.tb00536.x

National Association of Social Workers. (2015). *NASW standards and indicators for cultural competence in social work practice.* NASW Press. https://www.socialworkers.org/Practice/NASW-Practice-Standards-Guidelines/Standards-and-Indicators-for-Cultural-Competence-in-Social-Work-Practice

National Association of Social Workers, & Association of Social Work Boards. (2013). *Best practice standards in social work supervision.* National Association of Social Workers/Association of Social Work Boards.

National Board of Certified Counselors. (2016). *Code of ethics.* https://www.nbcc.org/assets/Ethics/NBCCCodeofEthics.pdf

Ogbeide, S. A., & Bayles, B. (2023). Using a Delphi technique to define primary care behavioral health clinical supervision competencies. *Journal of Clinical Psychology in Medical Settings*, 1–14. https://doi.org/10.1007/s10880-023-09964-2

Okech, J. E. A., Pimpleton, A., Vannata, R., & Champe, J. (2016). Intercultural conflict in groups. *Journal for Specialists in Group Work, 41*(4), 350–369. https://doi.org/10.1080/01933922.2016.1232769

Okech, J. E. A., Rubel, D. J., Jamaleddine, M., Hutchinson, C., & Redmond, L. (2023a). Applying the 10 principles of anti-oppression to group work supervision. *Journal for Specialist in Group Work, 48*(2), 90–108. https://doi.org/10.1080/01933922.2023.2190775

Okech, J. E. A., Rubel, D. J., & Kline, W. B. (2023b). *Interactive group work* (2nd ed.). American Counseling Association.

Overmier, J. B., & Seligman, M. E. (1967). Effects of inescapable shock upon subsequent escape and avoidance responding. *Journal of Comparative and Physiological Psychology, 63*(1), 28–33. https://doi.org/10.1037/h0024166

Owen, D. W. (2010). Spontaneous and guided imagery in counseling: Putting fantasy to work. *Turkish Psychological Counseling & Guidance Journal, 4*(33), 71.

Owen, J. (2013). Early career perspectives on psychotherapy research and practice: Psychotherapist effects, multicultural orientation, and couple interventions. *Psychotherapy, 50*(4), 496–502. https://doi.org/10.1037/a0034617

Patterson, O. (2018). *Slavery and social death: A comparative study, with a new preface.* Harvard University Press.

Perera-Diltz, D., & Moe, J. (2020). The wellness treatment plan. In W. W. Ishak (Ed.), *The handbook of wellness medicine* (pp. 45–55). Cambridge University Press. https://doi.org.proxy.lib.odu.edu/10.1017/9781108650182.005

Perryman, K. L., Houin, C. B., Leslie, T. N., & Finley, S. K. (2021). Using sandtray as a creative supervision tool. *Journal of Creativity in Mental Health, 16*(1), 109–124. https://doi.org/10.1080/15401383.2020.1754988

Peters, H. C. (2017). Multicultural complexity: An intersectional lens for clinical supervision. *International Journal for the Advancement of Counselling, 39*(2), 176–187. https://doi.org/10.1007/s10447-017-9290-2

Peters, H. C., Bruner, S., Luke, M., Dipre, K., & Goodrich, K. (2022). Integrated supervision framework: A multicultural, social justice, and ecological approach. *Canadian Psychology, 63*(4), 511–522. https://doi.org/10.1037/cap0000342

Peters, H. C., & Luke, M. (2021a). Social justice in counseling: Moving to a multiplistic approach. *Journal of Counselor Leadership and Advocacy, 8*(1), 1–15. https://doi.org/10.1080/2326716X.2020.1854133

Peters, H. C., & Luke, M. (2021b). Supervision of leadership model: An integration and extension of the discrimination model and socially just and culturally responsive counseling leadership model. *Journal of Counselor Leadership and Advocacy, 8*(1), 71–86. https://doi.org/10.1080/2326716X.2021.1875341

Peters, H. C., & Luke, M. (2022). Principles of anti-oppression: A critical analytic synthesis. *Counselor Education and Supervision, 61*(4), 335–348. https://doi.org/10.1002/ceas.12251

Peters, H. C., & Luke, M. (2023). Application of anti-oppression with group work. *The Journal for Specialists in Group Work*, *48*(2), 84–89. https://doi.org/10.1080/01933922.2023.2170508

Phillips, J. C., Parent, M. C., Dozier, V. C., & Jackson, P. L. (2017). Depth of discussion of multicultural identities in supervision and supervisory outcomes. *Counselling Psychology Quarterly*, *30*(2), 188–210. https://doi.org/10.1080/09515070.2016.1169995

Phillips, L. A., Logan, J. N., & Mather, D. B. (2021). COVID-19 and beyond: Telesupervision training within the supervision competency. *Training and Education in Professional Psychology*, *15*(4), 284–289. https://doi.org/10.1037/tep0000362

Pieterse, A. L., Evans, S. A., Risner-Butner, A., Collins, N. M., & Mason, L. B. (2009). Multicultural competence and social justice training in counseling psychology and counselor education: A review and analysis of a sample of multicultural course syllabi. *The Counseling Psychologist*, *37*(1), 93–115. https://doi.org/10.1177/0011000008319986

Pieterse, A. L., & Gale, M. M. (2023). There are no sidelines: A reaction to Legha's "getting off the racist sidelines: An antiracist approach to mental health supervision and training". *The Clinical Supervisor*, *42*(2), 263–279. https://doi.org/10.1080/07325223.2023.2251971

Pieterse, A. L., Utsey, S. O., & Miller, M. J. (2016). Development and initial validation of the anti-racism behavioral inventory (ARBI). *Counselling Psychology Quarterly*, *29*(4), 356–381. https://doi.org/10.1080/09515070.2015.1101534

Placeres, V., Davis, D. E., Gazaway, S., Williams, N., Mason, E., Hsu, W., Alsaegh, L., Rico, T. Q., & Glover, B. (2024). Multicultural competencies: A 30-year content analysis of American counseling association journals. *Teaching and Supervision in Counseling*, *6*(3), 54–66. http://doi.org/10.7290/tsc06mysq

Pope, M., Gonzalez, M., Cameron, E. R. N., & Pangelinan, J. S. (Eds.). (2020). *Social justice and advocacy in counseling: Experiential activities for teaching*. Routledge.

Prasath, P. R., & Copeland, L. (2021). Rationale and benefits of using play therapy and expressive art techniques in supervision. In *Techniques and interventions for play therapy and clinical supervision* (pp. 17–37). IGI Global.

Proctor, B. (1994). Supervision: Competence, confidence, accountability. *British Journal of Guidance and Counselling*, *22*, 309–318.

Pugh, M., & Margetts, A. (2020). Are you sitting (un) comfortably? Action-based supervision and supervisory drift. *The Cognitive Behaviour Therapist*, *13*, e17. https://doi.org/10.1017/S1754470X20000185

Purdie-Vaughns, V., & Eibach, R. P. (2008). Intersectional invisibility: The distinctive advantages and disadvantages of multiple subordinate-group identities. *Sex Roles: A Journal of Research*, *59*(5–6), 377–391. https://doi.org/10.1007/s11199-008-9424-4

Ramírez Stege, A. M., Chin, M. Y., & Graham, S. R. (2020). A critical postcolonial and resilience-based framework of supervision in action. *Training and Education in Professional Psychology*, *14*(4), 316–323. https://doi.org/10.1037/tep0000276

Ratts, M. J. (2009). Social justice counseling: Toward the development of a fifth force among counseling paradigms. *The Journal of Humanistic Counseling, Education and Development*, *48*(2), 160–172. https://doi.org/10.1002/j.2161-1939.2009.tb00076.x

Ratts, M. J., Singh, A. A., Nassar-McMillan, S., Butler, S. K., & McCullough, J. R. (2016). Multicultural and social justice counseling competencies: Guidelines for the counseling profession. *Journal of Multicultural Counseling and Development*, *44*(1), 28–48. https://doi.org/10.1002/jmcd.12035

Ray, D. C., Ogawa, Y., & Cheng, Y. J. (2022). Cultural humility and the play therapist. In *Multicultural play therapy* (1st ed., pp. 13–28). Routledge. https://doi.org/10.4324/9781003190073-3

Rhee, J. E. (2020). *Decolonial feminist research: Haunting, rememory and mothers*. Routledge.

Rigazio-DiGilio, S. A., & Anderson, S. A. (1995). A cognitive-developmental model for marital and family therapy supervision. *The Clinical Supervisor*, *12*(2), 93–118. https://doi.org/10.1300/J001v12n02_07

Rodney, R., Hinds, M., Bonilla-Damptey, J., Boissoneau, D., Khan, A., & Forde, A. (2024). Anti-oppression as praxis in the research field: Implementing emancipatory approaches for researchers and community partners. *Qualitative Research : QR*, *24*(4), 872–893. https://doi.org/10.1177/14687941231196382

Rogers, C. R. (1957). The necessary and sufficient conditions of therapeutic personality change. *Journal of Consulting Psychology*, *21*(2), 95–103. https://doi.org/10.1037/h0045357

Royster, R. (2021). Dolls4Peace memorial: Liberatory community art action and praxis. *Voices: A World Forum for Music Therapy*, *21*(1). https://doi.org/10.15845/voices.v21i1.3153

Sandeen, E., Moore, K. M., & Swanda, R. M. (2018). Reflective local practice: A pragmatic framework for improving culturally competent practice in psychology. *Professional Psychology: Research and Practice*, *49*(2), 142–150. https://doi.org/10.1037/pro0000183

Satir, V., Banmen, J., Gerber, J., & Gomori, M. (1991). *The Satir model*. Science and Behavior Books.

Schwartz, R. C. (2016). Dealing with racism: Should we exorcise or embrace our inner bigots? In *Innovations and elaborations in internal family systems therapy* (pp. 124–132). Routledge.

Schwartz, R. C., & Sweezy, M. (2019). *Internal family systems therapy*. Guilford Publications.

Seedall, R. B., Holtrop, K., & Parra-Cardona, J. R. (2014). Diversity, social justice, and intersectionality trends in C/MFT: A content analysis of three family therapy journals, 2004–2011. *Journal of Marital and Family Therapy*, *40*(2), 139–151. https://doi.org/10.1111/jmft.12015

Seligman, M. E. P., & Maier, S. F. (1976). Failure to escape traumatic shock. *Journal of Experimental Psychology*, *74*, 1–9. https://doi.org/10.1037/h0024514

Shaikh, A. N., Gummaluri, S., Dhar, J., Carter, H., Kwag, D., Ponce, J. E., Mason, E. C., & Peters, H. C. (2024). Application of the principles of anti—oppression to address marginalized students and faculty's experiences in counselor education. *Teaching and Supervision in Counseling*, *6*(3), 94–105. https://doi.org/10.7290/tsc06laio

Sheperis, C. J., & Bayles, B. (2022). Empowerment evaluation: A practical strategy for promoting stakeholder inclusion and process ownership. *Counseling Outcome Research and Evaluation*, *13*(1), 12–21. https://10.1080/21501378.2022.2025772

Sherbersky, H., Ziminski, J., & Pote, H. (2021). The journey towards digital systemic competence: Thoughts on training, supervision and competence evaluation. *Journal of Family Therapy*. https://doi.org/10.1111/1467-6427.12328

Shulman, L. S. (2005a). Signature pedagogies in the professions. *Daedalus*, *134*(3), 52–59. http://www.jstor.org/stable/20027998

Shulman, L. S. (2005b, February 6–8). *The signature pedagogies of the professions of law, medicine, engineering and the clergy: Potential lessons for the education of teachers*. Paper presented at the Math Science Partnerships (MSP) Workshop: "Teacher Education for Effective Teaching and Learning," Hosted by the National Research Council's Center for Education, Irvine, CA. http://hub.mspnet.org/media/data/Shulman_Signature_Pedagogies.pdf?media_000000001297.pdf

Singh, A. A. (2018). *The queer and transgender resilience workbook: Skills for navigating sexual orientation and gender expression*. New Harbinger Publications.

Singh, A. A. (2019). *The racial healing handbook: Practical activities to help you challenge privilege, confront systemic racism, and engage in collective healing*. New Harbinger Publications.

Singh, A. A., & Chun, K. Y. S. (2010). "From the margins to the center": Moving towards a resilience-based model of supervision for queer people of color supervisors. *Training and Education in Professional Psychology*, *4*(1), 36–46. https://doi.org/10.1037/a0017373

Singh, A. A., Nassar, S. C., Arredondo, P., & Toporek, R. (2020). The past guides the future: Implementing the multicultural and social justice counseling competencies. *Journal of Counseling and Development*, *98*(3), 238–252. https://doi.org/10.1002/jcad.12319

Skovholt, T. M., & Rønnestad, M. H. (1992). Themes in therapist and counselor development. *Journal of Counseling & Development*, *70*(4), 505–515.

Skovholt, T. M., & Rønnestad, M. H. (2003). Struggles of the novice counselor and therapist. *Journal of Career Development*, *30*(1), 45–58.

Smith, A., & Foronda, C. (2021). Promoting cultural humility in nursing education through the use of ground rules. *Nursing Education Perspectives*, *42*(2), 117–119. https://doi.org/10.1097/01.NEP.0000000000000594

Smith, E. B. (2019). Holding the tension of opposites: Counselors' experiences of the therapeutic internalization process. *Journal of Humanistic Counseling*, *58*(3), 204–222. https://doi.org/10.1002/johc.12120

Smith, E. B., & Luke, M. (2021). A call for radical reflexivity in counseling qualitative research. *Counselor Education & Supervision*, *60*(2), 164–172. https://doi.org/10.1002/ceas.12201

Smith, E. B., & Luke, M. (2023). Framing the call for radical reflexivity: Underpinnings of radically reflexive practice. *Journal of Creativity in Mental Health*. https://doi.org/10.1080/15401383.2023.2296965

Smith, L., Madon, N., Gordon, T., Asencio, C., Xu, O. Y., & Sheffey, M. (2023). Psychology, race, and "the politics of truth". *Journal of Theoretical and Philosophical Psychology*. https://doi.org/10.1037/teo0000249

Snow, K. C., Hays, D. G., Caliwagan, G., Ford, D. J., Mariotti, D., Mwendwa, J. M., & Scott, W. E. (2016). Guiding principles for indigenous research practices. *Action Research*, *14*(4), 357–375. https://doi.org/10.1177/1476750315622542

Spowart, J. K. P., & Robertson, S. E. (2024). Becoming a culturally responsive and socially just clinical supervisor. *Canadian Psychology = Psychologie Canadienne*. https://doi.org/10.1037/cap0000388

Springer, S. I., & Schimmel, C. J. (2015). Creative strategies to foster pre-service school counselor group leader self-efficacy. *Journal for Specialists in Group Work*, *41*(1), 1–17. https://doi.org/10.1080/01933922.2015.1111486

St.Pierre, E. A. (2021). Post qualitative inquiry, the refusal of method, and the risk of the new. *Qualitative Inquiry*, *27*(1), 3–9. https://doi.org/10.1177/1077800419863005

St.Pierre, E. A. (2023). Poststructuralism and post qualitative inquiry: What can and must be thought. *Qualitative Inquiry*, *29*(1), 20–32. https://doi.org/10.1177/10778004221122282

Steen, S., Melchior, S., Stone, T., & Melfie, J. (2023). Access to schools. In School counseling research: Advancing the professional evidence base (p. 27). Oxford University Press. https://doi.org/10.1093/oso/9780197650134.003.0002

Stein, E. S., & Cullen, J. A. (2024). Newer directions for parallel process in social work supervision. *Clinical Social Work Journal, 52*(2), 191–203. https://doi.org/10.1007/s10615-023-00903-0

Stoltenberg, C. D. (1981). Approaching supervision from a developmental perspective: The counselor-complexity model. *Journal of Counseling Psychology, 28*, 59–65. https://doi.org/10.1037/0022-0167.28.1.59

Stoltenberg, C. D., & McNeil, B. W. (2010). *IDM supervision: An integrative developmental model for supervising counselors and therapists* (3rd ed.). Routledge.

Stoltenberg, C. D., McNeil, B. W., & Delworth, U. (1998). *IDM supervision: An integrated developmental model for supervising counselors and therapists*. Jossey-Bass.

Storlie, C. A., Baltrinic, E., Fye, M. A., Wood, S. M., & Cox, J. (2019). Making room for leadership and advocacy in site supervision. *Journal of Counselor Leadership and Advocacy, 6*(1), 1–15. https://doi.org/10.1080/2326716X.2019.1575778

Storlie, C. A., Shannonhouse, L. R., Brubaker, M. D., Zavadil, A. D., & King, J. H. (2016). Exploring dimensions of advocacy in service: A content analysis extending the framework of counselor community engagement activities in Chi Sigma Iota chapters. *Journal of Counselor Leadership and Advocacy, 3*(1), 52–61. https://10.1080/2326716X.2015.1119071

Sue, D. W. (2016). *Race talk and the conspiracy of silence: Understanding and facilitating difficult dialogues on Race*. John Wiley & Sons, Inc.

Sue, D. W., Arredondo, P., & McDavis, R. J. (1992). Multicultural counseling competencies and standards: A call to the profession. *Journal of Counseling and Development, 70*(4), 477–486. https://doi.org/10.1002/j.1556-6676.1992.tb01642.x

Sue, D. W., Bernier, J. E., Durran, A., Feinberg, L., Pedersen, P., Smith, E. J., & Vasquez-Nuttall, E. (1982). Position paper: Cross-cultural counseling competencies. *The Counseling Psychologist, 10*(2), 45–52. https://doi.org/10.1177/0011000082102008

Swartz, D. (2012). *Culture and power: The sociology of Pierre Bourdieu*. University of Chicago Press.

Theoharis, G., Ashby, C., Franz, N., Gentile, S., Williams, C., Steuerwalt, B., & Devennie, M. (2022). Together, toward equity: A research-practice equity audit to understand high school opportunity gaps. *School-University Partnerships, 15*(1), 34.

Thrift, E., & Sugarman, J. (2019). What is social justice? Implications for psychology. *Journal of Theoretical and Philosophical Psychology, 39*(1), 1–17. https://doi.org/10.1037/teo0000097

Tinsley, M. (2022, July 14). Whiteness is an invented concept that has been used as a tool of oppression. *The Conversation*. https://theconversation.

com/whiteness-is-an-invented-concept-that-has-been-used-as-a-tool-of-oppression-183387

Toporek, R. L., & Daniels, J. (2018). *American counseling association advocacy competencies: Updated*. https://www.counseling.org/docs/default-source/competencies/aca-advocacy-competencies-updated-may-2020

Torres Rivera, E., & Torres Fernández, I. (2024). Decolonization is liberation: Operationalization of decolonial model of counseling using liberation psychology principles with the Latine population(s). *Journal of Multicultural Counseling and Development*. https://doi.org/10.1002/jmcd.12310

Tseng, W., & Streltzer, J. (2004). Culture and psychotherapy: Asian perspectives. *Journal of Mental Health*, *13*(2), 151–161. https://doi.org/10.1080/0963823041 0001669282

Tudge, J. R. H., Mokrova, I., Hatfield, B. E., & Karnik, R. B. (2009). Uses and misuses of Bronfenbrenner's bioecological theory of human development. *Journal of Family Theory & Review*, *1*(4), 198–210. https://doi.org/10.1111/j.1756-2589.2009.00026.x

Utay, J., & Miller, M. (2006). Guided imagery as an effective therapeutic technique: A brief review of its history and efficacy research. *Journal of Instructional Psychology*, *33*(1), 40–43.

Van Der Winjgaart, R. (2021). *Imagery rescripting: Theory and practice*. Pavilion Publishing & Media Limited.

Vidlak, N. W. (2002). Identifying important factors in supervisor development: An examination of supervisor experience, training, and attributes. *Dissertation Abstracts International: Section B: The Sciences and Engineering*, *63*(6-B), 3029.

Warde, B. (2012). The cultural genogram: Enhancing the cultural competency of social work students. *Social Work Education*, *31*(5), 570–586. https://doi.org/10.1080/02615479.2011.593623

Washington, A. R., Williams, J. M., & Byrd, J. A. (2023). Exposing blindspots and the hidden curriculum within counselor supervision models. *Counselor Education and Supervision*, *62*(2), 149–156. https://doi.org/10.1002/ceas.12260

Watkins, C. E. (2020). Relational humility and clinical supervision: On hypotheses, method, and measurement. *The Clinical Supervisor*, *39*(2), 148–167. https://doi.org/10.1080/07325223.2020.1744056

Watkins, C. E., Jr. (2023). Incorporación de la humildad cultural y las pautas de humildad cultural en la relación de supervisión de la psicoterapia: Un compromiso y una promesa. *Revista de Psicoterapia*, *34*(126), 9–18. [Incorporating cultural humility and cultural humility guidelines into the psychotherapy supervision relationship: A pledge and a promise]. https://doi.org/10.5944/rdp.v34i126.38689

Watkins, C. E., Jr., Hook, J. N., DeBlaere, C., Davis, D. E., Wilcox, M. M., & Owen, J. (2022). Extending multicultural orientation to the group supervision of psychotherapy: Practical applications. *Practice Innovations*, 7(3), 255–267. https://doi.org/10.1037/pri0000185

Watkins, C. E., Jr., Hook, J. N., Owen, J., DeBlaere, C., Davis, D. E., & Van Tongeren, D. R. (2019). Multicultural orientation in psychotherapy supervision: Cultural humility, cultural comfort, and cultural opportunities. *American Journal of Psychotherapy*, 72(2), 38–46. https://doi.org/10.1176/appi.psychotherapy.20180040

Watt, S. K. (2015). Privileged identity exploration (PIE) model revisited: Strengthening skills for engaging difference. In *Designing transformative multicultural initiatives* (pp. 40–57). Routledge.

Weck, F., Jakob, M., Neng, J. M. B., Höfling, V., Grikscheit, F., & Bohus, M. (2016). The effects of bug-in-the-eye supervision on therapeutic alliance and therapist competence in cognitive-behavioural therapy: A randomized controlled trial. *Clinical Psychology and Psychotherapy*, 23(5), 386–396. https://doi.org/10.1002/cpp.1968

Wei, M., Ku, T.-Y., & Liao, K. Y.-H. (2011). Minority stress and college persistence attitudes among African American, Asian American, and Latino students: Perception of university environment as a mediator. *Cultural Diversity & Ethnic Minority Psychology*, 17(2), 195–203. https://doi.org/10.1037/a0023359

Wells, V., Gibney, M., Paris, M., & Pfitzer, C. (2023). Student participation in a DEI audit as high-impact practice. *The Journal of Academic Librarianship*, 49(1), 102615. https://doi.org/10.1016/j.acalib.2022.102615

Whyte, M. K. W., & Toll, H. (2023). La créativité en tant qu'esprit : re-indigénisation et anti-colonialisme en art-thérapie [Creativity as spirit: Re-indigenization and anticolonialism in art therapy]. *Canadian Journal of Art Therapy*, 36(1), 2–11. http://doi.org/10.1080/26907240.2023.2213935

Wilcox, M. M., Barbaro-Kukade, L., Pietrantonio, K. R., Franks, D. N., & Davis, B. L. (2021). It takes money to make money: Inequity in psychology graduate student borrowing and financial stressors. *Training and Education in Professional Psychology*, 15(1), 2–17. https://doi.org/10.1037/tep0000294

Wilcox, M. M., Drinane, J. M., Black, S. W., Cabrera, L., DeBlaere, C., Tao, K. W., Hook, J. N., Davis, D. E., Watkins, C. E., & Owen, J. (2022a). Layered cultural processes: The relationship between multicultural orientation and satisfaction with supervision. *Training and Education in Professional Psychology*, 16(3), 235–243. https://doi.org/10.1037/tep0000366

Wilcox, M. M., Pérez-Rojas, A. E., Marks, L. R., Reynolds, A. L., Suh, H. N., Flores, L. Y., McCubbin, L. D., Wilkins-Yel, K. G., & Miller, M. J. (2024). Structural competencies: Re-grounding counseling psychology in antiracist and decolonial praxis. *The Counseling Psychologist*, 1–42. Advance Online Publication. https://doi.org/10.1177/00110000241231029

Wilcox, M. M., Winkeljohn Black, S., Drinane, J. M., Morales-Ramirez, I., Akef, Z., Tao, K. W., DeBlaere, C., Hook, J. N., Davis, D. E., Watkins, C. E., Jr., & Owen, J. (2022b). A brief qualitative examination of multicultural orientation in clinical supervision. *Professional Psychology: Research and Practice*, *53*(6), 585–595. https://doi.org/10.1037/pro0000477

Wilcox, M. M., Winkeljohn Black, S., Farra, A., Zimmerman, D., Drinane, J. M., Tao, K. W., DeBlaere, C., Hook, J. N., Davis, D. E., Watkins, C. E., & Owen, J. (2023). Cultural humility, cultural comfort, and supervision processes and outcomes for BIPOC supervisees. *The Counseling Psychologist*, *51*(7), 1037–1058. https://doi.org/10.1177/00110000231188337

Williams, M. T., Faber, S. C., Nepton, A., & Ching, T. (2023a). Racial justice allyship requires civil courage: Behavioral prescription for moral growth and change. *American Psychologist*, *78*(1), 1–19. https://doi.org/10.1037/amp0000940

Williams, M. T., McWilliams, J., & Abdulrehman, R. Y. (2023b). Antiracist supervision and training: Bringing change to mental health care. *The Clinical Supervisor*, *42*(2), 237–247. https://doi.org/10.1080/07325223.2023.2249464

Winkle-Wagner, R., Lee-Johnson, J., & Gaskew, A. N. (2019). *Critical theory and qualitative data analysis in education*. Routledge.

Wong, P., & Wong, L. (2020). Assessing multicultural supervision competencies. In D. L. Dinnel, D. K. Forgays, S. A. Hayes, & W. J. Lonne (Eds.), *Merging past, present, and future in cross-cultural psychology* (pp. 510–519). Taylor & Francis Group.

Wood, L. L. (2015). Eating disorder as protector: The use of internal family systems and drama therapy to help clients understand the protective function of their eating disorders. *Creative Arts Therapies and Clients with Eating Disorders*, 293–325.

Xia, M., Li, X., & Tudge, J. R. (2020). Operationalizing Urie Bronfenbrenner's process-person-context-time model. *Human Development*, *64*(1), 10–20. https://doi.org/10.1159/000507958

Yin, R. K. (2017). Case study research and applications: Design and methods (6th ed.). SAGE.

Yosso, T. J. (2005). Whose culture has capital? A critical race theory discussion of community cultural wealth. *Race Ethnicity and Education*, *8*(1), 69–91. https://doi.org/10.1080/1361332052000341006

Zalzala, A. B., & Gagen, E. C. (2023). Metacognitive reflection in supervision: The role of supervision in addressing health inequities. *Journal of Contemporary Psychotherapy*, *53*(1), 109–115. https://doi.org/10.1007/s10879-022-09561-8

Zhang, H., Watkins, C. E., Hook, J. N., Hodge, A. S., Davis, C. W., Norton, J., Wilcox, M. M., Davis, D. E., DeBlaere, C., & Owen, J. (2022). Cultural humility in psychotherapy and clinical supervision: A research review. *Counselling and Psychotherapy Research*, *22*(3), 548–557. https://doi.org/10.1002/capr.12481

Zhou, X., Zhu, P., & Miao, I. Y. (2020). Incorporating an acculturation perspective into the integrative developmental model (IDM) in supervising international trainees. *Training and Education in Professional Psychology*, *14*(4), 324–330. https://doi.org/10.1037/tep0000278

Zhu, P., & Luke, M. (2022). A supervisory framework for systematically attending to the outcomes in clinical supervision. *International Journal for the Advancement in Counselling*, *44*, 94–111. https://doi.org/10.1007/s10447-021-09455-9

Zilvinskis, J., Gillis, J., & Smith, K. K. (2020). Unpaid versus paid internships: Group membership makes the difference. *Journal of College Student Development*, *61*(4), 510–516. https://doi.org/10.1353/csd.2020.0042

# Author Index

# Subject Index

For Product Safety Concerns and Information please contact our EU
representative GPSR@taylorandfrancis.com
Taylor & Francis Verlag GmbH, Kaufingerstraße 24, 80331 München, Germany

www.ingramcontent.com/pod-product-compliance
Lightning Source LLC
Chambersburg PA
CBHW050332270326
41926CB00016B/3420

* 9 7 8 1 0 3 2 7 4 4 1 1 7 *